CW01203000

Occupational Health

Risk Assessment and Management

Occupational Health

Risk Assessment and Management

EDITED BY

Steven S. Sadhra BSc PhD Dip Occup Hyg MIOH MIOSH
Institute of Occupational Health
The University of Birmingham
Edgbaston
Birmingham B15 2TT
UK

Krishna G. Rampal MB BS MPH PhD FFOM(I) FFOM
Department of Community Health
Medical Faculty
National University of Malaysia (UKM)
Jalan Tenteram
Bandar Tun Razak
Kuala Lumpur 56000
Malaysia

FOREWORD BY
J. Malcolm Harrington

b

Blackwell
Science

Editorial Offices:
Osney Mead, Oxford OX2 0EL
25 John Street, London WC1N 2BL
23 Ainslie Place, Edinburgh EH3 6AJ
350 Main Street, Malden
MA 02148 5018, USA
54 University Street, Carlton
Victoria 3053, Australia
10, rue Casimir Delavigne
75006 Paris, France

Other Editorial Offices:
Blackwell Wissenschafts-Verlag GmbH
Kurfürstendamm 57
10707 Berlin, Germany

Blackwell Science KK
MG Kodenmacho Building
7–10 Kodenmacho Nihombashi
Chuo-ku, Tokyo 104, Japan

First published 1999

Set by Setrite Typesetters, Hong Kong
Printed and bound in Great Britain by
MPG Books Ltd, Bodmin, Cornwall

For further information on
Blackwell Science, visit our website:
www.blackwell-science.com

DISTRIBUTORS

Marston Book Services Ltd
PO Box 269
Abingdon, Oxon OX14 4YN
(*Orders*: Tel: 01235 465500
Fax: 01235 465555)

USA
Blackwell Science, Inc.
Commerce Place
350 Main Street
Malden, MA 02148-5018
(*Orders*: Tel: 800 759 6102
781 388 8250
Fax: 781 388 8255)

Canada
Login Brothers Book Company
324 Saulteaux Crescent
Winnipeg, Manitoba R3J 3T2
(*Orders*: Tel: 204 837-2987)

Australia
Blackwell Science Pty Ltd
54 University Street
Carlton, Victoria 3053
(*Orders*: Tel: 3 9347 0300
Fax: 3 9347 5001)

A catalogue record for this title
is available from the British Library

ISBN 0-632-04199-4

Library of Congress
Cataloging-in-publication Data

Occupational health: risk assessment and management/edited by Steven S. Sadhra, Krishna G. Rampal; foreword by J. Malcolm Harrington.
p. cm.
Includes bibliographical references.
ISBN 0-632-04199-4
1. Industrial hygiene. 2. Health risk assessment. I. Sadhra, Steven S. II. Rampal, Krishna G.
[DNLM: 1. Occupational Diseases—prevention & control. 2. Occupational Exposure—adverse effects. 3. Risk Assessment.
WA 44001491 1999]
RC967.0282 1999
616.9'803—dc21
DNLM/DLC
for Library of Congress 98-28848
CIP

Contents

List of contributors, viii

Foreword, xi

Section 1 Introduction

Chapter 1 Basic concepts and developments in health risk assessment and management, 3
Krishna G. Rampal and Steven S. Sadhra

Chapter 2 Organizing for risk assessment and management, 22
Michael K.B. Molyneux

Section 2 Risk assessment

Chapter 3 Toxicological basis of hazard identification, 41
Hilary J. Cross and Steven P. Faux

Chapter 4 Epidemiological basis of hazard identification, 56
David Koh and Adeline Seow

Chapter 5 Occupational hazard types and their characteristics, 78
Steven S. Sadhra

Chapter 6 Hazard identification techniques, 98
Steven S. Sadhra

Chapter 7 Standard setting in occupational health, 118
Leonard S. Levy

Chapter 8 Requirements of monitoring exposure to workplace contaminants, 129
Steven S. Sadhra and Kerry Gardiner

Chapter 9 Exposure modelling, 161
Christopher N. Gray

Chapter 10 Risk characterization, 177
Hani Raafat and Steven S. Sadhra

Section 3 Risk management

Chapter 11 Prevention and control of exposures, 197
Frank Gill

Chapter 12 Economics of risk management, 219
Ian Wrightson

Chapter 13 Emergency response, 246
Chris Whitmore

Chapter 14 Risk perception, 266
Anne Spurgeon

Chapter 15 Risk communication, 278
Frank Rose

Chapter 16 Health surveillance, 288
Tar-Ching Aw

Chapter 17 Auditing risk assessment and management, 315
Peter G. Nicoll

Chapter 18 Demonstrating compliance with the law, 344
Linda Goldman and Gillian S. Howard

Section 4 Applications of risk assessment and management in industry: case studies

Chapter 19 Agriculture (pesticides), 361
Ian Brown

Chapter 20 Assessment of exposure to isocyanates, 369
Iain MacKenzie

Chapter 21 Vibration, 379
Ian J. Lawson

Chapter 22 Risk management and manual handling, 390
Philip Wynn and Keith Pilling

Chapter 23 Risk management and display screen equipment, 405
Rodney J. Graves and Janice E. Jones

Chapter 24 Biological agents, 413
Jeremy R. Beach and Naveen Ratti

Chapter 25 Risk assessment and management of asbestos in Malaysian industry, 421
Lim Heng Huat

Chapter 26 Risk assessment for workers exposed to ionizing radiation, 428
John Hipkin, Eric Spence and Alexander Sutherland

Chapter 27 Stress, 438
Wilfred Howe

Chapter 28 Violence at work, 448
Stuart C. Whitaker

Appendices

1 Examples of UK legislation for different occupational hazard types, 459
2 Schedule 3 to RIDDOR 1995, 461
3 Information sources for the assessment and management of occupational health hazards, 471
Sheila Pantry, Steven S. Sadhra and Christine McRoy

Index, 479

List of contributors

T-C Aw MBBS, PhD, FFOM, FRCPC, FRCP
Institute of Occupational Health, The University of Birmingham, Edgbaston, Birmingham B15 2TT, UK

J R Beach MD, MRCP, MFOM
Institute of Occupational Health, The University of Birmingham, Edgbaston, Birmingham B15 2TT, UK

I Brown BSc (Agric), MB, BS, FFOM, RCP (Lond)
Department of Occupational Health and Safety, United Bristol Healthcare NHS Trust, Whitefriars Centre, Lewins Mead, Bristol BS1 2NT, UK

H J Cross BSc, PhD, MIBiol, CBiol
Institute of Occupational Health, The University of Birmingham, Edgbaston, Birmingham B15 2TT, UK

S P Faux BSc, PhD
MRC Toxicology Unit, Hodgkin Building, University of Leicester, Lancaster Road, Leicester LE1 9HN, UK

K Gardiner BSc, PhD, Dip Occup Hyg, MIOH, MIOSH
Institute of Occupational Health, The University of Birmingham, Edgbaston, Birmingham B15 2TT, UK

F Gill BSc, MSc, CEng, MIMinE, FIOH, MAIOH, FFOM (Hons), Dip Occup Hyg
Stone House, Bowyers, Farnham Road, Liss, Hampshire GU33 6LJ, UK

L Goldman LLB, BDS
7 Stone Buildings, Lincoln's Inn, London WC2A 3SZ, UK

R J Graves MA, MSc, FErgS, AFBPs, MIOSH, CPsychol
Department of Environmental and Occupational Medicine, University Medical School, University of Aberdeen, Foresterhill, Aberdeen AB25 2ZD, UK

C N Gray BA (Hons), MSc, PhD, CIH
Deakin University, School of Biological and Chemical Sciences, and Head of Occupational Hygiene Unit, Geelong, Victoria 3217, Australia

L Heng Huat MBBS, DIH, MPH, FAFOM, MFPHM
Mediviron Consultants, 8 Jalan 21/12, Seapark, 46300 Petailing, Jaya, Malaysia

J Hipkin BSc, PhD, MSRP
National Radiological Protection Board (NRPB), Northern Centre, Hospital Lane, Cookridge, Leeds LS16 6RW, UK

G S Howard LLB, Dip Comp Law (CANTAB)
34 Lyndale Avenue, Childs Hill, London NW2 2QA, UK

W Howe MBBS, MRCGP, FFOM
Conoco (UK) Ltd, Warwick Technology Park, Gallows Hill, Warwick CV34 6DB, UK

J E Jones MA, MSc, FBDO
Duncan and Todd Corporate Services, 14 Crown Terrace, Aberdeen AB11 6HE, UK

D Koh MBBS, MSc, PhD, FFOM, FAMS
Department of Community, Occupational and Family Medicine, National University of Singapore, Lower Kent Ridge Road, Singapore 0511

I J Lawson MB, BS, DRCOG, MIOSH, MFOM
Rolls-Royce plc, PO Box 31, Derby DE24 8BJ, UK

L S Levy MSc, PhD, FRCP, FFOM
Institute for Environment and Health, University of Leicester, 94 Regent Road, Leicester LE1 7DD, UK

I MacKenzie BA (Hons), Dip SH, MIOSH, RSP
Willis Corroon Limited, Queens Avenue, Bristol BS8 1SN, UK

C McRoy BA (Hons), ALA
Institute of Occupational Health, The University of Birmingham, Edgbaston, Birmingham B15 2TT, UK

M K B Molyneux MSc, PhD, FBIOH, CIH, FFOM (Hons), OBE
Shell International Ltd, Shell Centre, London SE1 7NA, UK

P G Nicoll BSc, ROH, CEA
Rio Algon Ltd, 120 Adelaide Street West, Toronto, Ontario, M5H 1W5, Canada

S Pantry OBE, BA, FLA, M Inst Inf Sci
Sheila Pantry Associates Ltd, 85 The Meadows, Todwick, Sheffield S26 1JG, UK

K Pilling BSc (Chem, Phy) MB, ChB, FFOM, MIOSH
Rover Group Ltd, International HQ, Warwick Technology Park, Warwick CV34 6RJ, UK

H Raafat BSc, MSc, PhD, CEng, MIMechE, FIOSH, RSP
Health and Safety Unit, Aston University, Aston Triangle, Birmingham B4 7ET, UK

K G Rampal MB, BS, MPH, PhD, FFOM(I), FFOM
Department of Community Health, Medical Faculty, National University of Malaysia (UKM), Kuala Lumpur 56000, Malaysia

N Ratti MRCP, AFOM
Institute of Occupational Health, The University of Birmingham, Edgbaston, Birmingham B15 2TT, UK

F Rose MBchB, FFOM, MRCGP
Vice President—Group Safety, Security, Health and the Environment, ICI Group Headquarters, 9 Millbank, London SW1P 3JF, UK

S S Sadhra BSc (Hons), PhD, Dip Occup Hyg, MIOH, MIOSH
Institute of Occupational Health, The University of Birmingham, Edgbaston, Birmingham B15 2TT, UK

A Seow MBBS, MMed, MFPHM
Department of Community, Occupational and Family Medicine, National University of Singapore, Lower Kent Ridge Road, Singapore 0511

E Spence BSc
National Radiological Protection Board (NRPB), Northern Centre, Hospital Lane, Cookridge, Leeds LS16 6RW, UK

A Spurgeon BSc, PhD, CPsychol
Institute of Occupational Health, The University of Birmingham, Edgbaston, Birmingham B15 2TT, UK

A Sutherland BSc
National Radiological Protection Board (NRPB), Northern Centre, Hospital Lane, Cookridge, Leeds LS16 6RW, UK

S C Whitaker PhD, RGN, RMN, OHNC, MIOSH, MMedSc
Institute of Occupational Health, The University of Birmingham, Edgbaston, Birmingham B15 2TT, UK

C Whitmore BA (Hons)
CW International Ltd, 71 Christchurch Road, Ringwood, Hampshire BH24 1DH, UK

I Wrightson PhD, DipSH, CChem, FRSC, FIOSH, RSP
Eagle Star Insurance Co. Ltd, Consultancy Services (Health and Safety), Engineering Department, 54 Hagley Road, Edgbaston, Birmingham B16 8QP, UK

P Wynn MBChB, MRCGP
Institute of Occupational Health, The University of Birmingham, Edgbaston, Birmingham B15 2TT, UK

Foreword

Risk assessment is the term most frequently on the lips of occupational health practitioners these days. Why? Because it is the term most frequently on the lips of visiting factory inspectors? That is perhaps a rather cynical answer but there is no doubt that assessing and managing risk is the central activity of occupational health and safety practitioners the world over. This is the driver for all our activities.

Yet many of us do not really know what these terms mean, let alone how we are supposed to implement the principles in our daily work. This is strange in a way because every one of us undertakes risk assessment in our daily lives—crossing the street, driving a car, engaging in leisure activities like football or sailing. What is different from these almost subconscious assessments to their place in occupational health? The answer really is not a lot *except* that here the well-being of populations of people (and the well-being of the employing enterprise) is to a large extent in our hands. Ultimately, health and safety is a management responsibility but it is we who provide the information advice and, indeed, structure of the process upon which management decisions will be based.

In the final analysis, risk assessment exists in order to provide the basis for valid decisions on control measures in the workplace to safeguard the health of work people. The prevention of illness and accidents at work is the backbone of occupational health practice. Yet few textbooks on occupational health devote much attention to the subject and fewer still provide a comprehensive account of processes required. This gap in the literature has been admirably filled by Steven Sadhra and Krishna Rampal in this book.

The introduction guides the reader through the basic concepts and begins the process of explaining hazard, risk, assessment, management, perception and communication. These topics are expanded further in subsequent chapters. Indeed, the section devoted to risk assessment covering toxicology, epidemiology, occupational medicine and occupational hygiene almost constitutes a textbook for occupational health *per se*.

In the risk management section, the psychology of risk perception and risk communications is addressed as well as the economic impact of the process. When all else fails, one still needs to have made provision for damage limitation exercises in the planning of emergencies. The final step in the process is to start again: audit the process, revise and improve.

Finally, there is an admirable collection of case studies to provide practical examples of how the various sections of the book can be put into practice, written by people who are experts in their field and have actually done what is required.

This outstanding collection of international contributors not only know their subject but they can write about it lucidily and with authority. Here for the first time is all you need to know about risk assessment and risk management. Now, after reading this book, you will feel confident to undertake these crucial processes in the prevention of ill health and accidents at work. In other words, competent to do what we are employed to do—protect the lives and livelihoods of others.

J. Malcolm Harrington CBE
Birmingham

Section 1 Introduction

Chapter 1 Basic concepts and developments in health risk assessment and management

Krishna G. Rampal and Steven S. Sadhra

Introduction

Risk assessment is not new. It is done each time we cross the street, participate in a sport or purchase new equipment for the home or business. On each occasion, we have pursued an activity in which we have, in some manner, assessed the associated risks, and decided that they are acceptable. The activities we are involved in can be continued as long as the risks associated with them are accepted, managed and maintained at that level. Do we, however, have a clear understanding of what risk assessment and the resultant options for managing the risks truly entail? Waterman (1993) wonders how many of us really know what risk assessment means, in spite of the term being in frequent use. This is more so when it involves not our health, but that of individuals for whom we are responsible; for example, for the employers, their employees, and for policy makers, society at large.

This chapter presents generalized definitions, terminology and concepts needed in understanding the field of occupational risk assessment and management. In conclusion, a framework is introduced which attempts to bring together and demonstrate the relationship between the fundamental tools used in the assessment and the management of workplace hazards. This framework (model) is the basis by which this book has been structured. A chapter has also been dedicated to examples of risk assessments for a range of workplace hazards, which highlight further the interface of the various components in the proposed model, as well as the practical issues.

The purpose of risk assessment

Risk assessment is a structured and systematic procedure which is dependent upon the correct identification of the hazards and an appropriate estimation of the risks arising from them, with a view to making inter-risk comparisons for purposes of their control or avoidance (Health and Safety Executive (HSE) 1995). It also provides the link between the scientific knowledge of the risks and the risk reduction measures to be taken. While risk assessment can be qualitative in nature, increasingly, the methods being used are becoming quantitative. Risk assessment aims to improve the quality of the decision-making process, and attempts to reduce the uncertainty as much as possible. It must be realized, however, that uncertainty does not disappear just because the risks are being assessed. The evaluation of risk is complex, especially when deciding whether the risks to the individuals or the public are acceptable.

In occupational health terms, the purpose of risk assessment is to enable a valid decision to be made about measures necessary to control exposure to substances hazardous to health arising in any workplace. It enables the employers to demonstrate that all factors pertinent to the work have been considered, and that a valid judgement has been reached about the risks. An important part of the assessment process is to define clearly the steps which need to be taken to achieve and maintain adequate control. In defining adequate control, one must decide on the acceptability of risks, which will depend on factors such as the legal requirements, costs and availability of controls, toxicity of the substance and the number of individuals exposed. The effort, detail and expertise required in conducting an assessment will depend on the nature and degree of risk, as well as the complexity and variability of the process. Clearly, risk assessment and risk management are two interrelated processes. It is commonly believed that risk assessment is based on scientific principles alone, whilst risk management also takes into consideration issues such as the technological feasibility, cost–benefit analysis, public perception and government policy. It is now not uncommon, however, to consider risk assessment as a component of overall risk management. The Royal Society Study Group on Risk Assessment (Royal Society Study Group 1992), in a follow-up of their earlier report (Royal Society Study Group 1983), highlighted that the notion to view risk assessment and risk management as overlapping, but separate, tasks, while attractive to scientists and technologists, is too simplistic. It also pointed out that risk management has become too fragmented, and there is a need for integration in managing risks faced by society.

Risk assessment and legislative developments

International developments have shown that legislation has been the main driving force behind formal risk assessments. Earlier legislation tended to be prescriptive, laying down specific sets of rules to follow, and has often been reactive following major incidents. For example, the Offshore Installation (Safety Case) Regulations 1992 was introduced after Lord Cullen's Report on the Public Inquiry into the Piper Alpha tragedy, which killed 167 people.

In the UK, an important move towards proactive health and safety management was made with the introduction of the Health and Safety at Work etc. Act (HSWA) 1974. HSWA 1974 contains an implied duty to carry out risk assessment by virtue of the phrase: 'so far as is reasonably practicable'. A more specific requirement for risk assessment was established in the Control of Lead at Work Regulations 1980. The requirement for the assessment of risk and proposal for ensuring safety (safety case reports) in some high-risk situations, such as major hazard sites and offshore oil and gas operations, is covered by the Control of Industrial Major Accident and Hazard (CIMAH) Regulations 1984 (amended by the 1990 CIMAH Regulations). The UK legislation, however, which probably made the biggest impact in terms of coverage and specific duties to undertake risk assessment, was the Control of Substances Hazardous to Health (COSHH) Regulations 1988 (now replaced by the 1994 COSHH Regulations). Examples of other UK legislation that contains definite requirements for risk assessments to be carried out include: Control of Asbestos at Work Regulations 1985; Ionizing Radiation Regulations 1985; Noise at Work Regulations 1989.

More recently, the concept of risk assessment has been introduced into a set of European Health and Safety Directives, the requirements of which were implemented in the UK in the so-called 'six-pack' of regulations. The specific requirements of these regulations have been brought together under an umbrella regulation implemented in the UK as the Management of Health at Work Regulations 1992, which require every employer to carry out 'a suitable and sufficient assessment of risk' to the health and safety of employees and to anyone else at work who may be affected by the work activity.

Paustenbach (1995) highlights the historical evolution of risk assessment in the USA, and how improvements made in this process have been the basis of both the environmental and occupational health regulations. The OSHA Act in the USA does not mention risk assessment *per se*, but focuses on the individual risk to employees exposed to agents at the permissible exposure limits (PELs) for a working lifetime. The workplace standards in the case of carcinogens were set as low as was deemed to be technically feasible and at reasonable cost. The 'benzene decision' by the Supreme Court in 1980 ruled that, before OSHA issues a standard, it must first demonstrate that the chemical poses a 'significant risk'. OSHA's attempt to set standards for 426 chemicals based on outside standards or to set standards based on general risk assessments, instead of a case-by-case demonstration of significant risks, was also struck down by the courts in 1992.

Worksafe in Australia has developed guidance on risk assessment in the workplace. The Occupational Safety and Health (Control of Industrial Major Accident and Hazard) Regulations 1996 have been enacted in Malaysia, with the equivalent of the UK COSHH Regulations being proposed as the Management of Chemicals Hazardous to Health Regulations. Risk assessment is an integral part of these regulations, and industry has been working towards achieving compliance. Intercountry differences and interagency differences within the same country exist in the methodology used to conduct risk assessments. Attempts continue to be made to standardize the approaches in risk assessment methodology; for example, in the UK, the Interdepartmental

Liaison Group on Risk Assessment reviewed the use of risk assessment within government departments (HSE 1996).

Terminology and key definitions

Attempts to standardize the methodology involved in conducting risk assessments will only be successful if the terminology used in risk assessment and management is consistent. Some success has been achieved with the development and use of standard safety and risk phrases. Obviously, it is essential for the practitioner to have a clear understanding of the key words and phrases used in the risk assessment field. Some of the general risk assessment terms relevant to the proposed risk assessment model (Fig. 1.1) are discussed below.

Hazard and hazard identification

A *hazard* is a substance, agent or physical situation with a potential for harm in terms of injury or ill health, damage to property, damage to the environment or a combination of these. Hazards can be physical, chemical, biological, ergonomic (including mechanical) and psychosocial. *Hazard identification*, the first step in the risk assessment, is purely

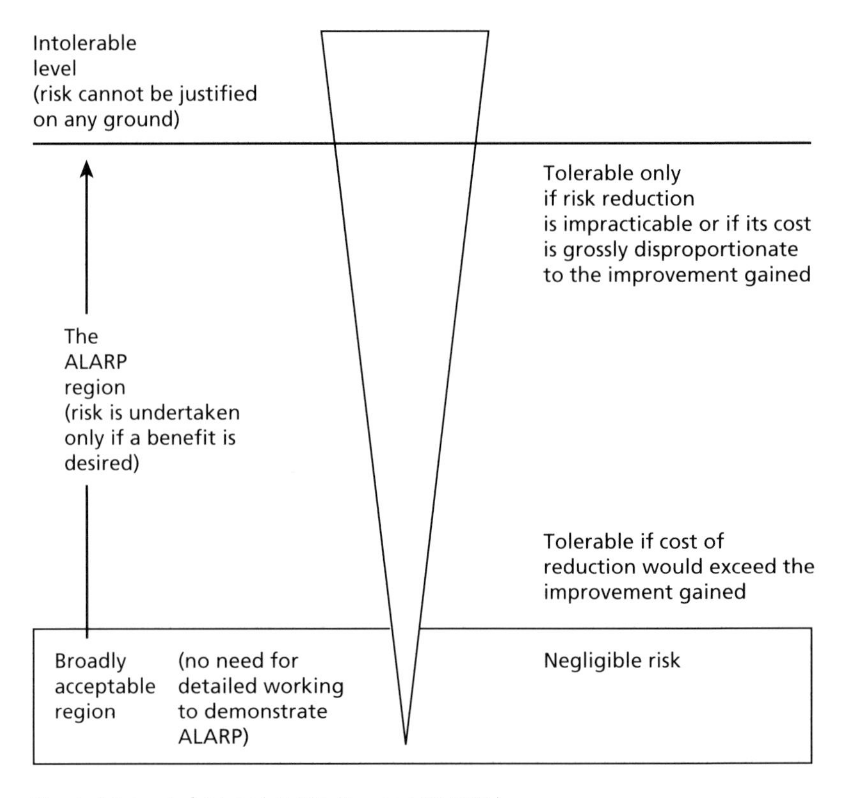

Figure 1.1 Level of risk and ALARP. (Source: HSE 1992.)

qualitative, and is defined as the process of recognizing that a hazard exists and defining its characteristics.

Risk and risk assessment

Risk is the likelihood of the harm or undesired event occurring, and the consequences of its occurrence. It is the probability that the substance or agent will cause adverse effects under the conditions of use and/or exposure, and the possible extent of harm. Hence, it is a function of both exposure to the hazard and the likelihood of harm from the hazard. The *extent of risk* covers the population which might be affected by the risk, i.e. the number of people who may be exposed and the consequences. *Risk assessment* is the overall process of estimating the magnitude of risk, and deciding whether or not the risk is tolerable or acceptable, taking into account any measures already in place.

Risk rating

When risks in the workplace or those faced by society need to be prioritized, attempts are made to rate or rank them. Although questions continue to be raised about the methodology involved in rating risks, it still dominates the risk assessments carried out by government agencies and safety and health professionals in industry. Whilst there are numerous methods to estimate risk, a common technique that continues to be used frequently employs a risk rating derived from a matrix based on the rating of the hazards in the workplace and the rating of the likelihood of exposure.

The risk rating is dependent on both the hazard rating and the likelihood rating, the equation used being: risk rating = hazard rating × likelihood rating. The hazard rating is based on the severity of harm and damage that can occur. Whether the harm caused is short or long term, the severity of harm needs to be evaluated. The severity categories can range from near miss/minor consequence (severity 1) to catastrophic consequences (severity 5). Wells (1996) noted that, whilst the harm done to persons would be placed into categories irrespective of the size of the company, similar financial loss could have different consequences on companies of varying size. The likelihood of exposure to the event also varies. This likelihood can vary from 1 to 10^{-5}. Acceptability of the consequences can also be based on the frequency or likelihood of the event. Consequences that are major or catastrophic are only acceptable when the likelihood or frequency of occurrence of the event is very small. The likelihood of the untoward events can be assessed using historical information or special techniques, such as fault tree analysis and event tree analysis.

The American Institute of Chemical Engineers has developed semi-quantitative guidelines for the ranking of risks, where Class I Risks are those considered to be of sufficient significance to warrant immediate shutdown until the hazard is mitigated. Under these guidelines, Class II Risks are those requiring immediate action to mitigate the risk, and a programme to provide a permanent solution should be initiated immediately; Class III Risks are those of a less serious nature, where the situation should be corrected as soon as possible. These risks are either related to the specific processes or the management systems. Class IV Risks are other areas where risk reduction or improvement in risk management is advised (Wells 1996).

Individual risk vs. societal risk

The most common question that is posed to risk assessors by the public and decision makers is: what is the risk to individuals and what is the risk to society at large? The risk to individuals is usually what members of the public desire to know, i.e. what is their risk from the hazard to which they are exposed, whilst policy makers who must decide on actions to be taken are more interested in societal risks. The HSE discussed these issues in detail in its document on the input of quantified risk assessment in decision making (HSE 1993a).

Individual risk is the risk of the agent harming a hypothetical person assumed to have representative characteristics of the population. It is the risk to a particular individual, and is the frequency at which that individual is expected to sustain a given level of harm from the hazard. An estimate of individual risk will depend on the frequency of harm or undesired event, the proportion of time an individual is exposed to the hazard and the vulnerability of the individual. The estimate of the individual risk of death from a particular cause is the chance in a million that a person will die from that cause in any one year, averaged over a whole lifetime. Risk estimates are made of those exposed to the risk.

Mathematically, individual risk can be calculated using the following formula:

$$\text{Individual risk} = F \times P_1 \times P_2 \qquad (1.1)$$

where F is the frequency of the undesired event, P_1 is the probability of the person being killed and P_2 is the probability of the person being exposed to the hazard.

Societal risk is the likelihood of the untoward events occurring in a group of people (usually three or greater). As in the measurement of individual risk, it is dependent on the frequency of the harm or undesired event, the proportion of time the group is exposed to the hazard and the vulnerability of the individuals forming the group. What is also included in its assessment is the number of persons in the group. The larger the group exposed, the greater the societal risk.

There are various kinds of societal risk, e.g. national, local or risks linking several communities, e.g. those exposed to a pipeline. Societal risks are normally evaluated when assessing risk from major industrial hazards which have the potential to cause large-scale injury and loss of life from a single event. Under the CIMAH Regulations, assessments are to be carried out by plant operators. In the context of these major industrial hazards, the *FN* curve is commonly used. The *FN* curve displays the experienced or predicted frequency (*F*) of an event killing more than a certain number of people (*N*). Quantitative risk assessments carried out to estimate the risk from these major hazards are only able to make an estimate of real risk within an order of magnitude.

Voluntary and involuntary risk

Both individuals and the society at large are known to be more willing to accept voluntary risk than involuntary risk. Each time someone wants to cross the road, climb a ladder or smoke a cigarette, the risk must be found to be acceptable. If an individual speeds to get to a place on time, the benefits must outweigh the risks taken. The risks of participating in a hobby, such as skiing or mountain climbing, are high. However, because these are made as a result of one's own choice, after balancing the pleasure derived and the risk of injury from it, they are accepted. Risks imposed on individuals without their knowledge and consent tend to be unacceptable, even though the risks may be lower than where involvement is voluntary.

Acceptable, tolerable and unacceptable risks

Hazards continue to exist, either because society does not know of the risks associated with them or it knows of the risks and accepts the levels of risk at which they exist. Are these risks acceptable or are they being tolerated because of the perceived or real benefit accrued from them? When attempts are made to measure and rank hazards in order of priority for the purposes of control, questions of acceptability of risks emerge repeatedly. What level of risk is deemed to be acceptable? These questions have led to risk comparisons being made. Risks are less likely to be acceptable if individuals or the community bearing the risks do not derive any benefit from them. Regulators develop standards of the levels of risks which employers must meet. These levels of risk range from those which are considered to be negligible, acceptable or tolerable to those that are unacceptable. These levels are used as guidance for action on control measures to be taken by employers. In order to ensure uniformity in the UK, the HSE defines the levels of risk that can be used as guidance for employers. Risks are considered to be negligible when the level of risk is such that no thought is given to their likelihood in the conduct of normal life. The risks are usually presumed to be below 1 in a million per annum of the occurrence of seriously adverse consequences. Acceptable risks or broadly acceptable risks are in the region of 1 in a million per annum of the occurrence of seriously adverse consequences, and where the conduct of life is not affected provided that reasonable precautions are in place. Broadly acceptable risks are those which are part of the background risk accepted as part of daily life. Those risks below the background level of risks already present and apparently acceptable to society are considered to be acceptable. This has led to the determination of estimates of the 'background risk', including risk from lightning, floods and driving a car. The question that emerged was: are these risks acceptable or are they being tolerated by society?

Tolerability does not mean acceptability. It refers to the willingness to live with a risk to secure certain benefits, and in the confidence that the risk is being properly controlled. Tolerable risks are a range of risks that are not negligible and which cannot be ignored, but which need to be reviewed and reduced still further if possible. These risks are undertaken on a regular basis for a benefit. The decision on what is a tolerable level of risk is usually political, taking into consideration the opinions given by various parties. Unacceptable risks are risks that are above the region of tolerability.

A comprehensive list of factors for judging the tolerability of societal risk has been presented by HSE (1993a). This list includes factors related to the nature of the hazard, consequential risks and benefits and the nature, purpose and limitation of the risk assessment. Economic factors, matters affecting the interests of a nation, the political aims of government and interest groups, public concern about the activity and public confidence in regulatory authorities, plant operators, experts and emergency services also need consideration.

The HSE (1988), reviewing the tolerability of risk from nuclear power stations, proposed levels that the regulators in the UK should apply. The HSE developed a three-tier system, shown in Fig. 1.1, where risks are divided into three groups: the acceptable region, the as low as reasonably practicable (ALARP) or tolerability region and the unacceptable region. The lower risk level is the level below which regulatory concern is not warranted, and for which no further action is necessary, except to ensure that the risk is maintained at the same level (1 in a million per person per year). The upper risk level is the level above which risks are not acceptable and cannot be justified on any grounds. The ALARP or tolerability region (risk level of 1 in 1000 per person per year for workers and 1 in 10 000 per person per year for the public) is the intermediate region between the broadly acceptable region and the intolerable risk region. The risks in this region are tolerable; however, there is a need to reduce the risks to as low as reasonably practicable. What this infers is that risks are tolerable only if risk reduction is impracticable, or if the cost of risk reduction is grossly disproportionate to the improvement gained.

The levels of tolerability of risk are different for working populations and for the general public. They also vary by country, industry and number of people at risk. Some industries tolerate risk less, e.g. the rail companies compared with those involved in forestry work and offshore operations. Each of these industries, however, continues to reduce the risks to as low as reasonably practicable. Industry wants to stay in business, and will close if it finds that it is not able to meet unwarranted demands on it. It has been suggested that the risk to individual members of the public from any major hazard should be at least 10 times lower than that of the workers, i.e. 100 per million or 1×10^{-4}, in the industry where the hazard exists. The level of risk to a member of the public should be equivalent to the risk of dying in a motor vehicle accident. The acceptable levels of risk in different agencies are given in Table 1.1.

Safety factors

A safety factor is the factor used by risk managers to decide what is an acceptable level of exposure. When setting standards, regulators rely on the inclusion of safety factors. In the USA, safety factors were used initially when acceptable daily intakes (ADIs) for food additives or contaminants were obtained by dividing the no observable adverse effect levels (NOAELs) in animals by a factor of 100. The 100-fold factor was used to allow for the increased sensitivity of humans relative to laboratory animals (factor of 10), and an additional factor of 10 for the range of biological sensitivity in humans. In the occupational situation, the approach of standard setting has not relied on the use of safety factors. There is a disparity between these assessment factors when risk assessment is approached for occupational and non-occupational situations. The European Centre for Ecotoxicology and Toxicology of Chemicals (ECETOC) Task Force (1995) suggests that due allowance should be given for the uncertainty, clearly making the distinction between the scientific and non-scientific elements. It has been suggested that there is a need to move away from using hypothetical 'maximally exposed individuals' to evaluate risks towards risks based on available data.

'Bright lines' are specific exposure concentrations or levels of risk that are considered to be safe or not safe. Sets of bright lines can be used to protect the general population and specific populations at risk, e.g. children and the elderly (Commission on Risk Assessment and Risk Management 1996). The provision for using safety factors may be easier for injury risks. For health outcomes where a threshold level exists, an

Table 1.1 Acceptable levels of risk.

Health and Safety Executive, UK		1×10^{-5}	Upper level
		1×10^{-6}	Acceptable level
		1×10^{-7}	Sensitive population
Du Pont		0.3×10^{-6}/year	?
UK Nuclear Power		1×10^{-6}/year	Upper level
Netherlands	$n = 10$	1×10^{-5}/year	Unacceptable
		1×10^{-7}/year	Acceptable
	$n = 100$	1×10^{-7}/year	Unacceptable
		1×10^{-9}/year	Acceptable

assessment factor is applied to the NOAEL to obtain an acceptable level of risk. When a threshold level cannot be determined, however, e.g. for carcinogens and mutagens, risk assessors could provide risk managers with information on the risks at different exposure levels, and let the risk managers decide on the action to be taken. Risk estimates have an element of uncertainty. Hence, before characterizing risk, the best estimate of the risk and the uncertainty associated with this estimate should be obtained. The uncertainty may be of one or two orders of magnitude, i.e. from 10^{-6} to 10^{-5} or 10^{-4}.

Quantitative risk assessment

Quantitative risk assessment (QRA) is often used in assessing and predicting risk from major hazards in plant and equipment during the design stage. It is, however, not legitimate to compare QRA-derived figures of risk from one hazardous situation to another or to base systems of control and countermeasures on these raw comparisons. With major hazards, it is important to be able to predict what could happen (how likely or unlikely), and then record what actually happened and how to control and reduce the risk (HSE 1993a). It must be realized that QRA is not a precise scientific exercise, and there are uncertainties involved in making these assessments. The decisions made on the action to be taken should not solely depend on the QRA, but also on other factors. The use of QRA must be selective.

A short-cut risk assessment method (SCRAM) can be conducted when carrying out a preliminary hazard analysis to determine whether a detailed risk assessment needs to be performed. It is felt that a QRA is better for making decisions associated with failures of technical equipment, rather than those of the management system. This is particularly true when the consequences of the failures are serious. Geyer (1996) advocates the use of well-established tools, such as SAFETI, RISKAT, RISKPLOT and SIREN, in determining individual and societal risk from plant accidents. In a climate of self-regulation, with the onus of proof on the employer, the employer must be able to demonstrate that the failure that occurred was extremely unlikely. Risk assessments allow for a better understanding of the work processes and hazards in the workplace. They also provide for an understanding of weaknesses in existing safety and health programmes, and assist in deciding the allocation of resources for safety and health.

Risk evaluation

Risk assessment methods used by policy makers and management must lead to the making of decisions on the prevention and control measures to be implemented. Risk assessment is not the end, but a means to an end. How these elements are applied varies, leading to various methods of performing risk assessments. Risk assessors must make tough choices in selecting the best available method that will suit their needs. Covello and Merkhofer (1993) provide an excellent discussion on the evaluation of risk assessment methods, which can be summarized as follows. The risk assessments carried out can be appraised using internal criteria of logical soundness, completeness and accuracy and external criteria of acceptability, practicability and effectiveness. The internal criteria assess the quality of the assessment and its results, while the external criteria provide standards for judging the application of the method in given situations. For the risk assessment to be logically sound, it should be able to be justified by theory, and its application is unlikely to violate theoretical assumptions. Logical problems arise when assumptions do not hold in specific applications. A risk assessment is complete when all relevant considerations are taken into account, and when using the risk assessment method does not lead to important omissions. Accurate risk assessments provide estimates of risk and uncertainties commensurate with available information. Risk assessments failing to account for uncertainties may provide risk estimates that appear to be more precise than they really are. Models, assumptions and calculations used in the risk assessment must be documented to allow for the verification of its accuracy.

Risk assessment is acceptable when it is understandable and is compatible with the attitudes and perceptions of potential users. The layperson may, however, have difficulty understanding risks explained in terms of probabilities. This is all the more so when the risk is small. Risk assessment is only practicable if it can be applied in the real world of limited resources and information. The objective of risk assessment is to determine an estimate of the risk that will guide decision making on the action to be taken. Hence, a risk assessment is effective when it is able to provide the risk manager with information on which to base his/her decision. Recommendations for decision makers include the development of flexible risk assessment guidelines and restraints that are designed to prevent overstandardization. Risk assessors should also provide a comprehensive statement of the uncertainties affecting the scope and interpretation of the assessment. Risk assessments need to be sound, objective and free of value judgements.

The majority of risk assessments can be undertaken in-house. However, an HSE evaluation of the COSHH Regulations (involving 536 employers in 1991–1992) found that 92% of employers had assessed at least one of their processes and 60% of employers had completed all or most of their assessments; 64% had sought outside help, with the majority (81%) from commercial consultants and 29% from employers' associations, and 56% from other sources, including their head offices and other employers (HSE 1993b).

Risk management

Risks are managed at the individual level, plant level and societal level.

Individuals regularly make decisions for themselves; employers are expected to make decisions for their employees and policy makers for society. The primary objective of managing risks is to prevent injuries and ill health from hazards. For example, for chemical substances, the decision on what strategy needs to be adopted in managing the risks depends on what alternatives are available for the substance in question and whether there are mechanisms for controlling the risk and permitting its safe use. The more severe the adverse health effects, the stronger the risk management strategy, always giving due consideration to the legal, scientific and public opinion aspects of risk management. Strategies that can be adopted include a complete ban of the substance or process, setting/complying with the established exposure standards, communicating information on risk to the stakeholders and, at the same time, using established prevention and control measures at workplaces. These control measures include substitution, engineering controls, improving the system of work and the use of personal protective equipment. The decision on the risk management strategy chosen quite often depends on what individuals or society are willing to pay to prevent injury, disease or death.

Establishing occupational exposure levels

One of the most common methods that has been used to manage risks at a societal level by regulatory agencies is to establish occupational exposure levels. Industry is then expected to comply with these standards. Although industry is expected to self-regulate, enforcement is crucial. There are intercountry differences in the terminology used for the exposure levels established (permissible exposure levels, maximum allowable concentrations, etc.) and also in their meaning. The setting of occupational exposure levels usually involves consultation with the interested parties. The degree of consultation varies from being integral, as in the rule-making procedure in the USA and Europe, to being policy maker driven with little consultation with the stakeholders. In developed countries, an opportunity is provided for scientific, technical and socioeconomic factors to be presented to policy makers. With more than 100 000 existing chemicals in the European Inventory of Existing Commercial Chemical Substances (EINECS), it was obvious to the Commission of the European Community that the rapid adoption of Community occupational exposure levels would not be easy. The steps for establishing standards under the Commission of the European Community Health and Safety (1993) include the preparation of a scientific dossier, a scientific review, recommendation to the Commission on a scientifically based occupational exposure level, evaluation of technical and policy aspects and proposal by the Commission on an occupational exposure level. There is then consultation with government authorities, the Advisory Committee and other interested groups on the Commission's proposal, and finally adoption of the directive. A more recent publication discusses the European Union's approach to setting occupational exposure limits for chemicals (Hunter *et al.* 1997).

Risk criteria

Risk criteria are usually determined by regulators. They determine how much risk is acceptable/tolerable. The criteria or standards set could be: comparative/equity based, involving what is acceptable in normal life or the amount of protection expected; cost–benefit analysis based, involving the balance between the risk of injury or disease and the cost of reducing the risk; or technology based, where the risk is reduced to a level which is satisfactory only when the best or state-of-the-art technology has been used to reduce the risk. The concept of tolerability combines both equity-based and cost–benefit analysis-based criteria, while the ALARP criterion is cost–benefit analysis based. Regulatory agencies in the USA are expected to control potential risks, e.g. for cancer, to a limit of less than 1 extra cancer death from a particular chemical per million persons exposed over a 70-year lifetime and, in the occupational setting, to 1 extra cancer death per 1000 workers exposed over a working lifetime. Samuels (1994), however, questions cost–benefit analysis in decision making, and states that fundamental mistakes continue to be made in an effort to skew the process in favour of easier and less contentious risk management.

Risk communication

Communicating information on risks to the stakeholders is imperative. It must be realized that employee and public opinion is a potent force that can be manipulated by the media and political interests. The public and media perceive risk differently. Their estimate of the seriousness of the risk is often influenced by personal benefit or loss, the information available to them on the risk and the familiarity with and understanding of the risk. Their perception may not be based on assessments by experts and, in some cases, they may even query the opinions of the experts on the real risks. Usually, their perception is also based on how the harm can affect what they value. The real risk and the perceived risk may be markedly different. People are generally afraid of the unknown, and can fall prey to those with secondary motives. Jungerman *et al.* (1996) found that men and women have a different perception of risk, and perception also depends on the kind of risk.

Communication on risk should aim to bridge the gap between perceived risks and real risks. This should lead to action being taken, demonstrating transparency in the decision-making process and management commitment in maintaining a safe and healthy workplace. Issues that need to be considered when communicating information to stakeholders include a clear objective of risk communication, language and literacy factors and the quality and quantity of the information available. It is important to inform those who are most affected, and to make sure that they understand what they are being told. When communicating with stakeholders, it is useful to show concern, involve them in the process and to acknowledge uncertainty when it exists. 'Take the jargon out of risk assessment and demystify risk assessment and make it more accessible to the public and decision makers' was a call made by David Eves of the HSE in 1992. Some risk managers, however, still feel that it is impossible or not necessary to communicate with the public. The OSHA Hazard Communication Standard 1983 in the USA led the way for the 'employee right to know', and employers have taken definite steps towards implementing this in their workplaces through hazard communication programmes.

In the context of chemical substances, the classification and labelling of chemicals may have different objectives. In some countries, it is an integral component of workplace hazard identification systems and is driven by the workers' right to know, while in others, such as the European Union, facilitating trade may be a major objective. In Canada, the Workplace Hazardous Materials Information System (WHMIS) is a national system to ensure that employers provide information and train employees in the use of hazardous materials. Information and labelling of controlled products and the provision of materials safety data sheets are defined under the Federal Hazardous Products Act 1985. In the European Community, most severe hazards are highlighted by symbols, and other hazards are specified in standard risk phrases and safety phrases that give advice on handling. Sowinski and Cavender (1993) clearly highlight the differences in the classification and criteria for toxicity, skin sensitization, skin irritant effect and carcinogenicity between OSHA in the USA, WHMIS in Canada and the European Commission. Efforts nevertheless continue to harmonize the systems.

Understanding the perceptions that people have of risk and communicating both risks and uncertainties clearly and in a manner that people can comprehend are crucial for risk management to be effective. Communication should be a specific component of all risk management plans, by setting aside about 10% of available resources for this purpose and holding risk managers accountable for meeting communication objectives.

Economics in risk management

Regulators conduct cost–benefit analysis before making new regulations. In the UK, this comes from the principle of 'reasonable practicability' under HSWA 1974. The Health and Safety Commission has required that cost–benefit assessments (CBAs) should be carried out for all proposals of health and safety regulations and Approved Codes of Practice since 1982. Cost–benefit assessments for regulators assist in making decisions about which chemicals or agents to target and in determining more effective ways to manage risks (Lopez 1996). Cost–benefit assessments must now be conducted for each individual maximum exposure limit proposal. In a CBA, the costs and benefits of the proposed level are measured in monetary terms. The aim of the CBA is to ensure that the proposals are worthwhile and consistent across the various industrial sectors. The key issues involved include determining the magnitude of the problem, quantifying the costs and benefits and placing a value on the benefits. At the plant level, CBA will involve the determination of the benefits obtained by ensuring that the risks are controlled. These gains could be health benefits, reduction in injury and ill health, increased productivity and decreased wastage. The quantum of risk is weighed against the sacrifice involved in averting the risk. This analysis requires that a financial value is placed on the prevention of death, injury, pain and suffering. There is always uncertainty in this exercise, but it is necessary to err on the side of safety when calculating costs and benefits. Benefits from activities which entail risks not accrued by the individual or a particular community are given less weight.

Prevention and control of hazards

For a large number of established risks from known hazards, there is specific legislation and standards. Risk control measures are then taken to achieve compliance. Standards keep changing, however, and safety and health managers need to keep abreast with these changes. Safe systems of work, standard operating procedures, permits to work and good practice manuals have emerged from risk assessments. Risks are reduced either by reducing the frequency of occurrence of the untoward event or by reducing the consequences of its occurrence. In spite of all the prevention and control measures being put into place, there is always a certain amount of residual risk.

Models of risk assessment and management

A model that has been accepted and widely used in the risk assessment area is a framework presented by the National Academy of Sciences Committee Report (National Research Council 1983). The four steps proposed in the risk assessment stage comprise: (i) hazard identification (determining the presence and quantity of contaminants that affect human health); (ii) dose–response assessment (the relationship between the concentration of the contaminants and the incidence of adverse health outcome); (iii) exposure assessment (determining the conditions of exposure and the doses received by those exposed); and (iv) risk characterization (estimating the likelihood of an adverse health outcome in exposed populations and the uncertainties associated with the estimate). Cornfield (1993) mapped the risks by identifying the hazards and controlling them by three lines of defence, including controlling the risks, maintaining the controls and dealing with breakdowns in the controls.

The Commission on Risk Assessment and Risk Management (1996), given a mandate by Congress in the USA, noted the different risk assessment strategies adopted by the various federal agencies. It proposed a framework, embracing collaborative involvement of stakeholders (making them partners in risk assessment and management), comprising six stages as shown in Fig. 1.2. The process starts with the step to formulate the problem in a broad public health and environmental health context. This is followed by the investigation and analysis of the risks, identification of the risk reduction options and evaluation of the potential consequences of each option (social, economic, ethical, legal). The responsible agency then makes a decision based on the stakeholders' input, implements the actions to reduce risks and finally carries out an evaluation. With new processes, technology and information, this risk management process is repeated if necessary. This proposed strategy is expected to improve the risk management approaches used by federal regulatory agencies in the USA. This framework is most appropriate and intended to reduce the risks to public health, safety and the environment at the macro level. There is no reason why the elements in the framework proposed by the Commission cannot be extrapolated to the company/plant level, and the approach, with some modifications, used to manage risks in the workplace.

Safety and health practitioners need to understand the factors considered in policy making and standard setting. They also need to assess and manage risks in their workplaces. We have proposed a model, shown in Fig. 1.3, which attempts to look at the decision-making process that occurs at the policy level, and which can also be used to perform risk

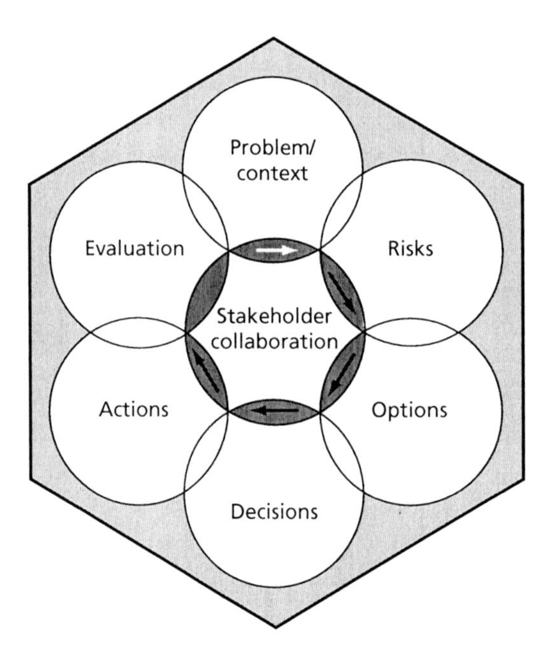

Figure 1.2 Risk management framework. (After The Commission on Risk Assessment and Risk Management, 1996.)

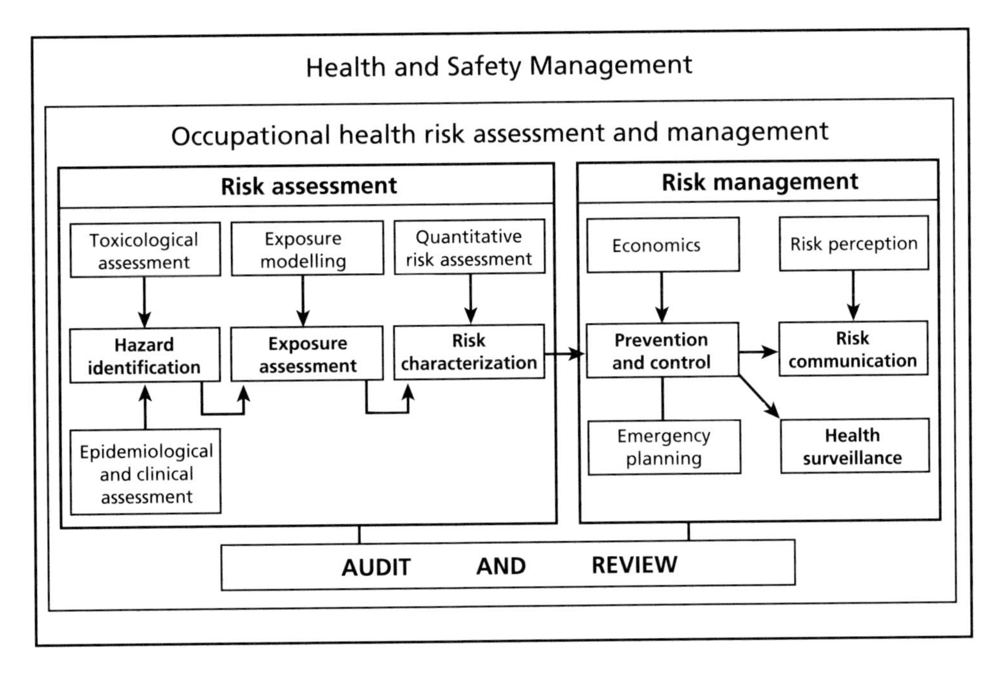

Figure 1.3 Model for risk assessment and management.

assessments and to manage the risks identified and prioritized. The process of risk assessment begins with hazard identification. Hazard identification for the risk manager includes all activities carried out in order to determine whether a substance, situation or activity has the potential to cause harm. Risk managers involved in policy making and the establishment of standards go through a detailed process, involving the assessment of the toxicological and epidemiological information available, to decide whether a particular substance, process or activity can cause harm and what harm it can cause. There is also a dependence on epidemiology to provide quantitative evidence of effects at low doses and of the relative susceptibility of humans (Doll 1995).

In the workplace, the risk assessor begins with an inventory of all the known hazards that exist. This inventory of hazards encompasses those that are present during normal and unusual work activity, involving breakdowns and maintenance. This inventory of hazards can be developed from a list of the chemicals purchased and used, through an understanding of the process in order to determine the intermediate and final products, by conducting a walk-through survey and by 'brainstorming' of those who work in specific areas. This hazard identification exercise can take place by studying each individual hazard, work process or work unit. A checklist of all known hazards is drawn up. Employee exposures and those at risk are assessed. This can entail simple walk-through surveys or detailed industrial hygiene surveys, depending on the nature of the hazard. Where exposures are not easily assessed, exposure modelling can be carried out. The objective of this exercise is to estimate and characterize the risk. The most appropriate method available is used so that the risks can be ranked and prioritized for the purposes of action to be taken. Prevention and control measures take into consideration the costs of the action and the benefits to be derived. Cost–benefit assessments are not only increasingly expected of regulators, but also of safety and health practitioners. The bottom line for management is profit: how will the measures taken to manage health risks improve the overall performance of the company, including the financial performance? Communication to employees and stakeholders on the risks they face and the steps taken to manage the risks needs to be highlighted. The correction of perception, transparency in decision making and a move away from keeping stakeholders in the dark should be followed by risk managers. The 'stakeholder right to know' is here to stay. Health surveillance measures are instituted when measures to prevent and control risks are associated with residual risks that are not acceptable. An increased use of biomarkers, indicative of the exposure, effects or susceptibility of individuals and populations at increased risk, has been advocated in risk assessment (International Program on Chemical Safety 1993). Health surveillance is also the litmus test of the effectiveness of control measures. The measures taken need to be continuously reviewed through a system of audits of the risk management programme. The model proposed forms the framework for this book, and each of the areas discussed forms the basis for chapters and case studies.

Conclusions

Risk assessment is a dynamic science that continually evolves as a result of both scientific developments and the concerns of different stakeholders. The concerns of stakeholders have, in recent years, led industries to revisit areas such as risk perception and risk communication. The way in which stakeholders perceive how risks are managed is crucial for the success of safety and health programmes in industry. The interests of the different stakeholders must be taken into consideration. Increasingly, safety and health practitioners will be expected to demonstrate how they have managed the risks, and how this has contributed to the overall performance of the company. While the methodology of assessing and managing risks may vary, the outcome should always be the same, i.e. the risks should be acceptable to the stakeholders.

References

Commission of the European Community Health and Safety (1993) *The Procedure for the Establishment of Occupational Exposure Levels in the European Community. Guidance Note*. European Commission Directorate-General (V), Luxembourg.

Commission on Risk Assessment and Risk Management (1996) *Risk*

Assessment and Risk Management in Regulatory Decision Making. Washington, DC.
Cornfield, T. (1993) Mapping out risk. *Occupational Safety and Health* **23** (9), 42–44.
Covello, V.T. & Merkhofer, M.W. (1993) *Approaches for Assessing Health and Environmental Risks.* Plenum Press, New York.
Doll, R. (1995) Assessment of risk from low doses: contribution of epidemiology. *Process Safety and Environmental Protection* **73** (Suppl.), S8–S11.
ECETOC Task Force (1995) *Assessment Factors in Human Health Risk Assessment.* Technical Report No. 68. ECETOC, Brussels.
Geyer, T. (1996) How great the risk the key. *Health and Safety Europe* **April**, 26–27.
HSE (1992) *The Tolerability of Risk from Nuclear Power Stations.* HMSO, London.
HSE (1993a) *Quantified Risk Assessment: Its Input to Decision Making.* HMSO, London.
HSE (1993b) COSHH—the HSE's 1991/92 evaluation survey. *Occupational Health Review* **July/August**, 10–15.
HSE (1995) *Generic Terms and Concepts in the Assessment and Regulation of Industrial Risks.* HMSO, London.
HSE (1996) *Use of Risk Assessment Within Government Departments.* HMSO, London.
Hunter, W.J., Aresini, G., Haigh, R., Papadopoulos, P. & Van der Hude, W. (1997) Occupational exposure limits for chemicals in the European Union. *Occupational and Environmental Medicine* **54**, 217–222.
International Program on Chemical Safety (1993) *Biomarkers and Risk Assessment: Concepts and Principles.* Environmental Health Criteria No. 155. World Health Organization, Geneva.
Jungerman, H., Pfister, H.R. & Fischer, K. (1996) Credibility, information preferences, and information interests. *Risk Analysis* **16**, 251–261.
Lopez, J. (1996) Taking chemicals to the limit. *Health and Safety at Work* **May**, 21–24.
National Research Council (1983) *Risk Assessment in the Federal Government: Managing the Process.* National Academy Press, Washington DC.
Paustenbach, D.J. (1995) The practice of health risk assessment in the United States (1975–1995): how the US and other countries can benefit from that experience. *Human and Ecological Risk Assessment* **1**, 29–79.
Royal Society Study Group (1983) *Risk Assessment.* The Royal Society, London.
Royal Society Study Group (1992) *Risk: Analysis, Perception and Management.* The Royal Society, London.
Samuels, S.W. (1994) An open systems approach to risk assessment. *American Journal of Industrial Medicine* **25**, 447–453.
Sowinski, E.J. & Cavender, F.L. (1993) Criteria for identifying and classifying toxic properties of chemical substances. In: *Patty's Industrial Hygiene and Toxicology* (eds. G.D. Clayton & F.E. Clayton), 4th edn., Vol. 2, Part A, Chapter 3, pp. 77–105. John Wiley, New York.
Waterman, L. (1993) What is a 'risk assessment' anyway? *Health and Safety at Work* **January**, 15–16.
Wells, G. (1996) *Risk Criteria. Hazard Identification and Risk Assessment.* Institution of Chemical Engineers, Rugby, UK.

Chapter 2 Organizing for risk assessment and management

Michael K. B. Molyneux

Introduction

The aim of this chapter is to identify the key issues which have a direct bearing on organization for the management of occupational health generally and health risk assessment specifically. On the one hand, it discusses high-level issues, such as management systems and policy, and on the other, it deals with the collection of basic work-related information for assessments.

Some readers may have the experience of introducing such a programme into a specific area of activity, thus having an insight into the organizational and technical issues that can arise. Others may be on the threshold of formulating and introducing a programme, in search of sensible ground rules on which they can rely. A third group may be students who need to form a view on the approach to defining the elements of a programme and gaining knowledge of the business environment within which it has to function. The information given and the views expressed will hopefully be of some value to all readers, based as they are on practical experience in industry.

Practising occupational health in a business environment

Given the task of introducing an occupational health programme into an organization, it is necessary to recognize the significance of three aspects of management which impinge directly on occupational health, i.e. management responsibility, business management and health management.

Recognizing line management responsibility

Historically, line management has delegated the management of health issues to the occupational health practitioner, largely through a lack of familiarity and knowledge of the subject. However, this is contrary to the generally accepted principle that the hazards and risks associated with the work activity need to be recognized, owned and managed by line managers. The occupational health practitioner's specialist role in this scheme is either as adviser or provider of specialist support services. It will be appreciated that, in a management role, e.g. as head of a health function within an organization, an occupational health practitioner would thereby assume line responsibility for that function. The relationship between line management control and the occupational health specialist is shown in outline in Fig. 2.1.

Fitting in with business quality management

In order to have a recognizable position in a business environment, the work of an occupational health function needs to be represented in a business plan, which identifies the customers, lists the services provided and identifies the goods which it has agreed to deliver. Costs and targets need to be stated, plus the means of recovering costs to ensure viability.

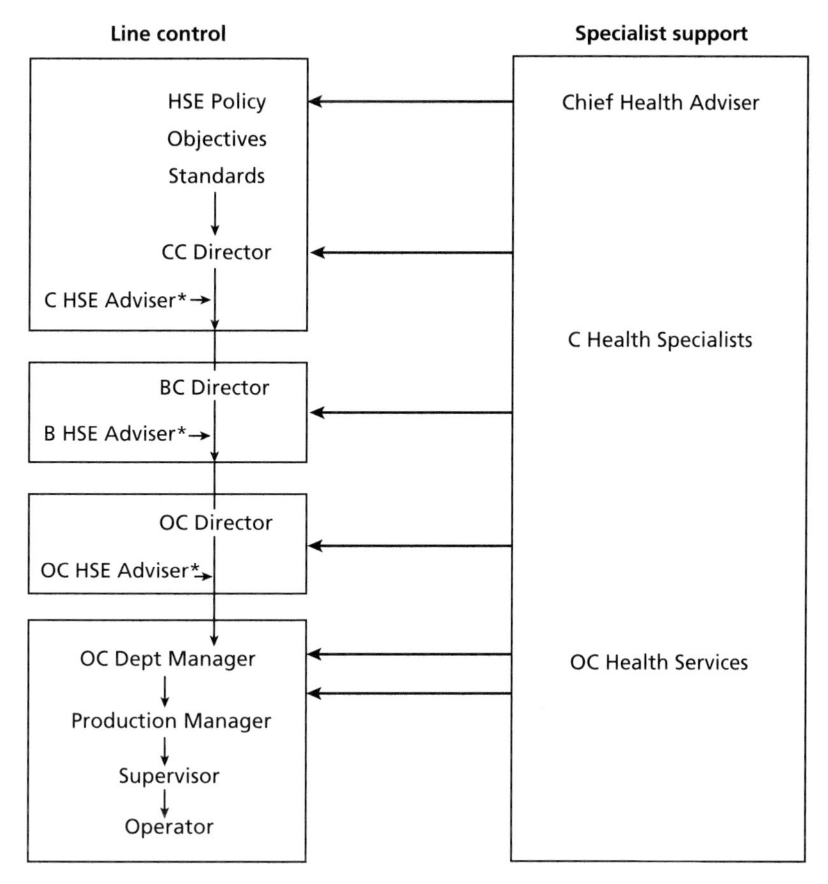

* may be trained non-specialist line management advisers

C Corporate

BC Business centre

OC Operating company

Figure 2.1 Outline of occupational health organization within a Health, Satety and Environment (HSE) management system.

This process leads to a clear view of individual tasks and targets and the extent to which they are achieved. There is provision in such a system for the detection of faults, for the appraisal of customer response and for improvement.

These are the elements of a Quality Management System (International Standards Organization (ISO) 1994), which can greatly facilitate and ensure the effectiveness of an occupational health function within an organization. Occupational health departments, which operate within a quality management environment in a business and which apply similar principles, are seen to be effective in achieving their objectives and commercial viability. The principles of business quality management are well recognized, and are seen to be fully compatible with the application of the principles of occupational health practice.

Introducing quality management into health

The discharge of the line manager's responsibility for health can be very much facilitated by a Health Management System, which is intended to operate parallel to, but is different from, the business management system referred to above. Such a system may embrace health, safety and environment (Health and Safety Executive (HSE) 1997; Chemical Industries Association (CIA) 1995; British Standards Institution (BSI) 1996), and may incorporate the infrastructure of an occupational health programme. For example, the CIA Responsible Care Management System for Health, Safety and Environment addresses health policy, the health organization, communication, hazard identification, risk assessment, operational procedures and controls and monitoring.

It can be seen that the organization of health matters and health risk assessment is such an intrinsic part of the management system that it would be inefficient to attempt to introduce an occupational health programme without first implementing the management system. Experience indicates that occupational health programmes which predate these more recent health management systems can have a much greater effectiveness within than without such a system. The quality management system promotes ownership of the programme by the line, improves understanding and increases awareness of health matters. When it is being introduced, the process can be greatly assisted by the occupational health practitioner who has a clear vision of the end product. When established, it assists the occupational health practitioner to fulfil the specialist role.

Adopting a structured approach

The words 'organization' and 'management' imply structure, at least sufficient to execute the tasks in hand. A basic structure for occupational health practice within an organization is shown in Fig. 2.2, which places policy, legislation, standards and procedures in key positions in

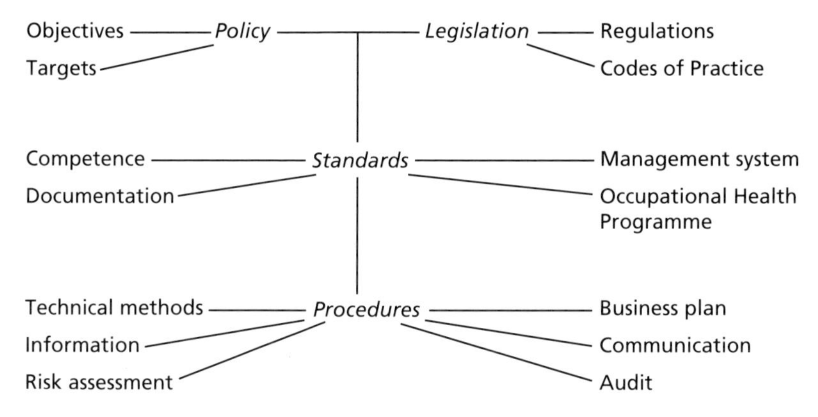

Figure 2.2 Basic structure for the management of occupational health practice.

the scheme. Standards would include an occupational health programme; procedures would embrace health risk assessment, the acquisition of information and the technical activities of fieldwork and laboratory analysis.

Using the driving forces

Policy and legislation occupy pivotal positions in the structure, as they have overriding influence on the health objectives of the organization, the former representing the wishes of the shareholders, the latter setting the external regulations and the rules for compliance. These are the principal driving forces which give impetus to all activity in occupational health. The absence of a health policy and weak legislation can effectively remove any impetus from a health programme. The task of introducing and implementing an occupational health programme in such a situation would be difficult.

Constructing an occupational health programme

There is no universal definition of an occupational health programme, but experience of one working model (Molyneux & Wilson 1990) can be used to demonstrate the scope and principles. In this model, there are nine programme elements, as shown in Table 2.1. As stated above, the responsibility for the implementation of such a programme falls on line management, and most of the effort may, at some stage in a mature organization, be properly and effectively delegated to non-specialist personnel. However, it is expected that practically all but the simplest of activities would benefit from an initial specialist input, and some may require continuing support, depending on the complexity and the degree of confidence in control.

Most of the elements include aspects of technical occupational health practice, i.e. hazard information, health risk assessment, competence,

Table 2.1 Elements of an occupational health programme.

Activity	Purpose
Communication	Co-ordination of programme
Health risk assessment	Development of control strategy
Competence	Provision of adequate resources
Records	Provision of data for review
Control of exposure	Implementation of improvement plan
Monitoring	Exposure evaluation
Health surveillance	Detection of harmful effects
Information, instruction, training	Maintenance of knowledge and skill
Audit, review	Assurance of compliance

control of exposure, exposure monitoring, health surveillance, training and audit. Experience has shown that the occupational health practitioner has a critical role to play in organization and communication, which can greatly enhance the effectiveness of a programme.

Developing a health policy

The health policy of an organization may be stated separately, but, as a high-level matter, it can be stated equally effectively in conjunction with safety and environment. In either case, it needs to be associated with objectives and targets. In general terms, policy sets the principles for reducing risk, objectives set longer term goals for risk reduction and targets state the intended improvement for the near future. Objectives and targets need to be quantifiable so that the implementation of policy can be verified (CIA 1995).

Obtaining the correct emphasis in the policy statement

An effective health policy for driving an occupational health programme would recognize health as an issue of prime importance and state the intention to avoid harm to the health of anyone who might be affected by the organization's activities. There would be a commitment to compliance with company and statutory provisions, and a statement that health was seen as an integral part of the business. The policy would be made available to employees and reviewed regularly.

Defining responsibilities for the implementation of policy

Individual responsibilities for health need to be defined, giving details of the roles of management, supervisors and staff with regard to:

- directing the implementation of the policy;
- monitoring performance;
- making available resources;
- developing objectives and targets;

- managing the health programme;
- maintaining procedures;
- compliance with standards and procedures;
- improving performance.

Stating objectives for the implementation of policy

Health objectives which would be expected to give effective support to the occupational health programme would address issues such as:

- implementation of a health management system;
- compliance with standards and procedures;
- employment of competent personnel;
- consultation with employees;
- emergency response capability;
- incident investigation;
- performance monitoring;
- improvement in performance.

Specifying targets for the implementation of policy

Health targets provide the practical means of achieving short-term goals, which would typically apply to issues such as:

- completion and maintenance of health risk assessments;
- implementation of improvement plans;
- installation of engineering controls;
- improved application of procedures;
- reduction in personal exposure;
- improvement in competence;
- auditing of performance.

The effective implementation of these targets determines the ultimate success of an occupational health programme. They would normally be included in the list of annual tasks and targets for individuals, and progress would be regularly assessed.

Documenting what the organization wants and does

The responsibilities, objectives and targets described above need to be underpinned by the criteria which describe the organization, its procedures and its methods. These criteria need to be documented and clearly understood, as it is against these that the organization will ultimately measure its health performance. For health, the documentation is comprehensive and would typically include the following.

- *Health manual*, including the policy, responsibilities, objectives and targets, the health programme and organization chart.
- *Annual health business plan*, including the scope of services, deliverables with targets, resources, costs and audit.
- *Procedures*, including measurement and calibration protocols, health

risk assessment, surveillance, audit, review methods, improvement planning, training schedules, reporting requirements, response to queries, emergencies and communication.
- *Plans for improvement*, including responsibilities, targets, resources and achievement criteria.
- *Records of data*, including results of surveys, tests, analytical quality assurance and calibration.
- *Reports*, including health risk assessments, exposure surveys, air and biological monitoring, health surveillance, control systems surveillance, audits, reviews, incident investigation, health statistics, non-compliances and prosecutions.
- *Reference documents*, including organization standard documents, limit values, legislative requirements and specialist and technical criteria.

It is worth noting that clear, up-to-date, complete and easily retrievable documentation can be taken as an indication of an organization's active participation in and commitment to occupational health. The pathways involved in the generation, analysis and review of health performance data, their cascade and feedback for control purposes, through an organization, are outlined in Fig. 2.3.

Organizing an occupational health programme

Primary purposes

All nine elements of the programme, which have been introduced previously, need to be organized in such a way as to achieve the primary purposes listed in Table 2.1. From this it can be seen that the primary purpose of communication is co-ordination; for health risk assessment, the development of a control strategy; for competence, the provision of adequate resources; for records, the ability to review; for control, the formulation of an improvement plan; for monitoring, exposure evaluation; for health surveillance, the detection of harmful effects; for information, instruction and training, the maintenance of knowledge and skill; for audit and review, the assurance that the policy is being implemented. The following issues have been selected for further discussion here.

Focal points as an aid to co-ordination

Although the occupational health practitioner may not have responsibility for the health of the workforce, the specialist skills of the experienced hygienist, physician and fellow practitioners can influence the direction and outcome of all aspects of the programme. The managers' awareness of health issues can be improved so that there is an understanding of the risks to health and the principles of prevention.

Site- or company-wide support for the implementation of a programme can be enhanced by close liaison with selected focal points

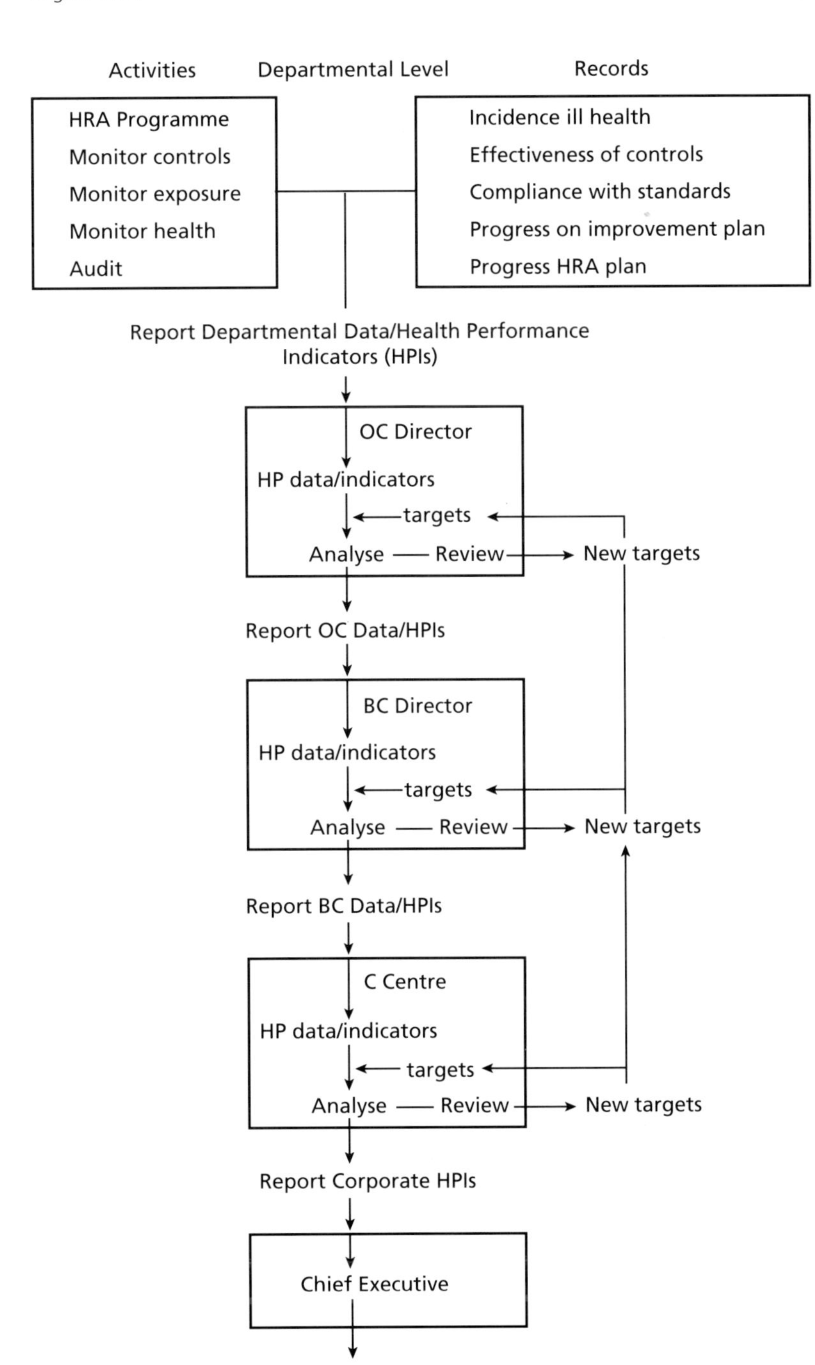

Figure 2.3 Outline of health data generation and reporting within a Health, Safety and Environment (HSE) management system.

having experience of company management and technical processes (Molyneux & Wilson 1990). Their participation in the management of health risk assessments, for example, creates strong, well-informed and productive relationships which enhance the effectiveness of a programme. This greatly facilitates the identification of priorities, the formulation of improvement plans and the allocation of resources. In time, the goal of integrating occupational health into the business process will have been achieved.

Health risk assessment as a core activity

It can be argued that the core activity of this scheme is health risk assessment, as it generates the strategy which determines the direction of the improvement plan for the control of exposure. It also specifies the need for monitoring and health surveillance to meet concerns on any residual risk to health. Experience indicates that assessments can be efficiently carried out if they focus on job type, taking a holistic view of the combined chemical, physical, biological and ergonomic agents which have a bearing on the health of the job holder (Molyneux & Wilson 1992). This is elaborated in a later section.

Identifying competence requirements

The aim is to ensure that all employees can competently deal with the health aspects of their job, whether they have management, supervisory, technical, operational or specialist supporting roles.

Clearly, the need for knowledge, skill and experience in occupational health practice will vary in scope, breadth and depth, depending on the demands of the job. Broadly speaking, there are two areas of practice to be addressed, one applying to the management, maintenance and use of control procedures, and the other applying to the skills of the specialists in hygiene and medicine. They are, of course, complementary.

For example, the director should be skilled in assessing compliance with the health policy and in evaluating performance in meeting health objectives; the manager should be skilled in managing a health programme, reviewing performance in a specified area, assessing health priorities and allocating resources; the supervisor should know the hazards in the work area and be skilled in the maintenance of safe systems of work and in keeping health-related records; the operator should know the hazards of each task, how to operate the control systems and be able to take appropriate action in abnormal situations. In contrast, the hygienist should know how to develop a risk control strategy, to assess risk and to evaluate exposure and control performance; the physician and related medical staff should know the hazards and possible harmful effects, apply appropriate surveillance strategies and promote health awareness and preventive measures.

All of these requirements need to be incorporated into personal development plans and training schedules to ensure that the risk to health is effectively managed and minimized.

Using audit as an educational tool

Audit is the primary means of assessing compliance with the criteria identified previously. Audits can be made to address the total range of issues from the policy statement downwards, and may be targeted at systems, such as the health management system, technical methods, such as those used in exposure evaluation, or documentation, such as records of data or reports of health surveillance (Molyneux 1994).

Experience suggests that, quite apart from this compliance role, audit is a powerful educational tool which can be used to demonstrate strengths and weaknesses, and thus promote progress. The process is assisted by the availability of concise criteria from which can be derived clear questions that can be phrased and systematically arranged in a questionnaire. Responses to such audits can be collated, analysed and reported promptly and anonymously if necessary. In the event that a programme is being newly implemented, such audits can be scheduled to monitor progress and to feed back findings while there is a high level of commitment and interest.

Organizing health risk assessment

The importance of health risk assessment as a primary influence in a risk control strategy has already been stated. It follows that, if assessment is properly introduced into an organization and effectively implemented, the programme is given a sound basis for the future.

Defining health risk assessment

The purpose of health risk assessment in the workplace, as referred to here, can be precisely defined, and lends itself to a structured approach (HSE 1989). The purpose is to assess risk to the health of individuals arising from activities in the workplace. The individuals at risk may be employees or any others who may be exposed. If the workplace activities affect persons outside the workplace, they will also be included in the assessment.

The assessment has three practical outputs, i.e. it specifies the need for additional controls in the workplace to give assurance of minimal risk, and, where there is doubt about the residual risk, it specifies the need for the monitoring of controls and for health surveillance. The assessment is only complete when these issues have been addressed.

The added value of health risk assessment

The first health risk assessment is a historical marker which gives an insight into previous risk, quantifies present risk and provides a baseline against which the impact of change on risk can be judged. It provides the workplace element of work history, as the jobs and tasks which are held in the assessment record can be linked with individuals. The principles can be applied to all hazards arising from the workplace, under the headings of chemical, physical, biological and ergonomic, thereby minimizing the duplication of effort. The intimate participation of managers, supervisors, operators and technical staff in the assessments ensures ownership by management, imparts knowledge of the agents and hazards and ensures direct involvement in the improvement and use of controls. All of these are of benefit to the organization.

Resources and competence for health risk assessment

The basic resources and competence required for assessments of the type defined above are determined by two pragmatic issues. The first is that the assessment is a tool which is intended to minimize risk in the workplace. It needs to be understood, owned and used by the employees who are at risk. It is logical that they should themselves take the lead in assessment, with specialist assistance if required. The second is that most assessments can be completed given an elementary knowledge of the processes and activities and by applying common sense and experience. Hence, the conclusion is that informed employees should themselves be capable of contributing to assessments within the range of their knowledge and experience.

The above observations are considered to be true subject to some qualifying remarks. The first is that small, simple job-type assessments require minimal skill and effort to effect adequate results. However, everything that is collated and acted upon should be recorded in an informative, concise and brief manner. The second is that many aspects of more complex assessments are within the capability of employees provided that they are prepared for the task, the assessments are structured, they are managed within an assessment programme and there is specialist support when appropriate.

Using external resources

Company employees have a unique contribution to make to health risk assessment because of their knowledge and experience. However, where internal resources are inadequate or overstretched, the services of external occupational health specialists may be required. Smaller companies or independent parts of large organizations can find themselves in either or both situations.

Problems can be faced and overcome on both sides. The employer with inadequate resources may not have the in-house experience to define the task, targets and the desired products, which renders a contract unmanageable. This can be overcome by employing a specialist who has the experience to define the requirement and effectively manage the contract. Failure to deal with these problems is the commonest cause of contract failure. The specialist, as an outsider, faces the task of undertaking assessments in novel business and technical environments. Given sufficient experience, novelty can be dealt with by the careful collection of background information and application of a structured approach and underlying principles. Pressures to take the lead away from line management should be resisted so that the assessments, once completed, are owned and used.

At the inception of risk assessment, when everyone is learning, specialist contractors of the necessary calibre are rare, but this can be reversed as skill and experience are acquired.

Guidance from the health practitioner

The occupational health practitioner will need to use judgement as to what, when and how much specialist support is required to assist the organization to define properly and complete its health risk assessment programme without diminishing ownership by the line. The practitioner needs to be alert to the possibility of a disproportionate amount of time and effort being directed at assessments in two directions, one being to make simple situations look difficult and complex, often associated with excessive documentation, the other being to make complex situations look simple. The former wastes effort and eventually discredits the process, and the latter gives a false sense of security. It is essential that resources are targeted where they are most needed, which requires an examination of the risks in order of priority. The informed view of the practitioner is of great value in striking the correct balance.

Execution and use of a health risk assessment

The technical content and scope of an assessment are addressed elsewhere in this book; for the purpose of understanding this issue, it is sufficient to note that there are four stages to the process, i.e. the identification of assessment units within which job types are to be assessed, the recognition of hazards, the evaluation of risks to health and, finally, the risk control strategy. The following comments can be sensibly applied in larger organizations where there are different job types, exposures of varying complexity and where implementation requires positive planning and resourcing. The key issues are the method of management, adoption of a common approach, training of non-specialist participants, team working, custody of and recording of key facts and recommendations.

Management

The prime concern of an organization will be to execute a plan which gives priority to and selectively applies resources to activities which are perceived to present the highest risk to health. This can be achieved by appointing a Central Assessment Team which has a broad knowledge of the whole range of activities and the potential risks. This would typically be led by a senior manager supported by a small team with supervisory, technical, hygiene and medical experience. The occupational health focal point would be a member of or work closely with this team. The team would specify and direct the programme and monitor the quality of the outputs.

Common approach
Quality is most likely to be achieved if assessments are carried out to a predetermined and agreed approach, which ensures that critical steps of the process are carried out on all assessments and that basic rules of reporting are followed. Some degree of standard documentation is desirable, but flexibility within the guidelines needs to be allowed.

Training
To non-specialist personnel, the risk assessment process is totally new, and some orientation is necessary. This is best provided by health practitioners who can explain the concept of agents, hazards and risks, with particular reference to the particular processes, and assist with the completion of model assessments which clearly demonstrate the methodology.

Team work
To ensure ownership by the line, the assessments should be carried out by Assessment Teams, the members of which are directly involved in the jobs and tasks being assessed. These teams operate as task forces, typically under the leadership of an area supervisor, and include operational personnel. They would be acquainted with and work with the hygienist and physician as necessary to complete each assessment. This is the best means of assuring that the information collected is real, and that the effort put into the assessment is appropriate to the risk.

Recording the assessment
The Assessment Team would collate, analyse and report the assessment to the agreed format, and submit it to the Central Assessment Panel for approval. The area manager would retain custody of the report and review it in response to potential changes in risk.

Implementing the assessment
The assessment only has value if its recommendations are translated into reality which is demonstrated to bring about the expected improvement. This is seen as the responsibility of the area manager, who would be expected to make proposals, formulate a plan, arrange for resources and see the work through to completion. The assessment would be updated accordingly.

Improving the control of exposure

As stated above, the health risk assessment provides the control strategy which is translated into a practical control improvement plan. The plan should have priorities and targets, and can be expected to address any combination of issues which are reflected in the traditional hierarchy of controls, i.e.:

- elimination of the hazard;
- substitution by a less hazardous agent;
- segregation of the hazard;
- enclosure of the hazard;
- application of exhaust ventilation;
- application of general ventilation;
- use of personal protective equipment.

All of the above can be used in any combination to achieve minimal exposure as far as is reasonably practicable. The following need to be applied in all work situations:

- adoption of safe methods of work;
- adherence to good personal hygiene;
- information, instruction and training appropriate to the job.

The higher in the hierarchy, the more reliable the method and the less the likelihood of failure. Hence, elimination, substitution, segregation and enclosure give a high degree of reliability. Personal protection and work method are more prone to failure. Thus the status and progress of a control regime can be judged on the basis of the methods applied.

Achieving the aim, targeting the resources

Avoiding overcomplication

The quality approach is recommended because it aids inputs to the various documentary elements of an occupational health programme; it is a good platform for encouraging improvement. However, the effort needs to be sharply focused on the critical activities. Good documentation is essential for the whole process, but the systems need to be simple and clear, both in terms of access and maintenance. Overelaboration leads to excessive cost, difficult application and, eventually, a lack of interest.

Placing resources in the right place at the right time

Resources in an organization are likely to be scarce and subject to competition. It is important to recognize that a number of demands are placed on the same individuals for quite valid reasons, and that the type of resource required changes with the life history of a programme (Molyneux 1992). There are a number of phases to consider:

- planning the programme and the systems;

- training and initial implementation;
- the period of initial assessment when the control strategy is being developed;
- the period during which controls are being improved and reassessed;
- the period of confirmed control with long-term surveillance in place.

Planning is essentially a desk top exercise requiring inputs at high levels; training and initial implementation are practical workplace exercises; assessment places heavy demands on line, technical services and advisory personnel; the introduction of improved controls requires detailed attention from the line and technical staff with capital expenditure; the final 'watch-dog' phase depends on the functioning of routine systems with specialist support as required.

Keeping the goal in sight

It is appropriate to end this chapter with two comments on the most important issues. One is that all the effort that goes into occupational health will be wasted if the goal of minimizing risk to health is not achieved. Another is that there is a great opportunity for diverting effort into systems and documentation which tend to become ends in themselves, but contribute little to the real goal of health protection.

Conclusions

The issues that have a direct bearing on risk assessment and the management of occupational health are the business environment, plus the aim of and commitment to the health policy. Policy is the main driving force, acting through line management. The specialist role of health practitioners is to advise, assist and give technical support within an organized management system. Progress is achieved through stated health objectives and targets which can be evaluated by audit. The documentation of standards, plans, procedures, data and records underpins the occupational health programme, the components of which are clearly definable. Co-ordination can be greatly assisted by focal points; effectiveness is directly dependent on competence in the line and in the specialist resource. Health risk assessment is seen as an essential core activity which needs to be structured, driven by line management, but effectively facilitated by the health specialist. Team work is an important feature of the process, culminating in a clear view of the risks, how they can be minimized and the need for surveillance.

Resources for all assessments need to be drawn from departmental employees, given adequate information and preparation. The contribution of the health specialist increases with the complexity of the task. The value of the assessment is in its influence over the development and implementation of the improvement plan, with targets, which ultimately leads to the control of risk.

References

BSI (1996) *Guide to Occupational Health and Safety Management Systems.* BS 8800. BSI, London.

CIA (1995) *Responsible Care Management Systems for Health, Safety and Environment.* Chemical Industries Association, London.

HSE (1989) *COSHH Assessments. Step by Step Guide to Assessment and the Skills Needed for it.* HMSO, London.

HSE (1997) *Successful Health and Safety Management*, 2nd edn. HSG (65). HSE Books, Sudbury, UK.

ISO (1994) *Quality Management Systems.* ISO 9001. British Standards Institution, London.

Molyneux, M.K. (1992) The implementation of COSHH. A case history. *Health and Safety at Work* **14**, 21–23.

Molyneux, M.K. (1994) *Occupational Health Auditing in Health Protection from Chemicals in the Workplace.* Chemical Industries Association, London.

Molyneux, M.K. & Wilson, H.G.E. (1990) An organised approach to the hazards of health at work. *Annals of Occupational Hygiene* **34**, 177–188.

Molyneux, M.K. & Wilson, H.G.E. (1992) Assessments and the assessor: a company approach to occupational health risks. *Annals of Occupational Hygiene* **36** (1), 71–78.

Section 2 Risk assessment

Chapter 3 Toxicological basis of hazard identification

Hilary J. Cross and Steven P. Faux

Introduction

Toxicology is the study of the adverse effects of chemicals on the body and other biological systems. Toxicology thus provides the basis for protecting the health of humans exposed to chemicals in the workplace.

The identification of hazards associated with a particular substance occupies an early stage in the risk assessment process. Once the hazard has been identified (see Chapter 6), the subsequent consideration of any dose–response relationship, together with available workplace exposure data, enables an assessment to be made of the associated risk, which will ideally lead to the introduction of an effective risk management strategy.

The aim of this chapter is to show how toxicology fits into the risk management process. The chapter begins with the clarification of some basic toxicological terms and principles, followed by an outline of the procedures for assessing the toxicity of new and existing substances; finally, it considers how toxicological data are made available for use in risk assessment.

This chapter focuses entirely on occupational toxicology, i.e. health effects associated with chemical exposures in the workplace. The physicochemical properties of chemicals, which form another part of the hazard assessment process, are addressed in Chapter 5. The consideration of effects in the general public resulting from environmental exposure to chemicals and the effects of chemicals on ecosystems are beyond the scope of this chapter.

Some toxicological terms and fundamentals

Hazard identification

Hazard identification is the identification of the adverse effects which a substance has an inherent capacity to cause. The term *hazard* encompasses not only toxicological properties, which are the focus of this chapter, but also physicochemical and ecotoxicological properties. The toxicological property, for example, might be skin irritation. For another substance, it might be cancer. Information on hazards, the dose–response relationship and exposure data provides the three essential elements in the assessment of risk.

Dose–response relationship

The dose–response relationship refers to the relationship between the dose of a chemical and the response that it elicits. As the dose of a substance increases, e.g. the amount of substance ingested or absorbed through the skin, or the airborne concentration of a gas, the response increases. The response may be expressed in terms of either the severity of a graded response or the percentage of the population affected by an adverse effect, and may range from no measurable response to maximal response. A graded response could, for example, be irritation caused by exposure to chlorine gas. This response could range in severity from slight irritation of the nasal passages to pulmonary oedema and bronchial constriction. The typical dose–response relationship is represented by a cumulative frequency distribution curve, illustrated in Fig. 3.1. In this figure, the response is expressed as the percentage of a population responding. The curve demonstrates the small proportion of the population who respond to a low dose (sensitive individuals), the small proportion of the population who only respond to a high dose (resistant individuals), and the majority who respond around the mid-point, the median effective dose (ED_{50}). In the acute toxicity test, which is described later in this chapter, the response measured is death, and the dose–response relationship can be used to derive the median lethal dose (LD_{50}).

In risk assessment, the dose–response relationship provides the basis for estimating the response associated with the predicted exposure. Implicit in the dose–response relationship is that, for most substances, there will be a dose below which no response is detectable, i.e. a *threshold*. The threshold may also be referred to as the no observable adverse effect level (NOAEL). The identification of the threshold or NOAEL plays an important part in the establishment of occupational

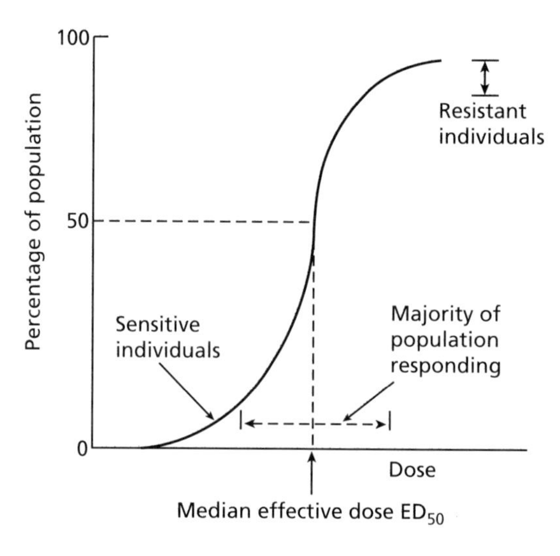

Figure 3.1 Typical dose–response curve.

exposure limits (OELs), and this issue is addressed in Chapter 7. For certain substances, however, such as those known to cause cancer involving a genotoxic mechanism of action, it is generally recognized that there is no threshold, or that a threshold cannot be identified with any certainty. This means that, at any dose, no matter how small, a response may still occur in a sufficiently large population. This is also the case for some respiratory sensitizers.

Toxicokinetics

Toxicokinetics is the study of the absorption, distribution, metabolism and excretion of substances. These processes are described below.

Absorption is the process by which a substance enters the body. In the workplace, the most likely routes of exposure are inhalation or skin absorption and, less commonly, ingestion. A knowledge of the likely route(s) of exposure for a specific substance is an important aspect of both the assessment and management of risks, providing an indicator of the most appropriate means of monitoring worker exposure and also of how exposure may best be controlled. For substances that are absorbed mainly by inhalation, exposure is usually assessed using environmental monitoring methods, i.e. by measuring the concentration of the substance in air (see Chapter 8). Airborne concentrations may then be reduced by, for example, installing a ventilation system or by enclosing part of a process as discussed in Chapter 11. Particular substances may penetrate the skin and become absorbed into the body. Determining the airborne concentration of such substances will provide a poor indicator of an individual's internal dose. In such cases, biological monitoring methods, such as the measurement of the levels of the substance or its metabolites in urine or blood samples, are likely to offer a more accurate indicator of the subject's internal dose. (For further details on biological monitoring, see Chapter 16.)

In some animal experiments, alternative exposure routes are sometimes employed, such as intraperitoneal, intravenous or subcutaneous injection, intratracheal instillation or intramuscular implantation. There may be valid reasons for using these routes of exposure in particular experiments, such as ensuring that a known concentration of the substance reaches a particular target tissue. However, interpreting the results emanating from such experiments and extrapolating these data to humans in the occupational setting require careful consideration. Issues relating to the extrapolation of animal data are addressed later in this chapter.

Distribution refers to the process by which a substance, once it has been absorbed, or its metabolites partition within the body. The distribution of a substance can give an indication of any likely target organ(s), and also the potential for accumulation.

Metabolism is the process by which a substance absorbed into the body is changed into one or more chemically different substances (metabolites). The metabolic process may be enzyme mediated or non-enzymatic. Metabolism may result in one of two outcomes: bioactivation, in which a non-toxic substance is metabolized to toxic metabolites; or detoxification, where a toxic substance is metabolized to non-toxic metabolites. For many substances, several metabolic pathways exist, representing both bioactivation and detoxification; for such substances, toxicity may only ensue if a detoxification pathway fails or becomes saturated. Examples of some substances that undergo bioactivation, and their toxic metabolites, are presented in Table 3.1.

Excretion is the process by which a substance that has been absorbed and/or its metabolite(s) is eliminated from the body. Different substances may be excreted from the body by different routes and at different rates. The most common excretory routes are the urine, faeces and breath. Other routes of excretion include sweat, saliva and tears. Inorganic mercury compounds, for example, are excreted mainly in the urine, and the measurement of urinary levels of mercury is a recognized biological monitoring method for assessing exposure. In contrast, carbon monoxide is exhaled unchanged in the breath, and this provides one biological monitoring method for assessing carbon monoxide exposure.

Information on the toxicokinetics of a substance is critical to our understanding of the mechanisms of toxicity, and thus plays an important role during the evaluation of toxicological data. Studying toxicokinetics enables identification to be made of species, strain and/or gender differences, all of which are key elements when extrapolating from animal experiments to humans. Understanding the toxicokinetics of a substance may also lead to the development of biological monitor-

Table 3.1 Some substances that undergo bioactivation.

Substance	Toxic metabolite(s)	Toxic effect
Acetaminophen (paracetamol)	Benzoquinoneimine	Liver necrosis
Bromobenzene	Bromobenzene epoxide	Liver toxicity
1,3-Butadiene	Epoxybutene, diepoxybutane	Leukaemia
2-Butoxyethanol	Butoxyacetic acid	Haematotoxicity
2-Chloroethanol	Chloroacetaldehyde	Systemic effects, involving liver and nervous system; possible mutagenicity
Chloroform	Phosgene	Liver and kidney toxicity
n-Hexane	2,5-Hexanedione	Peripheral neuropathy
Tetrachloroethylene	Trichloroacetic acid (mouse) Thioketene intermediate (rat)	Liver cancer (mouse) Renal cancer (rat)
Vinyl chloride	Chloroacetaldehyde	Liver cancer

ing methods as an alternative means of assessing exposure to taking air measurements. The examples of inorganic mercury and carbon monoxide have already been reported. 2-Butoxyethanol (2-BE) provides another example. 2-Butoxyethanol is a glycol ether that is widely used as an industrial surface cleaner. It enters the body by inhalation and by skin absorption, is metabolized principally to butoxyacetic acid (BAA), a metabolite which appears to be responsible for 2-BE-induced haematotoxicity, and is excreted in the urine as BAA. The measurement of BAA levels in end-of-shift urine samples is recommended as an indicator of exposure to this glycol ether.

Target organs

Different substances may affect different organs in the body in different ways, and the *target organ* or *target tissue* is the organ or tissue where the adverse effect occurs. The reason for this difference may be that a particular chemical has a tendency to accumulate in a specific tissue. Cadmium and its inorganic compounds, for example, accumulate in the kidneys and, with repeated exposure, can cause tubular dysfunction and associated proteinuria. Alternatively, the target organ may be the site where a substance is metabolized to toxic metabolites. The liver is the principal site for the metabolism of many exogenous substances and, consequently, is the target organ for several chemicals. Examples of hepatotoxicants include carbon tetrachloride, *N,N*-dimethylformamide (DMF) and halothane. In all cases, the severity of the effect depends on the concentration of the substance or its metabolite in the target organ. For some substances, there may be more than one target organ. Exposure to tetraethyl lead, for example, is associated with effects on blood synthesis, liver and kidney damage and neurotoxicity. Exposure to inorganic mercury compounds, as another example, can lead to renal toxicity and central nervous system toxicity. Table 3.2 summarizes some target organs that are associated with particular substances.

Types of toxic effect

Chemical exposures can lead to a variety of toxic effects that may be described in several ways. Toxic effects may be described according to:
- duration of exposure (acute or chronic);
- site of tissue damage (local or systemic);
- occurrence of effect in relation to time of exposure (immediate or delayed);
- reversibility of effect (reversible or irreversible);
- target organ (e.g. hepatotoxicity, renal toxicity, neurotoxicity, haematotoxicity);
- nature of toxic effect (e.g. whether functional, biochemical or morphological);
- specific toxic effect (e.g. carcinogenesis, sensitization, mutagenesis).

Table 3.2 Target organs associated with some substances.

Target organ	Substance
Skin	Chromium(VI) compounds, soluble nickel salts
Eyes	Ammonia, chlorine, iodine, glutaraldehyde, silver compounds, *N,N*-dimethylamine
Respiratory tract	Acid anhydrides, ammonia, azodicarbonamide, cadmium, chlorine, chromium(VI) compounds, cobalt, glutaraldehyde, iodine, isocyanates, kaolin, silica, talc, hardwood and softwood dust
Blood	Aniline, benzene, 2-butoxyethanol, lead, 4-nitroaniline, tetraethyl lead
Liver	Carbon tetrachloride, *N,N*-dimethylformamide, halothane, 2-nitropropane, tetraethyl lead
Kidney	Cadmium, chloroform, lead, mercury and inorganic mercury compounds, tetraethyl lead
Central nervous system	Acrylamide, dichloromethane, lead, mercury and inorganic mercury compounds, styrene, tetraethyl lead, trichloroethylene
Peripheral nervous system	Acrylamide, *n*-hexane
Heart	Carbon disulphide
Reproductive system	2-Ethoxyethanol, isoflurane, 2-methoxyethanol, 2-methoxyethylacetate, phthalate esters

Duration of exposure

Probably the most useful way to describe toxic effects for the purpose of hazard identification is according to the *duration of exposure*. Patterns of exposure in the workplace can be divided into two broad categories. The first category involves a short period of exposure, e.g. seconds or minutes, and may involve high levels of exposure. This exposure pattern may be a typical occurrence in some industrial processes. In the steel-making industry, for instance, certain areas are associated with high carbon monoxide levels, and the exposure of workers is controlled by limiting the amount of time spent in these areas to short periods. Alternatively, this type of exposure may only occur in unexpected circumstances, such as when leakages or accidental spillages take place. Toxic effects that are caused by short periods of exposure to high concentrations of a substance are termed *acute effects*.

The second category of exposure is that of repeated or prolonged exposure, typically involving relatively low levels of a substance, which may continue day after day, week after week, throughout the working life of an individual. Effects resulting from this pattern of exposure are described as *chronic effects*, *long-term effects* or *effects of repeated/prolonged exposure*.

When considering the hazards associated with a specific substance, it is essential to recognize that the two different exposure patterns described above can give rise to substantially different effects. With toluene exposure, for example, the acute effects are irritation of the eyes and respiratory tract, whereas the chronic effects are primarily central nervous system toxicity. The recognition of the difference between acute and chronic toxicity provides the rationale for the two types of OEL which form part of the strategy for controlling exposures in the workplace in many countries: a short-term limit and a long-term limit. The assessment and prevention of acute and chronic toxicity may therefore require substantially different approaches in terms of monitoring exposure, as discussed in Chapter 8, and also different strategies in the risk management process.

Local or systemic effects

The terms *local effect* and *systemic effect* refer to the site of tissue damage. A *local effect* is one that occurs at the site of first contact with the substance. Examples of substances which cause local effects are chlorine, which causes irritation of the eyes, skin and respiratory tract, and chromic acid, which has a corrosive effect on the skin. In contrast, a *systemic effect* occurs at a site distant from the initial point of contact, and takes place after a chemical has been absorbed into the body. An example of a systemic toxicant is the industrial solvent DMF. It enters the body either by inhalation of vapours or by absorption through the skin. It is then distributed via the blood to the liver, where it is metabolized to a toxic intermediate, which is responsible for the tissue damage at this site.

Immediate and delayed effects

Immediate effects are toxic effects that develop soon after exposure occurs. Narcosis resulting from exposure to high concentrations of 1,1,1-trichloroethane is a typical example of an immediate effect. With some substances, toxic effects only become apparent some time after exposure has taken place, e.g. months or years later. These effects are termed *delayed effects*. A typical example of a delayed effect is cancer, which may occur many years after first exposure to a substance. Identifying the causative agent is clearly much easier when an immediate effect is involved, rather than a delayed effect.

Reversible and irreversible toxicity

Toxic effects that subside once exposure ceases are termed *reversible effects*, whereas those that remain following the cessation of exposure, and may even progress, are termed *irreversible effects*. Irritation of the eyes, skin and respiratory tract, resulting from exposure to chlorine gas, is an example of a reversible effect; these effects recede once exposure ceases. Cancer provides a typical example of an irreversible effect. *n*-Hexane provides an example of a substance which can cause irreversible or reversible toxicity, depending on the level and duration of exposure. Repeated exposure to *n*-hexane can cause peripheral neuropathy, an irreversible effect characterized by a loss of sensation and function in the limbs. Short-term exposure to high concentrations of *n*-hexane can lead to narcosis, due to a depressive effect on the central nervous system. The narcotic effects recede when exposure stops. Clearly, in this case, irreversible toxicity is a more serious outcome than reversible toxicity. A knowledge of whether a substance may induce reversible or irreversible toxicity, and under what conditions, is an important issue when devising a risk management strategy.

Some specific toxic effects

Respiratory sensitizers (or asthmagens) are substances that induce a state of specific airway hyper-responsiveness in particular individuals. When the airways have become sensitized to a substance, further exposure, even to minute amounts, can cause respiratory effects. The mechanism involved in respiratory sensitization may be immunological or irritant. *Skin sensitizers* are substances that induce an immunologically mediated skin reaction, allergic contact dermatitis, in certain individuals as a result of skin contact. Subsequent exposure, even to tiny amounts, can evoke a skin response in sensitized subjects.

Carcinogenicity is a multistage process whereby exposure to a substance results in genetic damage within a cell, leading ultimately to the uncontrolled proliferation of cells and the induction of tumours. Carcinogenic substances may be divided into those which cause cancer by a genotoxic mechanism (i.e. the substance or metabolite causes direct damage to deoxyribonucleic acid (DNA)) and those which cause cancer by a non-genotoxic mechanism.

Mutagenicity refers to a permanent change in the genetic material of a cell, involving either a single gene, a block of genes or an entire chromosome, which may be passed on to the next generation of cells. If a substance causes mutations in the genetic materials of germ cells (reproductive cells, including sperm or ova), the genetic damage may be passed on to the offspring. If a substance causes mutations in somatic cells (non-reproductive cells in the body), this could provide the basis for the development of cancer.

Hazard identification

The process of hazard identification essentially involves the assessment of the toxicity of a substance and the evaluation of the toxicological data resulting from this assessment. In the European Community (EC), the approach to hazard identification differs according to whether a substance is an existing substance or a new substance. *Existing substances* are substances that are listed in the European Inventory of Existing Commercial Chemical Substances (EINECS); EINECS contains over 100 000 substances that were in use in the EC between 1971 and 1981. Any substance not listed in EINECS is called a *new substance*.

Toxicological assessment of new substances

The assessment of the toxicity of new substances takes place before the substance is placed on the market, and involves animal experiments and *in vitro* assays. The statutory requirement for testing new substances for toxicological, physicochemical and ecotoxicological properties is contained in the Dangerous Substances Directive (Council Directive 67/548/EEC 1967). In the UK, this requirement is implemented by the Notification of New Substances (NONS) Regulations 1993. Guidelines for the conduct of tests investigating these properties have been drawn up and agreed by international competent organizations, such as the Organization for Economic Co-operation and Development (OECD), with the aim of ensuring that the data generated conform to an accepted standard. Guidelines for the following tests are contained in Annex V of the Dangerous Substances Directive (Council Directive 67/548/EEC 1997a):

- acute toxicity (oral, inhalation or dermal);
- acute toxicity (skin or eye irritation);
- skin sensitization;
- subacute (28-day) toxicity (oral, inhalation or dermal);
- mutagenicity;
- subchronic (90-day) toxicity (oral, inhalation or dermal);
- carcinogenicity;
- reproduction toxicity.

The extent of testing that is required for a new substance will depend, to a large degree, on the amount of substance that is to be placed on the market. Early indications that a substance may cause serious toxicity, such as mutagenicity, carcinogenicity or effects on reproduction, can also trigger additional testing requirements.

The toxicity tests are intended to provide information on the toxicological properties of a new substance, such as the target organ(s), toxic effects and the reversibility of such effects, information on the dose–response relationship and whether further testing is required. Some of the more frequently used toxicity tests for new substances are briefly described in the following paragraphs, with an indication of how a substance might be classified and labelled on the basis of the test results.

The *acute toxicity test* is intended to provide a preliminary indication of toxicity following the administration of a single dose of a substance. The substance is administered to animals either orally, dermally or by inhalation, depending on which route is the most likely exposure route in humans, and lethalities and toxic effects are recorded during the subsequent 14-day period. This test is generally used to derive the LD_{50} value, which represents the median lethal dose; that is, the dose that is lethal to 80% of the animals. In the case of inhaled substances, the median lethal concentration (LC_{50}). A modified version of the test, called the fixed-dose procedure, has been developed which attempts to avoid using death as the end-point. This test focuses on 'evident toxicity' in preference to death. On the basis of the results from either acute toxicity test, a substance may be classified as 'harmful', 'toxic' or 'very toxic'. Table 3.3 summarizes how results from the acute toxicity test are used to classify and label a substance.

Tests for *skin and eye irritation* also come under the heading of acute toxicity tests. The *skin irritation test* involves the application of a single dose of a substance to the shaved skin of experimental animals, generally the rabbit. The test is intended to determine the potential of a substance to cause skin irritation and the severity of the skin response, and to indicate the reversibility of the effect. On the basis of the results of this test, a substance may be classified as either 'irritant' or, for those substances causing severe and irreversible effects, 'corrosive'.

In the *eye irritation test*, effects on the cornea, iris and conjunctiva are observed following a single application of substance to the eye. Generally, the test is conducted on the rabbit. As with the skin irritation test, the severity of the response and the reversibility are both assessed. Depending on the severity of the response in this test, a substance may be classified as 'irritant' and may carry the label 'irritating to the eyes'

Table 3.3 Classification and labelling of a substance using acute toxicity data.

		Label	
Test result	Classification	Symbol (indication of danger)	Risk phrase
LD_{50} (oral) $\leq 25\ mg\ kg^{-1}$	Very toxic	T+ (very toxic)	R28. Very toxic if swallowed
LD_{50} (dermal) $\leq 50\ mg\ kg^{-1}$	Very toxic	T+ (very toxic)	R27. Very toxic in contact with skin
LC_{50} (inhalation) $\leq 0.25\ mg\ l^{-1}/4\ h$ (aerosols or particulates); $\leq 0.5\ mg\ l^{-1}/4\ h$ (gases or vapours)	Very toxic	T+ (very toxic)	R26. Very toxic by inhalation
LD_{50} (oral) $> 25, \leq 200\ mg\ kg^{-1}$	Toxic	T (toxic)	R25. Toxic if swallowed
LD_{50} (dermal) $> 50, \leq 400\ mg\ kg^{-1}$	Toxic	T (toxic)	R24. Toxic in contact with skin
LC_{50} (inhalation) $> 0.25, \leq 1\ mg\ l^{-1}/4\ h$ (aerosols or particulates); $> 0.5, \leq 2\ mg\ l^{-1}/4\ h$ (gases or vapours)	Toxic	T (toxic)	R23. Toxic by inhalation
LD_{50} (oral) $> 200, \leq 2000\ mg\ kg^{-1}$	Harmful	Xn (harmful)	R22. Harmful if swallowed
LD_{50} (dermal) $> 400, \leq 2000\ mg\ kg^{-1}$	Harmful	Xn (harmful)	R21. Harmful in contact with skin
LC_{50} (inhalation) $> 1, \leq 5\ mg\ l^{-1}/4\ h$ (aerosols or particulates); $> 2, \leq 20\ mg\ l^{-1}/4\ h$ (gases or vapours)	Harmful	Xn (harmful)	R20. Harmful by inhalation

or 'risk of serious damage to the eyes'.

Animal tests are available to assess the potential of a substance to cause *skin sensitization* in humans. The tests are conducted on guinea pigs, and involve an induction phase, when animals receive repeated intradermal or topical doses of the substance, followed by challenge with a non-irritating dose of the substance applied topically. The skin response and the proportion of animals responding are observed. Animal data from this test can be used to support human evidence, which may lead to a substance being classified as 'sensitizing', and thus labelled with 'may cause sensitization by skin contact'.

Repeated-dose toxicity tests, which are either of 28 days' duration (subacute toxicity) or, if there are indications of particular toxicity, 90 days' duration (subchronic toxicity), provide a means of assessing the toxic effects resulting from repeated exposure to a substance. Animals are treated daily either orally, dermally or by inhalation, depending on the most likely exposure route for humans. During the treatment period, animals are investigated for clinical effects, functional changes in the nervous system or other organs and histopathological changes in tissues. The reversibility of any effects is determined. Results from a 28-day or 90-day test may lead to a substance being labelled with the risk phrase 'danger of serious damage to health by prolonged exposure'.

A range of tests are available to assess the *mutagenic potential* of a substance, each test investigating a specific genetic end-point. The tests include *in vitro* tests, using bacterial cells or mammalian cells, and *in vivo* tests, using whole animals. The extent to which a new substance is tested for mutagenicity will depend on the results of preliminary tests for mutagenicity, the physicochemical properties of the substance and information from other toxicity studies. As a minimum requirement, new substances should be tested in assays for gene mutations in bacteria, structural chromosome aberrations in mammalian cells and, in an *in vivo* assay, for structural chromosomal damage. The results from these assays are intended to provide an indication of the carcinogenic potential of the substance and may indicate the need for further investigation. Additional *in vivo* mutagenicity tests are available which can indicate the substance's potential to cause heritable genetic damage, i.e. damage to the DNA that can be expressed in the offspring. Such substances would be classified as 'mutagenic', either category 1 or category 2, and labelled with 'may cause heritable genetic damage'.

In the case of new substances, a *carcinogenicity test* is only required if there are indications from other tests, including mutagenicity tests, that the substance may have carcinogenic potential. In the carcinogenicity test, animals are treated daily with the substance for the major part of their lifespan (18 months for mice or hamsters; 24 months for rats). The route of exposure used should be the most likely route of exposure for humans. At the end of the study, the animals are thoroughly investigated for cancer incidence and for other signs of toxicity. Animal carcinogenicity tests provide information which, together with human evidence, may result in a substance being classified as 'carcinogenic'. 'Carcinogenic' substances are divided into one of three categories, depending on the strength of the available evidence.

Reproductive toxicity tests are intended to detect developmental toxicity and effects on male and female fertility. The assessment of developmental toxicity involves treating pregnant females with the substance during the period of organogenesis, and examining the effect on the uterus and fetuses. Effects on fertility are assessed in one- or two-generation studies, in which male and female animals are treated. The females are treated before and during pregnancy, and also during lactation. The effects on the resulting offspring are examined. On the basis of the results of animal tests, together with epidemiological data, a substance may be classified as 'toxic to reproduction'. Three categories exist, depending on the strength of the evidence, and different labels are used according to whether the substance impairs fertility ('may impair fertility') or causes developmental toxicity ('may cause harm to the unborn child').

Toxicological assessment of existing substances

The toxicological assessment of existing substances involves the consideration of the available toxicity data that will not have been generated using the systematic and rigorous procedures required for new substances. The animal and *in vitro* data that may exist for such substances may have been generated using test methods that differ substantially from the recommended methods specified in Annex V. The adequacy of such data for the purpose of classification and labelling, or for the preparation of safety data sheets, as described later in this chapter, must be judged on a case-by-case basis. The availability of human data from epidemiological investigations, studies conducted in human volunteers or from case reports may make a significant contribution to the toxicological assessment in this respect (see Chapter 4). The assessment of all available data may reveal important gaps in the toxicological database. Further testing of the substance using recommended methods may therefore be required, and a recommendation for further testing may be one outcome of the assessment.

For some new and existing substances, it may be possible to predict the toxicological properties on the basis of the known toxicity associated with other chemically similar compounds. This is the basis of the structure–activity relationship (SAR), which provides an important, alternative source of toxicity data for some substances.

Evaluating toxicological data

For new substances and for many existing substances, most if not all of the toxicological data are generated in species other than humans. Animal experiments and *in vitro* assays are generally conducted under carefully controlled conditions, and involve clearly defined exposure to the test substance. Under such conditions, the causal relationship between the substance exposure and any response is relatively easy to define. However, the data obtained from such experiments need to be extrapolated to humans. Extrapolation plays an essential step in the risk assessment process, and entails a careful consideration of all the available data to determine whether there is likely to be any difference in the response to a substance between the experimental model used and humans. A number of factors need to be taken into consideration when extrapolating from animals to humans, including:

- possible species variation;
- potential sex differences;
- use of different routes of exposure;
- different patterns and levels of exposure.

Different species may vary considerably in their response to a substance. These variations may arise as a consequence of differences in metabolism, qualitative and/or quantitative, or variations in the absorption, distribution and/or excretion of a substance. Toxicokinetic investigations provide a fairly reliable means of identifying such species differences, and therefore play a crucial role in the evaluation of toxicity data.

Tetrachloroethylene provides one example where interspecies variability in metabolism leads to marked differences in toxicity. Tetrachloroethylene is widely used as a solvent in the dry-cleaning industry, and has been shown to produce liver tumours in mice and kidney tumours in rats. An evaluation of the animal toxicity data involves a consideration of whether these tumours are relevant to humans. Toxicokinetic data for tetrachloroethylene show that it is metabolized by several different pathways. One metabolic pathway involves the oxidative metabolism of tetrachloroethylene to trichloroacetic acid, a metabolite which causes liver tumours by a non-genotoxic mechanism called peroxisome proliferation. Peroxisome proliferation only occurs in mice. Another metabolic pathway involves the formation of a glutathione conjugate that undergoes enzymatic cleavage in the kidney to form a reactive thioketene intermediate, which appears to be responsible for the development of kidney tumours in rats. This metabolic pathway only occurs in rats. Therefore neither the mouse liver tumours nor the rat kidney tumours appear to be relevant to humans, and current understanding is that tetrachloroethylene does not present a carcinogenic risk for humans. The main health effect associated with tetrachloroethylene in humans is considered to be sensory irritation, and the OEL is designed to protect against this effect. Potential reproductive effects are still under investigation.

Another important factor involved in extrapolating data from animal experiments to humans is that the exposure conditions used in the animal tests are likely to be very different from those that occur in the workplace. Animal tests are frequently conducted under conditions that involve high levels and short durations of exposure, constant exposure levels, constant temperature and minimal physical activity. Typical occupational exposures are rarely like this and, in extrapolating data, these differences should be taken into account.

The extrapolation of toxicity data from animal experiments to humans is beset with many difficulties, some of which have been described. In the absence of data indicating the contrary, the most cautious, and thus most appropriate, approach is to assume that humans are more sensitive to the substance than animals. This approach involves the application of *safety factors*. Safety factors or uncertainty factors may also be applied to allow for deficiencies in the data.

How toxicological data are used

Under current EC legislation, suppliers of substances or preparations, which are defined as 'dangerous', are required to provide information on the hazardous properties so that users can take the necessary precautions to protect their own or their employees' health. The information on hazardous properties is provided by classifying and labelling substances and preparations, and by preparing safety data sheets. The statutory requirements to provide this information are contained in the Dangerous Substances Directive (Council Directive 67/548/EEC 1967) and the amended version of the Directive (Council Directive 92/32/EEC 1992), referred to as the Seventh Amendment. A further use of toxicological data involves the development of OELs, which form an important part of the strategy for controlling exposure to harmful substances in the workplace. The philosophy underlying OELs and the practice of establishing OELs are discussed in Chapter 7. Data which specifically relate to the carcinogenic properties of substances are also used in the International Agency for Research on Cancer (IARC) evaluation of the carcinogenic risk of chemicals to humans, described in Chapter 4.

Classification and labelling

Classification involves the 'identification of the properties of substances and preparations that may constitute a hazard during normal handling and use' (Health and Safety Commission (HSC) 1997). Classification involves a consideration of the available data relating to toxicological, physicochemical and ecotoxicological properties, and a comparison of these with clearly defined criteria. The outcome of this process is that, once a substance has been classified, it will be labelled accordingly. The label is intended to provide essential information to the user about any hazardous properties which, together with more detailed information contained in the safety data sheet, will enable the user to take precautionary measures. The classification process and labelling criteria are contained within Annex VI to the Dangerous Substances Directive (Council Directive 67/548/EEC 1997b) and, in the UK, are presented in the Approved Guide to the Classification and Labelling of Substances and Preparations Dangerous for Supply (HSC 1997).

Safety data sheets

Suppliers of substances and preparations that are considered to be dangerous also have a responsibility by law to produce safety data sheets. Safety data sheets contain, in addition to toxicological data, information on the identity of the substance, recommendations for handling, storage and disposal, physicochemical properties, first aid and fire-fighting measures and transport information. Safety data sheets are intended to provide users of a substance with sufficient information about the hazardous properties of the substance which, together with the labelling information described previously, enables the user to conduct a risk assessment.

Conclusions

Toxicology plays an important role in the risk assessment and risk management process, contributing data which may be used in a number of different ways. Toxicological data may be used in the preparation of safety data sheets, substance hazard classification and labelling and in the development of OELs and biological monitoring methods. All of these applications have the potential to make a significant contribution to the protection of the health of humans in the workplace.

References

Council Directive 67/548/EEC (1967) *Directive on Classification, Packaging and Labelling of Dangerous Substances.* OJ number 196, 16.8.1967. EC Publication, Luxembourg.

Council Directive 92/32/EEC (1992) *Updated Version of Directive 67/548/EEC.* OJ number L 154, 5.6.1992. EC Publication, Luxembourg.

Council Directive 67/548/EEC (1997a) *Annex V. Methods for the Determination of Physico-chemical Properties, Toxicity and Ecotoxicity.* EC Publication, Luxembourg.

Council Directive 67/548/EEC (1997b) *Annex VI. General Classification and Labelling Requirements for Dangerous Substances and Preparations.* EC Publication, Luxembourg.

HSC (1997) *Approved Guide to the Classification and Labelling of Substances and Preparations Dangerous for Supply; CHIP 97; Guidance on Regulations.* HSE Books, Norwich.

Chapter 4 Epidemiological basis of hazard identification

David Koh and Adeline Seow

Introduction

Epidemiological studies have been the mainstay for the identification of hazards and the provision of information for the classification of hazards and the setting of exposure levels. This chapter provides an overview of epidemiological studies and how they contribute to the process of hazard identification.

What is epidemiology?

Last (1988) defines epidemiology as: 'the study of the distribution and determinants of health-related states or events in specified populations, and the application of this study to control of health problems'. In other words, it is a study of 'how' and 'why' diseases are distributed in groups of people.

The application of epidemiology can be illustrated by how some questions in the occupational health setting are answered (at least partly) by the epidemiological approach. These include the following examples.

Is there a connection between certain occupations and diseases? If so, how can these diseases best be prevented?
For example, in the study of occupational diseases, the questions asked might include: 'is work as a chimney sweep connected with scrotal cancer?'; and 'do vinyl chloride monomer workers have an increased risk for angiosarcoma of the liver?'.

The epidemiological approach can also be applied to the study of work-related diseases which are multicausal in nature, such as low back pain and coronary heart disease, where workplace factors, such as manual handling and psychological stress, play important roles, but are not the sole factors in the development of the disease.

How do we evaluate whether or not a substance is harmful to humans?
The assessment of the toxic potential of a substance depends both on the results of animal toxicological studies and human data collected in epidemiological studies (see Chapter 3). As an example, the International Agency for Research on Cancer (IARC) has reviewed hundreds

of chemicals and exposures for their carcinogenic potential. The classification of the substances reviewed into categories, such as carcinogens (Group 1), probable carcinogens (Group 2A), possible carcinogens (Group 2B) or unclassifiable (Group 3), depends on both experimental toxicological and epidemiological evidence. The epidemiological approach is particularly useful in the assessment of the carcinogenic potential of mixtures or exposure circumstances.

How can exposure standards be set on a scientific basis?

As discussed in Chapter 7, occupational exposure limits (OELs) in various countries are set on the basis of a variety of factors. Scientific reasons form only part of this basis. However, the starting point in the setting of standards is often based on scientific evidence. This gathered evidence is dependent, to a moderate or large extent, on the epidemiological approach applied in studies of human populations. For example, in setting standards for exposure to benzene, one would take into consideration toxicity studies in animals and in *in vitro* test systems. However, attempts to understand and quantify the health effects of benzene on humans would require well-conducted epidemiological studies measuring outcomes such as the immunological effects, leukaemogenesis or mortality. Several studies have been carried out among chemical workers exposed to varying levels of benzene, and the results have been used to make recommendations for the setting of OELs for this compound.

How often should workers exposed to prescribed hazards be subjected to medical examinations, and which are the best tests to be performed?

Workers exposed to prescribed hazards may require statutory health monitoring (see Chapter 16). How often should such workers be tested? What is the cost effectiveness of the monitoring? How does the prognosis of cases detected early compare with cases detected at a late stage? Such questions can be answered in occupational health services' research, again using the epidemiological approach.

Data for epidemiological studies

Epidemiological studies use two major sources of data from occupational settings: (i) *data collected routinely for other purposes*, such as vital registration data, official employment records or hospital discharge information; and (ii) *data collected specifically for the evaluation of health outcomes of certain exposures*, such as an epidemiological study performed to evaluate the potential cancer risk of benzene among petroleum workers.

In acquiring data for use in epidemiological studies, the two most important groups of measurements are exposure assessments and outcome measures.

Exposure assessments
As discussed in Chapters 8 and 16, a valid means of determining the extent of exposure to the putative risk factor is required. This may take the form of actual biological measurements (e.g. blood lead levels), measurement of ambient levels (e.g. asbestos fibre counts) or the use of surrogate measures, such as the length of time in a particular occupation which is known to involve exposure to the agent under study.

For example, in a study of the occurrence of respiratory cancer among workers exposed to chloromethyl ethers, different jobs in a plant were rated on a scale of 0–6 in order of increasing potential exposure to the compounds (Gowers *et al.* 1993). The periods during which each individual had worked in these jobs were obtained from personnel records, and the ratings for each job were summed to give the cumulative dose in units of rating-years.

Outcome measures
In order to measure risk, a valid assessment of whether or not the outcome has occurred must be included in the data collection. Outcomes include discrete events, such as death and the onset of disease, as well as sickness absence rates, or changes in health status, such as the improvement or deterioration in neurobehavioural test scores, quality of life indices, etc. Some of the rates used to express the occurrence of these outcomes are discussed below.

In most epidemiological studies, a rigorous protocol, which includes clearly defined criteria for assessing exposure and outcome, should be in place before the commencement of the study. Wherever possible, these criteria should be objective, and the ascertainment should be performed 'blind' to the other aspects of the study. For example, a research assistant whose task is to determine an improvement in symptomatology from case records should be unaware of the treatment status of each patient, so that potential biases (see later) can be eliminated.

The use of rates as epidemiological measurements

Epidemiology is a quantitative discipline, using numerical measures of disease occurrence and distribution to describe an illness. The simplest unit of measurement is a count of events, such as accidents or diseases. The following are examples of counts.

- There were 67 serious road traffic accidents among bus drivers in a town, and 30 serious road traffic accidents among taxi drivers in a town last year.
- Eighty out of 100 cases of a new and puzzling occupational disease in an industrial estate were from the electronics industry.

Counts, however, are of limited use, as they cannot be used to answer questions such as: 'which job, bus driving or taxi driving, has a higher risk of accidents?'. Neither can they be used to arrive at conclusions such as: 'as 80% of the occupational diseases are from the electronics industry, surely this must be a high-risk occupation for the disease'. Obviously, the number of persons at risk for the accidents or disease is important.

In order to make meaningful comparisons, rates, or the proportion in a group with the event or disease, need to be computed. A rate comprises a numerator and denominator. The numerator is the total number of events measured. The denominator, or population at risk, consists of all those in whom the event can happen. In the above examples, the number of bus and taxi drivers in the town and the proportion of workers in the industrial estate working as electronics workers would be important.

The main advantage of using rates is that the event or disease occurrence in two or more groups can be compared. Two common rates are the prevalence and incidence rates.

Prevalence rate

The *prevalence rate* measures how much a disease or condition prevails in a given population at a designated time. *Point prevalence* refers to the number of persons with the disease or attribute at a specified point in time, divided by the total number of persons in the group. The numerator for *period prevalence* is the number of persons with the disease or attribute at any time in a specified period, while the numerator for *lifetime prevalence* is the number of persons with the disease or attribute for at least part of their life (Last 1988).

Incidence rate

The *incidence rate* is the rate at which new events occur in a population. The numerator is the number of new events in a given period, while the denominator is the population at risk during the period. The denominator is sometimes expressed as person-time (the sum of the units of time contributed by each person who is subject to the exposure of interest). These two types of incidence rate have been termed *cumulative incidence* and *incidence density*, respectively.

The incidence rate quantifies the likelihood or *risk* of a person developing the event or disease in a given period of observation.

Relationship between prevalence and incidence

For a given disease, the incidence and prevalence are related by the expression:

$$\text{Prevalence} \propto \text{Incidence} \times \text{Duration of disease} \qquad (4.1)$$

The situation is analogous to a reservoir, being supplied by streams and emptied through a dam. The amount of water in the reservoir, the prevalence, is dependent upon the water flowing in from the streams (the incidence) and the water flowing out through the dam (people who recover from the disease or die).

Prevalence and incidence should not be used interchangeably, as they measure different things. It follows that they cannot be compared with each other. For example, let us consider the scenario given below.

In a large multinational company, the prevalence of coronary heart disease is higher than the prevalence of the common cold. Yet, more work days are lost each year because of the common cold than because of coronary heart disease. Does this mean that coronary heart disease is less disabling than the common cold, or that people use the common cold as an excuse to stay away from work?

In this situation, the prevalence of coronary heart disease, a long-lasting disease, is large compared with its incidence. The reverse is true for the common cold. It has a low prevalence, but a high incidence. The number of work days lost reflects the incidence rate, consequent upon the new development of the disease. This should not be compared with the prevalence rate of the disease.

Other types of rates

In occupational settings, comparisons between industries or over time become meaningful only when the denominators include a consideration of the duration of exposure or, more specifically, the working time. Accident rates and sickness absence rates are commonly used to assess hazards and behavioural characteristics, respectively, of working groups. They are also important tools in the study of working conditions, such as the effect of shift work. For purposes of comparison, these rates can be expressed as relative measures, commonly given as *frequency* and *severity* rates.

Sickness absence rates

The frequency and severity rates used in sickness absence reporting are commonly expressed as follows.

The *sickness absence frequency rate* is expressed as the mean spells of absence per person, or:

$$\frac{\text{Total number of new spells of absence in a defined period}}{\text{Average population at risk in that same period}} \quad (4.2)$$

The *sickness absence severity rate*, on the other hand, is expressed by the mean number of days of absence per person, or:

$$\frac{\text{Total days of absence in a defined period}}{\text{Average population at risk in that same period}} \quad (4.3)$$

Accident rates

The presentation of accident statistics, as outlined in the International Labour Office (ILO) encyclopaedia (Brancoli 1983), can also be in the form of frequency and severity rates. The *accident frequency rate* is given by the number of accidents in relation to the man-hours worked, i.e.:

$$\frac{\text{Total number of accidents} \times 1\,000\,000}{\text{Total number of man-hours worked}} \quad (4.4)$$

Where the denominators are not readily available, it is suggested that an incidence rate is used. This is expressed as:

$$\frac{\text{Total number of accidents} \times 1000}{\text{Average number of persons exposed}} \quad (4.5)$$

The *accident severity rate* indicates the time lost as a result of accidents, and is given by:

$$\frac{\text{Total number of days lost} \times 1000}{\text{Total number of man-hours worked}} \quad (4.6)$$

For example, a study of occupational injuries among furniture workers in Finland (Aaltonen 1996) recorded 214 accidents during the 1-year study period. The overall disabling injury rate (an incidence rate) was 14.4 per 100 workers per year. The severity rate (days of sick leave per injury) was 9.1 in small companies (20–49 workers) and 16.2 in large companies (> 200 workers).

The use of rates is an important concept in hazard identification. Relationships between exposure and outcome are often expressed in terms of rates of death, disease or disability across various exposure groups. There is very little justification for conclusions to be based on numerator data alone. In addition, when evaluating epidemiological studies, one should consider whether the rate chosen is appropriate; for example, the incidence density would provide a more accurate estimate of risk if the denominator (i.e. the size of the population at risk) changes throughout the observation period.

Linking disease with exposures

One of the important uses of epidemiology is to test the hypothesis that a certain exposure, e.g. to dust, may increase the risk of a health outcome, e.g. lung cancer. This necessitates the measurement of the likelihood of this outcome in both exposed and unexposed groups. If the likelihood of the outcome is statistically dependent on the extent of exposure, an association is said to exist between the two.

Comparing rates—relative risk

The commonest way of comparing the risk between exposure groups is to obtain the relative risk or rate ratio. This is defined as:

$$\text{Relative risk (RR)} = \frac{\text{Incidence rate in exposed}}{\text{Incidence rate in unexposed}} \quad (4.7)$$

Using the relative risk, one is able to compare the rates of several groups with that of a single standard reference group. For example, in a study comparing the risk of lung cancer among workers exposed to varying levels of benzo[a]pyrene (BaP) in the iron and steel industry, the risk among men exposed to a cumulative total of BaP between 0.85 and 3.2 $\mu g\,m^{-3}$ per year was 1.6 times that of those in the unexposed group, and the risk among men exposed to $\geq 30\,\mu g\,m^{-3}$ per year was 1.8 times that of those in the unexposed group (Xu *et al.* 1996). This pattern of increase in risk with increasing levels of exposure is known as a dose–response relationship, and provides empirical support for a causal relationship between the exposure and outcome.

The difference in rate between those exposed and those not exposed to the putative risk factor is a measure of the rate of the disease that can be attributed to the exposure. This rate difference is also known as the *attributable risk*, and is a measure of the impact of the exposure on an individual's disease risk.

Adjustment of rates

In comparing rates of disease or death from specific causes between two occupational groups, it is important to remember that other factors, apart from the occupational exposure, can influence disease rates. For example, age is a principal determinant of many diseases. Differences in disease rates between two groups may be the result of differences in the age distribution rather than the exposure of interest.

In order to obtain a valid comparison between groups, it is often necessary to remove the influence of age. This can be done by using age-specific rates (e.g. death rates from lung cancer for men aged 40–49 years are compared between coke oven workers and the general population). It is more useful, however, to have a summary statistic of such comparisons that takes into account the differing age structures of the two populations. Two commonly used statistics are the age-adjusted (or age-standardized) death (or incidence) rates and the standardized mortality (or incidence) ratio.

In the *direct method* of age adjustment, the age-specific rates of the two populations, e.g. in two adjacent cities, being compared are applied to a standard population. This procedure gives the expected rate that would have occurred if these cities had the same age distribution, i.e. that of the standard population. A valid comparison between these two computed rates, which are now adjusted for the effect of age, can then be made.

Occupational studies commonly seek to compare the number of deaths or health outcomes in a given occupational group (e.g. textile factory floor workers) with the general population, or with a second occupational group (e.g. office staff in the same industry). The standardized mortality (or morbidity) ratio (SMR) is another method of age adjustment. This is the *indirect method* of standardization, and has the advantage that a knowledge of the age-specific death rates is not necessary. The SMRs can be computed using the age distribution and the total number of deaths in the occupational group, and the age-specific death rates for the comparison group.

This technique can be used to adjust for factors other than age which may affect the outcome (see 'Confounding', later). As an example, a study of perinatal deaths among children of men employed in the printing industry, and exposed to lead plus solvents, recorded 117 deaths among these children. When compared with children born to all married couples in the same city, adjusting for maternal age, year of birth, sex and birth order, an SMR of 1.6 was obtained. This suggests that children born to the exposed group were 1.6 times more likely to die in the perinatal period than those born to the general population, adjusted for differences in the distribution of maternal age and the other factors listed between the two groups (Kristensen *et al.* 1993).

Types of epidemiological study

Epidemiological studies generally fall into two broad groups: *observational* studies, in which the investigator measures a phenomenon such as an exposure and/or a disease, and *experimental* studies, in which an intervention, either therapeutic or preventive, is introduced and the effect of this intervention is studied.

Observational studies can be further classified into *descriptive studies*, which serve to document or evaluate 'what is happening' (such as the trends in the incidence of occupational asthma over time, or the occurrence of a cluster of cases of hepatitis in a particular factory), and *analytical studies*, which are designed to test cause and effect relationships (such as the link between the exposure to allergens in the worker's environment and the risk of asthma).

Figure 4.1 outlines the types of epidemiological study.

Case studies and case series

A case study is an example of an observational study confined to a single individual in whom an unusual occurrence is described. A case study is often a starting point for further epidemiological studies.

For example, Toren and Jonsson (1996) reported a case of vibration white finger in an autopsy assistant. Autopsy assistants have to prepare corpses for autopsy, including the sawing of skulls with an electric saw. Vibration measurements during skull sawing showed a frequency-weighted acceleration level of $8.9\,m\,s^{-2}$, and this was postulated as a possible cause of blanching of the fingers.

A single case report, however, cannot answer a question because there is no comparison group against which the hypothesis may be tested.

The case study can be expanded to a description of several cases, when it becomes a case series. Studying the characteristics of a group of

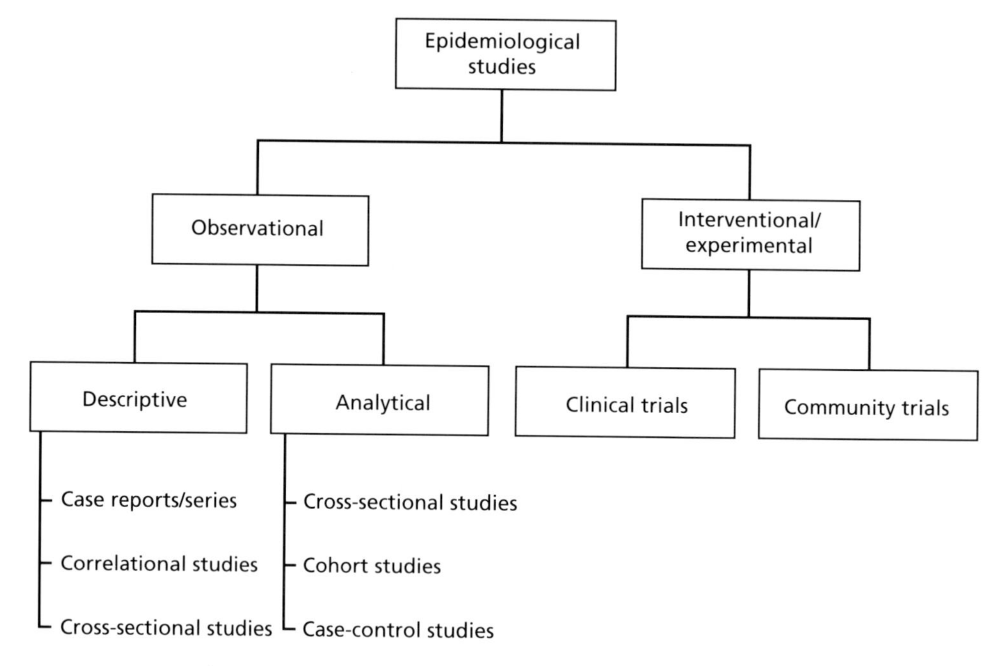

Figure 4.1 Classification of epidemiological studies.

similar occurrences may help to document common features, describe the natural history of the illness or signal the emergence of something new.

Cross-sectional studies

The cross-sectional study provides a snapshot of what is happening in a population. It is usually carried out as a single examination of a cross-section of the population at a particular point in time, and provides prevalence data for a disease or attribute.

For example, how many persons in a population of cotton textile factory workers have byssinosis? Sometimes relationships or associations can be uncovered in cross-sectional studies. In the case of byssinosis in cotton textile factory workers, it may be found that workers in a dusty section have higher prevalence rates of byssinosis compared with workers in less dusty sections. Could cotton dust, then, be the cause of byssinosis?

In the case study example given above (Toren & Jonsson 1996), an analytical investigation to examine the relationship between skull sawing and white finger could take the form of a cross-sectional study. From the initial case study, the investigators proceeded to send a questionnaire to 17 autopsy assistants who were exposed to local vibration, and 18 medical examiners (who were not exposed to vibration) as a comparison group. Eleven of the assistants (85%) and one of the examiners (6%) reported a history of blanching of the fingers provoked by cold. The result was statistically significant, indicating an association between the exposure and the health effect.

The main advantages of cross-sectional studies are that they are cheap and relatively quick and easy to conduct. The main disadvantage of this type of study is that the study may be conducted on a 'survivor' population, left behind after the affected or ill workers have departed. Taking the earlier example of byssinosis, many of the workers with byssinosis might have left the job because of the illness, or have been transferred to easier and lighter jobs in the factory. In this case, a cross-sectional study might find that workers in the dusty sections in the factory have a lower prevalence of byssinosis compared with workers in the less dusty sections.

Case control studies

The case control study examines *cases* of the disease, and compares the characteristics of the cases with a group of *controls* who do not have the disease. The study examines persons after the disease has developed (cases), and looks back (retrospectively) in an attempt to determine which factor is associated with the disease. A group of non-diseased persons (controls) is similarly studied.

For example, persons with gliomas in the central nervous system (cases) can be studied in relation to a particular exposure, e.g. lead compounds, and compared with a control group of persons without the disease (how many people in the non-diseased group were previously exposed to lead at work?). The strength of the association, in this case, between work with lead and the disease, is measured in terms of odds ratios. For a rare disease, the odds ratio approximates to the relative risk for the disease.

A case control study of myocardial infarction, restricted to males aged between 30 and 74 years in Sweden (Gustavsson *et al.* 1996), showed a relative risk (compared with a random sample of the population base) of 1.53 (95% confidence interval (CI) 1.15–2.05) for bus drivers in Stockholm. Taxi drivers in Stockholm had a relative risk of 1.65 (95% CI 1.30–2.11), while truck drivers did not show any marked excess risk.

The case control study is relatively inexpensive to conduct, fairly quick to perform and is especially relevant for cases of rare diseases. However, it is not able to provide the exact risk of developing the disease. This type of study only demonstrates the association with the disease, and does not imply causation. Other major problems include recall bias and the choice of an appropriate control group. Sometimes, matching is performed for the control group, e.g. age- and sex-matched controls, to make the two groups more comparable (see 'Confounding', later).

Cohort studies

The cohort study begins with the characterization of the factor in question (e.g. exposure or non-exposure to radon daughters at work) in a given population (cohort). The suspected factor, in this case exposure to radon daughters, is identified first before the group is followed up. All members enrolled in the cohort must be free of the outcome of interest.

The cohort is then followed up over a period of time, and studied to determine whether the outcome of interest (e.g. lung cancer) develops in both the exposed and unexposed groups. This follow-up could be a prospective process. Alternatively, a historical cohort assembled in the past (e.g. persons employed in a bus company over the last 20 years) could be followed up from the commencement of their enrollment to the present.

The comparison group may comprise similar, but unexposed, workers. For example, the question to be answered may be: 'does the group of workers exposed to radon daughters have a higher rate of lung cancer compared with an unexposed group in the same industry after a follow-up period of 25 years?'.

The general population may also be used as a comparison group. A cohort of 7887 male and 576 female Danish asbestos cement workers employed from 1928 to 1984 were followed up for deaths, emigrations and incident cancer cases during the period 1943–1990 (Raffn *et al.* 1996). The incidence of lung cancer among the workers was then compared with that of the general population in Denmark. Among the male workers, the lung cancer incidence was 1.7 times higher than that of the general population. The standardized morbidity ratios were increased for all histological types of lung cancer: 2.6 for adenocarcinoma, 1.7 for squamous cell carcinoma and 1.5 for anaplastic carcinoma.

Smaller cohorts can also be studied for shorter periods. Nielsen *et al.* (1996) reported five cases of malignant melanoma among a cohort of 837 lithographers followed in the Danish Cancer Register from 1974 to 1989. The relative risk of melanoma among lithographers was 3.4 (95% CI 1.2–7.5). The authors agreed that the risk for developing melanoma was multifactorial, sun exposure probably being the most important factor. However, they felt that the chemical compounds used in lithography, notably hydroquinone (which has a biological effect on melanocytes), could have acted in combination with sun exposure to increase the risk of malignant melanoma in lithographers.

The cohort study is an expensive and time-consuming undertaking. However, it provides strong evidence for a cause and effect relationship, particularly because the exposure is documented at the start of the follow-up period, and its temporal relationship to the outcome is not in question, a problem that sometimes arises in case control studies.

Nested case control studies

A nested case control study is a cost-effective way of utilizing the data within a large cohort study. In this design, both cases and controls are drawn from a cohort that is being followed up, the cases being those developing the disease of interest during the course of the study.

For example, a cohort of workers belonging to a large telephone company was followed up, and workers developing leukaemia were compared with controls selected from the remaining pool of employees without the disease. The job histories of both groups were compared

Table 4.1 Types, uses, advantages and disadvantages of epidemiological studies.

Type of study	Uses	Advantages	Disadvantages
Cross-sectional studies	Assess the health status of a defined population Provide a basis for health planning and evaluation Definition of normal values Generate hypotheses of disease aetiology	Quality of data easily controlled by standardizing techniques, ensuring uniform diagnostic criteria Can study association of disease with a wide range of factors simultaneously Quick and relatively inexpensive; require fewer subjects than cohort studies	Unsuitable for rare diseases Difficult to interpret temporal sequence (?cause before effect) Do not measure directly the risk of developing the disease
Case control studies	Test hypotheses of disease aetiology Investigate source of disease outbreak	Efficient design for rare diseases Can study wide range of risk factors in relation to the disease of interest	More difficult to establish temporal relationship between cause and effect Particularly prone to selection and measurement bias
Cohort studies	Test hypotheses of disease aetiology Investigate source of outbreak Describe course of disease or survival of a group of patients	Able to distinguish temporal sequence of cause and effect Can measure disease incidence (risk) directly in exposed and unexposed groups Can study more than one outcome in relation to the factor chosen Less susceptible to bias (e.g. in subject selection)	Expensive Require long follow-up periods, especially for rare diseases May require large number of subjects Loss to follow-up may introduce bias Drift in standard of outcome ascertainment over time

with respect to the extent of their exposure to electric and magnetic fields during the course of their work (Matanski *et al.* 1993).

Such a study design has the advantage of saving on the resources needed to compute job–exposure matrices for an entire database of employees, and is an efficient method of utilizing the information available in a prospective study, while, at the same time, removing many of the potential biases normally encountered in case control studies.

Table 4.1 summarizes the uses, advantages and disadvantages of the different types of epidemiological study. Figure 4.2 illustrates the case control, cohort and nested case control studies in a pictorial diagram.

There are obviously many limitations on the types of study that may be carried out in occupational health settings to evaluate safety and risks. Chief among these are ethical and logistical constraints. As a rule, risk assessments should be based on all the available data at that time; in some cases, data available from humans may be descriptive or cross-sectional in origin. The maxim 'some data are better than no data at all' applies as long as the limitations of the various study designs are given due consideration in the review process.

Meta analysis of epidemiological studies

Meta analysis has been described as the process of using statistical methods to combine the results of different studies (Last 1988). This is performed by the systematic, organized and structured evaluation of the problem of interest, using information from a number of independent studies of the problem. This type of analysis includes aspects of an overview as well as the pooling of data, but implies more than either.

Meta analysis has a qualitative component, in the application of predetermined criteria of quality before a study is selected for inclusion in the analysis. It also has a quantitative component, in the process of integration of the numerical information of the different studies into a whole. Meta analysis is also subject to several biases. One such bias is publication bias, where studies with 'negative' or 'non-significant' results are less likely to be published.

One example of a meta analysis involves a review and pooling of studies to examine occupational electric and magnetic field (EMF) exposure and the risk of brain cancer (Kheifets *et al.* 1995). The meta analysis concluded that there was a small elevation of risk, but a considerable heterogeneity of the results. The authors concluded that: 'However, because of the lack of adequate exposure information and a clear dose–response pattern, it is not possible to conclude that EMF is causally associated with the observed excess of brain cancer in workers employed in electrical occupations'.

Another meta analysis examined studies on asbestos and colorectal cancer, and reported an overall relative risk of 0.99 for the 30 studies that were reviewed. The author (Weiss 1995) concluded that: 'the evidence does not meet the important criteria for a judgement of causality

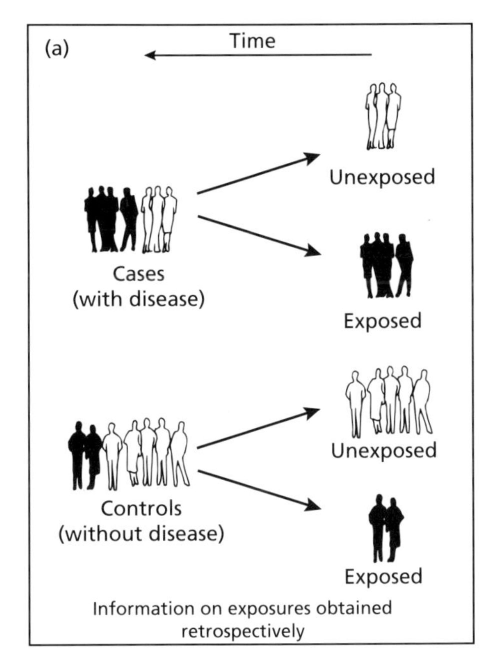

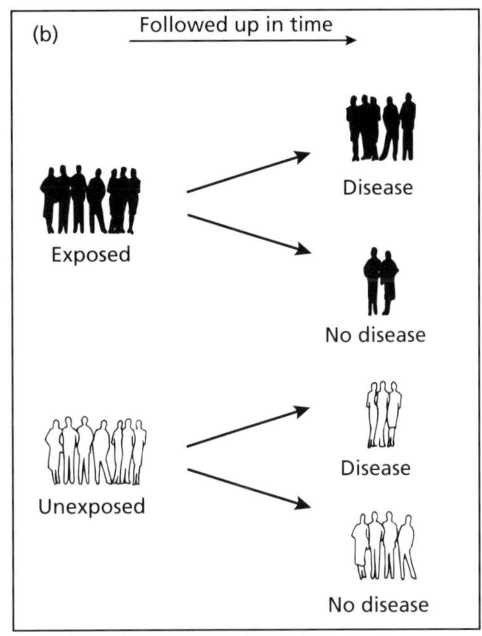

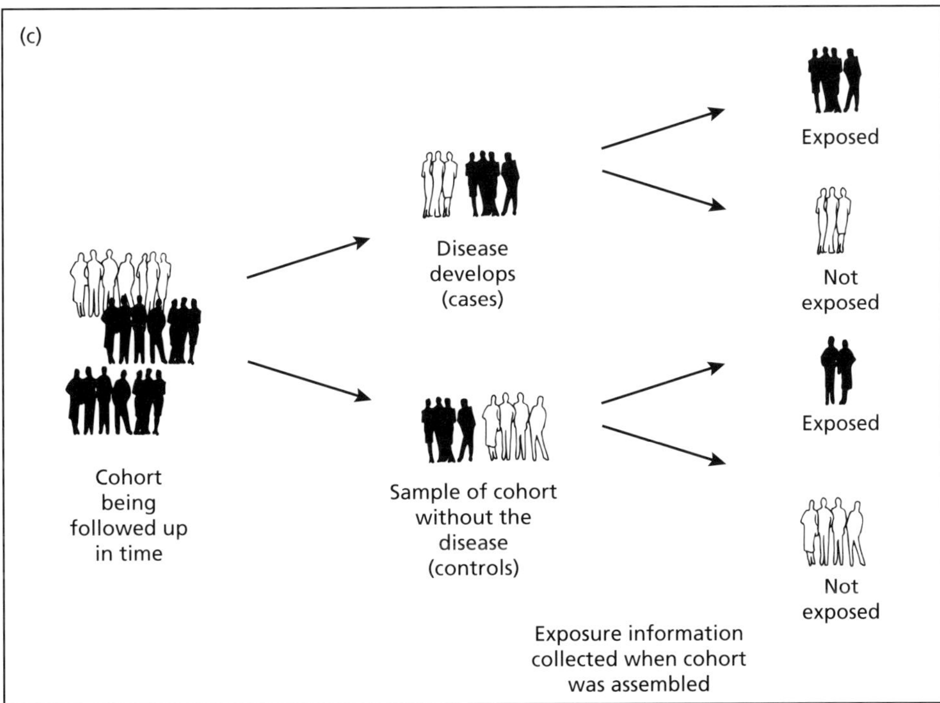

Figure 4.2 Schematic diagram to illustrate case control (a), cohort (b) and nested case control (c) studies.

because the relative risk is not consistently elevated, weak in the two studies with a statistically significant elevation of SMR, and limited data do not support a dose–response relationship'.

Association and causation

Most epidemiological studies examine associations between variables. Associations are relationships which exist between the occurrence of one variable (such as an exposure or risk marker) and the occurrence of another variable (usually the outcome of interest, e.g. an accident or a disease). Associations can be positive (the factor and outcome occur together), negative (the factor and outcome tend not to occur together), or there may be no association. If an association is found between the exposure and the outcome, the next question is whether the association is spurious or real.

Spurious associations

Spurious associations are often due to chance, bias or confounding.

Chance

Epidemiological studies are often carried out on samples from a population rather than on the entire population. This gives rise to sampling variation or random error. Statistical testing is used to determine the likelihood of a chance association in epidemiological studies. The results of epidemiological studies may be expressed in terms of confidence intervals (CIs), e.g. the relative risk (RR) for a disease in a group of exposed workers is 3.0 (95% CI 1.7–5.7) compared with that in a group of unexposed workers. This means that the point estimate of the relative risk in the study sample is 3.0, and there is a 95% likelihood that the population relative risk is in the range 1.7–5.7. Alternatively, tests of statistical significance are presented, e.g. relative risk = 3.0 ($P < 0.05$). In this case, the 'P value' denotes the probability that the observed relative risk arose purely by chance. A P value of less than 0.05 is said to imply a 'statistically significant' association between the exposure and outcome under study.

Bias

In epidemiological terminology, bias does not imply a partisan point of view. Bias refers to an unintentional error, caused by any trend in the assembly of the study population, or in the collection and analysis of the data, that can lead to conclusions systematically different from the truth. Bias may be either liberal, in which the observed effect is greater than the true effect, or conservative, in which the effect appears smaller than it really is. Many types of bias have been described. The best safeguard against biases is to be aware of them, and to consciously avoid them in all stages of the study.

Selection bias occurs when the study subjects are selected in a way that can misleadingly increase or decrease the magnitude of an association (Friedman 1994). For example, a cohort of workers may be selected to study the effects of a health promotion programme on certain health outcomes. Two groups, one voluntarily enrolled in the programme and another who refused to be enrolled, may be followed up for 10 years. Regardless of the true effect of the health promotion programme, the health outcomes would, in all likelihood, be more favourable for the group that voluntarily enrolled into the programme. The people in this group would generally be healthier, more health conscious and tend to take better care of themselves.

Information bias occurs when the method of data collection makes the information obtained from two or more groups differ in some misleading way (Friedman 1994). A good example of this type of bias is the recall bias in case control studies of adverse reproductive outcomes and parental environmental exposures to workplace toxins. The parents with adverse reproductive outcomes would have thought a lot about the possible causes, and would be more likely to recall adverse environmental influences compared with parents with normal deliveries. This may lead to the erroneous conclusion that such influences are, in fact, more common among the former group.

Another example of information bias is interviewer bias. For example, a research assistant whose task is to determine symptomatology among exposed and unexposed workers might unconsciously be more rigorous in searching for symptoms in the exposed group. To avoid this, the research assistant should be unaware of the exposure status of each subject in the study.

Confounding

A *confounder* is a factor which is associated with the exposure under study, such that it is unequally represented in the two groups being compared. At the same time, it is also causally associated with the development of the disease. It should, however, not be an intermediate step in the exposure–outcome sequence. In this way, the confounder may account for part of the observed effect of the exposure on the disease.

For example, a study examined the relationship between lung function (expressed as forced expiratory volume in 1 s (FEV_1)) in fire-fighters and the duration of work (as an indication of cumulative smoke exposure). Age is likely to act as a confounder, as the duration of work is associated (increases) with age, and age, by itself, has a negative effect on lung function. Thus, older workers may have a poorer lung function that is due to a combination of the effect of age and their longer working exposure. If the confounding is not recognized and controlled for, this relationship may be wrongly attributed entirely to the effect of work.

The effects of confounding can be minimized by careful study design.

In the example above, the investigators could choose to restrict the study to workers in a particular age range. Another method more commonly applied in case control studies comparing 'exposed' and 'unexposed' groups of workers would be to match on the confounder in order to equalize its distribution between the groups. For example, the entry of a case in a certain age range would lead to the selection of one or more controls in that same age range. In interventional studies, the technique most often used to control for confounding is randomization, or the random allocation of subjects into intervention and control groups.

Unlike bias, confounding can also be accounted for in the data analysis stage of a study. The use of standardization techniques has been described briefly above. Currently, statistical methods for multivariate analysis are often utilized to control for confounding factors. Some degree of familiarization with such techniques and the interpretation of results produced by these analyses is helpful in the critical assessment of epidemiological studies.

Effect modification

Effect modification (unlike bias and confounding) is not a source of error, but an important qualifier of the relationship being studied. An effect modifier is any factor that affects the relationship between the putative cause and its outcome. For example, the relative risk of lung cancer after asbestos exposure is different between smokers and non-smokers. In this case, smoking status is said to be an effect modifier of the relationship between asbestos exposure and lung cancer.

Statistically, effect modification (also known as '*interaction*') is detected when the effect measure (e.g. relative risk or odds ratio) changes across varying levels of the factor. Age is often cited as an example of an effect modifier, and relationships which hold true for the young may not necessarily be valid for an older population.

In contrast with confounding, when the presence of a confounder needs to be 'adjusted for', any significant effect modification should *not* be adjusted for. Instead, it should signal the need to analyse and report the data *separately* for each stratum.

In the above example on asbestos and lung cancer, it would be clearly erroneous to attempt to combine the data for smokers and non-smokers by 'adjustment', and more meaningful instead to report the relative risk estimates for these groups separately.

Causal associations

Causation is difficult to prove. While several studies may point to the existence of a statistical relationship between a particular exposure and a health outcome, each of these needs to be evaluated with regard to the extent to which it supports an actual cause and effect. This evaluation includes an assessment of how well the role of bias and confounding has been excluded from the observed relationship. The type of study is also of importance.

In the hierarchy of epidemiological information, a well-conducted interventional or experimental study represents the 'gold standard' that the relationship is causal. If a particular exposure is linked with disease causation, the reduction or abolition of new cases of the disease with the removal of the exposure is convincing evidence of the fact. Several lists of criteria have been proposed to aid in the establishment of causality (Hill 1965; Susser 1991). Important considerations include the following.

1 *The consistency of the association*: has it been demonstrated in several studies in various contexts?
2 *The strength of the association*: is the size of the relative risk of a reasonable magnitude?
3 *The existence of a dose–response pattern*: does the risk increase with the extent of exposure?
4 *The existence of a temporal relationship between exposure and outcome*: have the studies shown that exposure consistently precedes the outcome?
5 *The biological plausibility of the relationship*: is there a biological explanation for the observed phenomenon, or is it compatible with pre-existing theory and knowledge?

Pitfalls in epidemiology

As with other disciplines, epidemiology has its shortcomings. The common problems encountered in epidemiological studies are as follows.

1 Poor response rates in a study.
2 High turnover of the study population.
3 The healthy worker effect (where the comparison group of non-workers or other workers may have a different general health status compared with that of the exposed study group).
4 Poor quality of exposure measurement data.
5 The problem of multiple exposures.
6 Poor quality of health effect (outcome) data.
7 Having a study period shorter than the latency period of the health effect.
8 Problems associated with the study of small populations.

These problems are not always insurmountable. However, a knowledge of these pitfalls will enable one to appraise better the results of epidemiological studies and interpret their relevance in a more realistic manner.

Appraising an epidemiological study

Although not all occupational health practitioners may be involved in conducting epidemiological surveys, it is important that they are able to read and assess their quality. The validity, reliability and usefulness of most epidemiological studies can be assessed by considering the questions listed in Table 4.2.

International Agency for Research on Cancer (IARC) classification for carcinogens

The process undertaken by the IARC in its classification of carcinogens is a good example to demonstrate the use of epidemiology in hazard identification and risk assessment. In this process of the evaluation of the carcinogenicity of over 700 agents (IARC 1992a), mixtures or exposures, the body of evidence is considered as a whole. Epidemiological studies in humans, experimental results on animals and data on the possible mechanisms of action are reviewed, summarized and evaluated.

The IARC has stated that its use of the term 'carcinogenic risk' reflects the qualitative notion that exposure to an agent may lead to cancer in humans. The evaluation by the IARC is with regard to the strength of the evidence that an agent is carcinogenic, based on the available data, and does not include its carcinogenic potency. The four groups (IARC 1992b) are described below.

Group 1

The agent (mixture) is carcinogenic to humans. The exposure circumstance entails exposures that are carcinogenic to humans. Examples of

Table 4.2 Checklist of questions in the assessment of an epidemiological study.

1. Has the research question been clearly defined?
2. Is the study design appropriate to answer the question?
3. What is the quality of the exposure data collected in the study?
4. What is the quality of the health effect data?
5. Is the study population (depending on the study design, it could include cases and/or control groups) valid?
6. If sampling has been performed, has the correct sampling strategy been used?
7. What is the response rate? If the response rate is low, has a subset of the non-respondents been studied to ascertain if they are similar or dissimilar to the responders?
8. Have the effects of confounders been considered and adjusted for?
9. What statistical methods have been used for data analysis? Are these the appropriate methods?
10. For positive results, have association–cause issues been discussed?
11. For negative results, have power estimations been made? For example, could the negative results be due to a small sample size?
12. Have unwarranted extrapolations or generalizations been made?
13. How do the results affect current knowledge?

Group 1 agents include arsenic, asbestos, benzene, chromium(VI) compounds, 2-naphthylamine, nickel compounds and vinyl chloride. Mixtures in Group 1 include alcoholic beverages, untreated and mildly treated mineral oils, soots and tobacco smoke. Exposure circumstances classified in Group 1 include aluminium production, furniture and cabinet making and iron and steel founding.

Agents, mixtures and exposure circumstances in Group 1 are definitely carcinogenic, based so far on actual evidence from epidemiological studies.

Group 2

Group 2 is subdivided into Groups 2A and 2B.

Group 2A

In Group 2A, the agent (mixture) is probably carcinogenic to humans. The exposure circumstance entails exposures that are probably carcinogenic to humans. Examples of Group 2A agents are benzo[a]pyrene, cadmium, formaldehyde, silica and styrene oxide. Group 2A mixtures include diesel engine exhaust and polychlorinated biphenyls. Petroleum refining is one example of a Group 2A exposure circumstance.

Group 2B

Group 2B agents (mixtures) are possibly carcinogenic to humans. The exposure circumstance entails exposures that are possibly carcinogenic to humans. Examples of Group 2B agents include acetaldehyde, acrylamide, antimony trioxide, ceramic fibres, 2,4-diaminotoluene, lead and lead compounds, phenyl glycidyl ether and styrene. Group 2B exposure circumstances include carpentry and joinery and the textile manufacturing industry.

The classification of agents into Groups 2A and 2B is based on available epidemiological, experimental carcinogenicity and other relevant biological data. The IARC has stated that: 'In the absence of conclusive epidemiological data, it is prudent, as well as biologically plausible, to regard, for public health purposes, those agents for which there is sufficient evidence of carcinogenicity in experimental animals, as if they presented a carcinogenic risk to humans'.

Group 3

The agent (mixture or exposure circumstance) is not classifiable as to its carcinogenicity to humans. Examples of Group 3 agents include styrene–butadiene copolymers, sulphur dioxide, talc not containing asbestiform fibres, titanium dioxide, toluene and xylene. Group 3 mixtures include crude oil, jet fuel, petroleum solvents and highly refined mineral oils. Exposure circumstances in Group 3 include leather goods manufacture, lumber and sawmill industries and paint manufacture.

Group 4

The agent (mixture) is probably not carcinogenic to humans. One example is caprolactam.

Conclusions

Epidemiology as applied to hazard identification and health risk assessment is useful in many occupational health situations.

Although many factors must be considered during the course of hazard identification and risk assessment, results from epidemiological studies are one of the cornerstones in the process. Their main advantage is that the evidence is based on experience in human populations. Pitfalls include inadequate exposure characterization, health effect measurement and other biases and confounders.

The occupational health practitioner needs a sound understanding of epidemiology as part of his/her training in order to appreciate the principles of hazard identification and risk assessment, and to keep up to date with the professional literature. This will ensure a competent and effective practice in occupational health.

References

Aaltonen, M.V.P. (1996) Occupational injuries in the Finnish furniture industry. *Scandinavian Journal of Work, Environment and Health* 22, 197–203.

Brancoli, M. (1983) Accident statistics. In: *Encyclopaedia of Occupational Health and Safety* (ed. L. Parmeggiani), 3rd edn., Vol. 1, pp. 32–35. International Labour Office, Geneva.

Friedman, G.D. (1994) *A Primer of Epidemiology*, 4th edn. McGraw-Hill, New York.

Gowers, D.S., DeFonso, L.R., Schaffer, P., *et al.* (1993) Incidence of respiratory cancer among workers exposed to chloromethyl-ethers. *American Journal of Epidemiology* 137, 31–42.

Gustavsson, P., Alfredsson, L., Brunberg, H., *et al.* (1996) Myocardial infarction among male bus, taxi and lorry drivers in middle Sweden. *Occupational and Environmental Medicine* 53, 235–240.

Hill, A.B. (1965) The environment and disease: association or causation. *Proceedings of the Royal Society of Medicine* 58, 295–300.

IARC (1992a) *IARC Monographs on the Evaluation of Carcinogenic Risks to Humans. User's Guide.* WHO, IARC, Lyon.

IARC (1992b) *IARC Monographs on the Evaluation of Carcinogenic Risks to Humans. Lists of IARC Evaluations.* WHO, IARC, Lyon.

Kheifets, L.I., Afifi, A.A., Buffler, P.A. & Zhang, Z.W. (1995) Occupational electric and magnetic field exposure and brain cancer: A meta-analysis. *Journal of Occupational and Environmental Medicine* 37 (12), 1327–1341.

Kristensen, P., Irgens, L.M., Daltveit, A.K. & Andersen, A. (1993) Perinatal outcome among children of men exposed to lead and organic solvents in the printing industry. *American Journal of Epidemiology* 137, 134–144.

Last, J.M. (1988) *A Dictionary of Epidemiology*. Oxford University Press, Oxford.

Matanski, G.M., Elliott, E.A., Breysse, P.N. & Lynberg, M.C. (1993) Leukemia in telephone linemen. *American Journal of Epidemiology* 137, 609–619.

Nielsen, H., Henriksen, L. & Olsen, J.H. (1996) Malignant melanoma among lithographers. *Scandinavian Journal of Work, Environment and Health* **22**, 108–111.

Raffn, E., Villadsen, E., Engholm, G. & Lynge, E. (1996) Lung cancer in asbestos cement workers in Denmark. *Occupational and Environmental Medicine* 53, 399–402.

Susser, M. (1991) What is a cause and how do we know one? A grammar for pragmatic epidemiology. *American Journal of Epidemiology* 133, 635–648.

Toren, K. & Jonsson, P. (1996) Is skull sawing by autopsy assistants overlooked as a cause of vibration-induced white fingers? *Scandinavian Journal of Work, Environment and Health* **22**, 227–229.

Weiss, W. (1995) The lack of causality between asbestos and colorectal cancer. *Journal of Occupational and Environmental Medicine* 37 (12), 1364–1373.

Xu, Z., Brown, L.M., Pan, G.W., *et al.* (1996) Cancer risks among iron and steel workers in Anshan, China, Part II. Case-control studies of lung and stomach cancer. *American Journal of Industrial Medicine* 30, 7–15.

Chapter 5 Occupational hazard types and their characteristics

Steven S. Sadhra

Introduction

Hazards in the working environment may be divided into five main categories: chemical, physical, biological, ergonomic and psychosocial. These hazard types (examples listed in Table 5.1) may produce an immediate or delayed response, dictated largely by their inherent characteristics and the intensity and frequency of exposure. The characteristics of the hazards will also depend on the process type, process conditions and the environment in which they are generated. Regulations introduced to control risks arising from specific occupational hazards are not discussed in this chapter, but examples are listed in Appendix 1.

This chapter provides a brief overview of the different hazard types, their characteristics and examples of occupations in which they occur. Further examples of workplace hazards associated with particular work activities and occupational diseases can be found in specific regulations on reportable and prescribed (compensatable) occupational diseases. In the UK, work activities and the associated occupational diseases are listed in Schedule 1 of the UK Social Security (Industrial Injuries) (Prescribed Diseases) Regulations 1985 and in Schedule 3 (see Appendix 2) of the Reporting of Injuries, Diseases and Dangerous Occurrences Regulations (RIDDOR) 1995 (Health and Safety Executive (HSE) 1996). This chapter does not cover the toxicological classifications of chemicals, which are discussed in Chapter 3.

Table 5.1 Occupational hazard types.

Hazard category	Examples
Chemical	Dusts, fibres, fumes, mists, gases, vapours, liquids
Physical	Noise, vibration, ionizing and non-ionizing radiation, extremes of temperature and pressure, electricity, illumination and visibility
Biological	Viruses, bacteria, fungi, protozoa, nematodes
Ergonomics and mechanical	Overexertion, repetitive actions, posture traps, impact, contact, entanglement, ejection
Psychosocial and organizational	The individual, work demand and conditions, work environment, organization

Chemical hazards

Chemicals are the most common airborne contaminants encountered in the workplace, and include gases, vapours, mists or solids in the form of dusts, fibres or fumes. In addition to presenting inhalation hazards, some of these materials may be toxic by absorption through the skin or may act as skin irritants. As well as health hazards, the physical hazards of chemicals should be considered, i.e. their potential to be flammable, explosive and reactive.

In the UK, the principal regulations dealing with the classification of hazardous chemical substances are the Chemicals (Hazard Information and Packaging for Supply) Regulations 1994 (known as the CHIP 2 Regulations) (HSE 1995). The CHIP 2 Regulations cover, in particular, the requirements for the classification, packaging and labelling of both substances and preparations which are dangerous for supply, and the information to be provided in safety data sheets. They prescribe a system of symbols, categories of danger and risk phrases (see Chapter 3) for identifying the nature of any hazard associated with the contents of a package or container.

'Substances hazardous to health' in the UK are defined under the Control of Substances Hazardous to Health (COSHH) Regulations 1994 (HSE 1997) as any substance (including any preparation) which falls into one of the following categories:

- a substance listed in Part 1 of the Approved Supply List under CHIP 2 as 'very toxic, toxic, harmful, corrosive or irritant';
- a substance which has been assigned an occupational exposure limit (OEL);
- a biological agent;
- dust of any kind when present at a 'substantial' concentration in air;
- any substance not mentioned above which creates a hazard to health of any person which is comparable with the hazard created by the substances mentioned above.

Note. If a substance has not been assigned an OEL, then 'substantial concentration' is taken as $10\,mg\,m^{-3}$, 8-h time-weighted average, of total inhalable dust, or $4\,mg\,m^{-3}$, 8-h time-weighted average, of respirable dust.

Aerosols

'*Aerosol*' is a scientific term which applies to any dispersed system of liquids or solid particles suspended in air. Aerosols occur widely in the workplace environment, arising from industrial processes and workplace activity, and take many different forms; a summary classification of a range of typical aerosols is given in Fig. 5.1. It contains examples of both workplace aerosols and, for comparison, some naturally occurring and synthetic aerosols found in the outdoor atmospheric environment. Some aerosols of interest, i.e. dusts, fibres, fumes, mists and smoke, are discussed below.

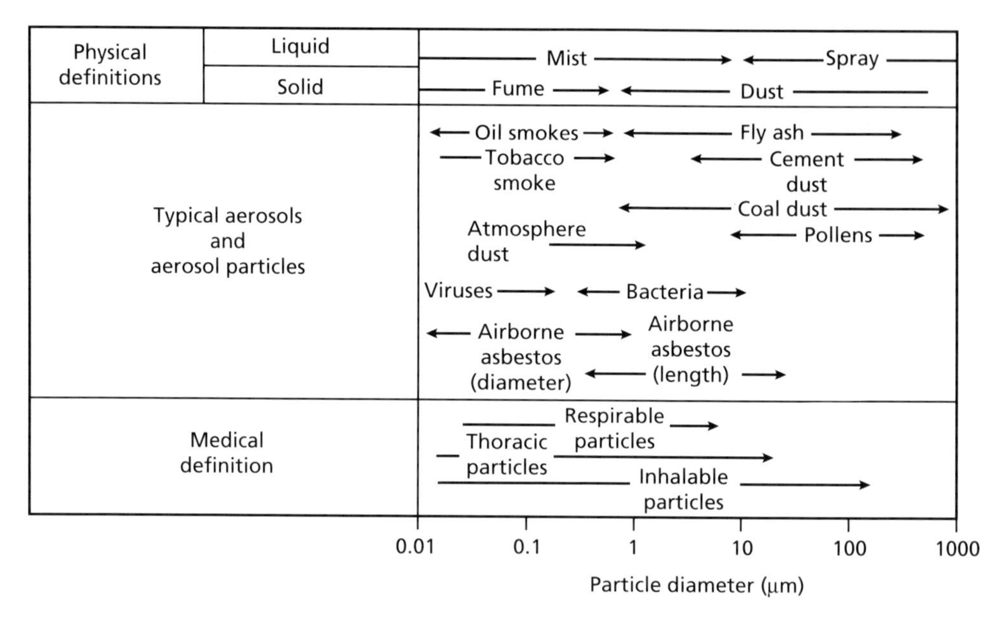

Figure 5.1 Classification of typical aerosols ('medical' definition refers to particle size fractions, where exposure to the various parts of the human respiratory tract is possible). (From Harrington and Gardiner 1995.)

Dusts are generated from solid materials by mechanical processes, such as grinding, crushing, milling and sanding, or are released by handling or other disturbances. Dusts can be derived from inorganic minerals, such as asbestos, coal and silica, and various organic sources, such as wood dust, flour, cotton and grain dust. Dusts can also be derived from animal dander, insects, mites, fungal spores and pollen.

Once inhaled, the fate of a particular particle depends on its size, density and shape. Heavier particles tend to be deposited by sedimentation or impaction within the upper respiratory tract; those with a smaller mass penetrate into the lower, alveolar region before being deposited; those of smallest size and weight remain airborne to be exhaled or retained on lung surfaces through diffusion. Different particle types may settle at the same rate, and hence be deposited in the same part of the respiratory system. Such particles are said to have the same aerodynamic diameter. The aerodynamic diameter is defined as the diameter of a theoretical sphere of unit density ($10^3\,kg\,m^{-3}$) which settles at the same speed as the particle in question. Particles of different size, shape and density are therefore compared in terms of their aerodynamic diameter. The aerodynamic diameter relates most closely to the ability of particles to penetrate to various depths of the respiratory tract, and their likelihood of deposition at critical target sites (Vincent 1990). Three particle size fractions are distinguished: (i) the inhalable fraction, which constitutes the mass fraction of total airborne particles inhaled through the nose and/or mouth; (ii) the thoracic fraction, which constitutes the mass fraction of inhaled particles penetrating the respiratory system beyond the larynx; and (iii) the respirable fraction, which constitutes the mass fraction of inhaled particles penetrating to the unciliated airways of the lungs (the alveolar region). Figure 5.1 shows the typical size ranges for these three fractions.

In occupational hygiene, a respirable *fibre* is defined as a fibre that is greater than 5 μm in length, with a length to breadth ratio of at least 3:1 and a diameter of less than 3 μm. Fibres can be generated from minerals, such as asbestos, and man-made sources, including fibreglass, mineral wools and ceramic fibres. Asbestos is the collective term used to describe several naturally occurring fibrous, hydrated silicate minerals, which have been exploited for their useful properties of flexibility, resistance to chemical attack, high tensile strength, low combustibility and low thermal conductivity. Asbestos is found in two mineral species: serpentine and amphibole. Serpentine asbestos includes chrysotile (white asbestos), and amphibole asbestos includes actinolite, amosite (brown asbestos), anthophyllite, crocidolite (blue asbestos) and tremolite. The greatest quantity of asbestos is used in the manufacture of asbestos cement, followed by the manufacture of floor tiles and as a component of brake pads and clutch plates.

Fumes are solid particles, usually generated by condensation from the gaseous state, generally after volatilization from molten materials. The formation of the fume is often accompanied by a chemical reaction, such as oxidation. Examples include lead oxide from smelting, iron oxide from arc welding, hot asphalt and volatilized polynuclear aromatic hydrocarbons from coking operations. When a metal is heated, the atoms disperse into the air and form a gaseous mixture. These atoms then combine rapidly with oxygen and recondense, forming extremely fine fumes with diameters usually in the range 0.001–1.0 μm. Fume particles often flocculate to produce larger aggregates.

Mists are finely divided liquid droplets suspended in air. Mists may be formed by the atomization of liquids by bubbling, boiling, spraying, splashing or agitation. Examples of mists include oil mist from coolants used in metal cutting, acid mists from electroplating and pesticide mists from spraying operations. The droplet sizes vary depending on the conditions and liquid composition, and are usually in the range 0.01–150 μm. *Fog* is a term used to describe a mist that has a particle concentration high enough to obscure visibility.

Smoke is produced by the incomplete combustion of carbonaceous materials, such as wood, coal, oil and tobacco. The particle size is generally below 0.5 μm in diameter. Particles may agglomerate into chains. Situations in which smoke is produced also tend to lead to the production of gases which may contain droplets.

The term *bioaerosol* refers to a wide range of airborne particles (solid or liquid) derived from living matter. Bioaerosols include microorganisms (e.g. viruses, bacteria, allergens), with sizes ranging from submicrometre viruses to fungal spores which may exceed 100 μm in diameter.

Gases and vapours

A *gas* is a formless fluid which occupies a space or enclosure, and can only be changed to the liquid or solid state by the continued effect of increased pressure and/or decreased temperature. Thus, gases do not usually exist as liquids or solids at normal room temperature and pressure. Irritant gases are an important example of respiratory toxins, and the site of injury is related to the solubility of the gas. For example, gases that are highly water soluble, such as hydrogen fluoride and ammonia, tend to dissolve in the moist lining of the upper respiratory tract, often producing immediate irritation. Less soluble irritant gases, such as nitrogen dioxide, ozone and phosgene, reach the bronchioles and alveoli, where they dissolve slowly, and may cause pneumonitis and pulmonary oedema hours later. Gases may also act as asphyxiants by interrupting the supply of oxygen (simple asphyxiants) or by inhibiting tissue oxygenation (chemical asphyxiants). Examples of simple asphyxiants include carbon dioxide, methane and nitrogen, which may cause sudden death by displacing oxygen from the inspired air, and therefore may present a problem for those working in confined spaces. Chemical asphyxiants block the delivery or use of oxygen at the cellular level. Examples of chemical asphyxiants include carbon monoxide, a product of incomplete combustion, cyanide, in electroplating and fires, and hydrogen sulphide, which is found in sewers, coal mines, petrochemical refineries and rubber manufacturing plants. Some vapours, such as isocyanates, may cause allergic responses that damage the lung directly or impair gaseous exchange.

Vapour is a gaseous form of a substance that occurs in the solid or liquid state at standard temperature (293 K) and pressure (760 mmHg) (STP). The vapour can be changed back to the solid or liquid state by either increasing the pressure or decreasing the temperature. A knowledge of the vapour pressure (VP) of a chemical can be extremely valuable, as it relates to the propensity for the chemical to volatilize and pose an inhalation hazard. The relationship of VP to temperature is not linear; however, VP data are normally given as a single point value, e.g. 20°C. The Clapeyron equation is often used for extrapolation to other temperatures, but the more accurate equation is that derived by Antoine:

$$\ln P_o = A - (B/T + C) \quad (5.1)$$

where P_o is the partial pressure, T is the absolute temperature (K) and A, B and C are constants, the values of which can be obtained from most chemistry reference books, such as the *CRC Handbook of Chemistry and Physics* (Lide 1996). As a guide, volatile compounds normally have a VP value of greater than 1 mmHg at ambient temperature, and exist entirely in the vapour phase, semivolatile compounds have a VP value of 10^{-7}–1 mmHg, and can be present in both the vapour and the particle phases, and non-volatile compounds have a VP value of less than 10^{-7} mmHg (Riggins & Petersen 1985).

In order to take into account the toxicity of the material, as well as its volatility, the VP values can also be used to calculate the vapour hazard ratio (VHR), which is defined as:

$$VHR = SC/OEL \tag{5.2}$$

where OEL is the relevant occupational exposure limit for a substance (in parts per million (ppm)) and SC is the saturation concentration (also in ppm). SC is defined as:

$$SC = VP_{STP} \times 10^6/BP \tag{5.3}$$

where BP is the barometric pressure (760 mmHg).

Another important physical property of gases and vapours is their density. The vapour density is defined as the weight of gas or vapour in relation to the weight of an equal volume of air. Thus, if the vapour density is less than unity, the material will be lighter than air, and will rise and dissipate in the air if unconfined, e.g. hydrogen. If the vapour density is greater than unity (i.e. heavier than air), the gas will linger near the ground and collect in spots, e.g. carbon dioxide, chlorine and trichloroethylene. However, this is not a problem in most industrial premises as there is usually sufficient mixing to prevent stratification.

Most organic chemicals (solids, liquids and gases) are flammable in the right combination with air and in the presence of an ignition source (hot surface, electrical spark, frictional spark or direct flame). Most inorganic substances are not flammable, with the exception of hydrogen, phosphorus, sulphur, magnesium, aluminium and titanium. The combustion characteristics of solids and liquids are based on their ignition energies, and are defined below.

- Flammable limits: the lower (LEL) and upper explosive limits (UEL) are the lowest and highest concentrations of gas or vapour in air, respectively, that are capable of igniting. The flammable range is the numerical difference between LEL and UEL.
- Flash point: the minimum temperature at which sufficient vapour is given off to form a mixture with air which is capable of igniting.
- Autoignition temperature: the lowest temperature at which the material will ignite spontaneously.
- Fire point: the lowest concentration at which the heat from the combustion of a burning vapour is capable of producing sufficient vapour to sustain combustion.

The properties of some flammable substances are given in Table 5.2. Many solid particulates, particularly organic materials, in the right combination with air and in the presence of an ignition source can also form an explosive mixture. The most severe dust explosions occur with particle diameters of between 10 and 50 μm. Coarser particles, with diameters greater than 200 μm, present a far lower explosive risk. Some of the most serious dust explosions have been associated with relatively harmless dusts created during the processing of sugar and starch, as well as metals, such as zinc and aluminium. Other materials, such as coal,

Table 5.2 Properties of some flammable substances.

Substance	Flash point (°C)	Ignition temperature (°C)	Flammable range (% v/v in air)
Acetic acid	40	485	4–17
Acetone	−18	535	2.1–13
Acetylene	−18	305	1.5–80
Ammonia	Gas	630	1.5–27
Benzene	−17	560	1.2–8
n-Butane	−60	365	1.5–8.5
Carbon disulphide	−30	100	1–60
Carbon monoxide	Gas	605	12.5–74.2
Cyclohexane	−20	259	1.2–8.3
Ether	−45	170	1.9–48
Ethanol	12	425	3.3–19
Ethylene	Gas	425	2.7–34
Hydrogen	Gas	560	4.1–74
Methane	Gas	538	5–15
Toluene	4	508	1.2–7
Vinyl chloride	−78	472	3.6–33

wood, grain and many plastics, can also form explosive dust clouds. The lower explosive concentrations ($mg\,m^{-3}$) of certain substances are as follows: sugar, 350; coal, 550; wood, 400; zinc, 4800; polystyrene, 150; magnesium, 200; methyl methacrylate, 200. Most dust explosions occur at specific sites within a plant, such as cyclones, settling chambers, powder silos, milling plant, pneumatic conveying equipment and dust collection systems.

Some gases and vapours have a distinctive odour which may provide a warning sign of their presence (Table 5.3). Chemicals are considered to have adequate warning properties if the odour threshold is below their OEL. Moore and Hautala (1983) compared the odour thresholds of 214 industrial chemicals with their threshold limit values (TLVs) and volatilities, and derived odour safety factors for each compound. The odour thresholds are usually based on population averages in smell sensitivities; however, individual odour sensitivities can differ quite markedly due to a variety of physiological conditions. Furthermore, continuing exposure to an odour usually results in a gradual diminution or even disappearance of the smell sensation, a phenomenon known as olfactory fatigue. An example of a chemical which is known to cause olfactory fatigue is hydrogen sulphide.

Physical hazards

Physical stressors include extremes of temperature, lighting, noise, vibration, changes in atmospheric pressure and radiation.

A convenient division of the radiation spectrum is between ionizing and non-ionizing radiation. *Ionizing radiation* is defined as radiant

Table 5.3 Examples of irritation and odour thresholds. (After Ness 1991.)

Compound	Irritation threshold (ppm)	Odour threshold (ppm) (odour description)
Acetic acid	10–15	0.2–24 (vinegar)
Acetone		100 (nail polish remover)
Ammonia	55–140	0.32–55
Benzene		4.68 (aromatic)
Butyl acetate	300	0.037–20 (fruity)
Carbon disulphide		0.21
Chlorine	1–6	0.01–5 (bleach)
Chloroform	>4096	50–307
Dimethylamine		0.047 (fishy, ammonia)
Epichlorohydrin	100	10–16
Ethyl ether	200	0.33
Formaldehyde	0.25–2	0.1–1.0
Hydrogen sulphide	50–100	0.00001–0.8 (rotten egg)
Isoamyl acetate	100	0.002–7 (banana oil)
Isopropyl alcohol	400	7.5–200
Methyl methacrylate	170–250	0.05–0.34
Phosgene		1 (hay-like)
Phosphine		0.021 (oniony, fishy)
Styrene (uninhibited)	200–400	0.047–200
Sulphur dioxide	6–20	0.47–5
Toluene	300–400	0.17–40
1,1,1-Trichloroethane	500–1000	20–40 (chloroform)
Turpentine	200	200
Xylene	200	200

energy which produces ionization of the matter through which it passes. As ionizing radiation penetrates matter, it collides with atoms and molecules, giving rise to ions and free radicals.

The amount of energy absorbed in unit mass of tissue is called the absorbed dose and is measured in joules (J) per kilogram (kg). The unit for the absorbed dose (D) is called the gray (Gy), and is defined as an energy deposition of one joule per kilogram ($1\,J\,kg^{-1}$):

$$D = \text{Absorbed dose (Gy)} = \text{Energy absorbed (J)/Absorbing mass (kg)} \tag{5.4}$$

However, in biological systems, the same absorbed dose of different types of radiation gives rise to different degrees of biological damage. To allow for this, the absorbed dose of each type of radiation is multiplied by a quality factor (Q), which reflects the ability of the particular radiation to cause damage, and is known as the dose equivalent. The dose equivalent is measured in sieverts (Sv). The dose limits for the body are usually quoted in millisieverts (mSv), which can be related to the gray as follows:

$$\text{Dose equivalent} = \text{Absorbed dose} \times Q \times N \tag{5.5}$$

where N is a further correction factor which accounts for other parameters, such as the absorbed dose rate and fractionation.

Sources of ionizing radiation can be divided into two main groups: electromagnetic radiation, such as X-rays and γ-rays, and particulate radiation, such as α-particles, β-particles and neutrons. Biological damage caused by ionizing radiation may occur at different levels: damage to the body as a whole, damage to individual cells and damage to cellular constituents, such as chromosomes. For the purposes of radiological protection, two types of radiation effect are distinguished: (i) stochastic effects (e.g. mutagenic, carcinogenic and teratogenic), for which the risk increases progressively with the dose received, and there is no detectable threshold; and (ii) non-stochastic effects (e.g. erythema of the skin, cataract of the eye lens, skin ulceration and impaired fertility), which vary in severity with the level of radiation dose received, but are not detectable until a threshold dose has been received. Workers who may be exposed to ionizing radiation include:

- atomic energy plant workers;
- radiologists and radiotherapists;
- radiographers (examining the integrity of structures, such as welds);
- dental workers;
- cathode ray tube makers;
- thorium ore producers;
- uranium miners;
- X-ray diffraction apparatus operators;
- luminous dial painters;
- researchers using radioactive isotope tracers;
- pharmaceutical workers (sterilize dressings).

Electromagnetic radiation with wavelengths greater than 10 nm emits insufficient energy to ionize biologically important atoms or molecules. This radiation is called *non-ionizing*. Categories of non-ionizing radiation which are important in occupational health include ultraviolet (UV), infrared (IR), microwave and radiofrequency (MW/RF) and lasers. The term laser is the acronym for Light Amplification by Stimulated Emission of Radiation. Laser wavelengths range from the IR to the UV and include visible light. Some lasers are potentially very hazardous because of their high radiance, high energies and long range. The most susceptible organ to lasers is the eye, which may focus relatively wide beams on a small area of the retina to cause irreversible damage. A hazard classification scheme for lasers IEC 825-1 (International Electrotechnical Commission 1993) has been developed, which is used to establish safe working practices appropriate to the classification of the laser being used. Ideally, lasers of class 1 or 2 should be used as these present little hazard potential. Lasers are used in the construction industry (for reference lines), in welding and cutting processes and in medical and scientific equipment. The effects of UV radiation are mainly photochemical, and injuries may occur in occupations involving drying and curing processes, arc welding, plasma torch operations, lasers, as well as natural sunlight. IR radiation is emitted by all hot bodies; industrial exposure occurs in glass blowing, metal forging and, to a lesser extent, in metal cutting and welding. Microwaves are emitted at extremely high radiofrequencies, and may be used in certain drying processes, radar equipment, communication systems and scientific equipment.

Noise is defined as unwanted sound. It can be a nuisance, resulting in disturbance, loss of sleep and fatigue. Noise can also distract attention and concentration, mask warning signals or interfere with work. The loudness of a noise source is directly related to the sound pressure level (SPL). The SPL is defined as:

$$\mathrm{SPL} = 10 \times \log(P_a/P_r)^2 \tag{5.6}$$

where P_a is the sound pressure of the sound being considered and P_r is the reference, i.e. the sound pressure at the threshold of hearing: $2 \times 10^{-5}\,\mathrm{N\,m^{-2}}$ (pascals, Pa).

Occupational noise exposure may be divided into three categories.

1 Continuous noise: normally defined as broadband noise of approximately constant level and spectrum to which employees may be exposed for a period of 8 h per day, 40 h per week.

2 Intermittent noise: defined as exposure to a given broadband SPL several times during a normal working day.

3 Impact noise: defined as exposure to a sharp burst of sound which is generally less than 0.5 s in duration. Noise resulting from widely spaced impacts, such as noise from a drop hammer or a cartridge operated hand tool, is termed 'impulse noise'. Impulse or impact sounds can be characterized in terms of their rise time, peak sound level and pulse duration.

With continuous noise, the likelihood of noise-induced hearing loss (NIHL) is determined by the noise level and frequency, duration of exposure and individual susceptibility. The occurrence of NIHL generally results from damage to the hair cells located within the cochlea, a sensorineural loss which may be temporary or permanent. Permanent losses cannot be corrected by conventional surgical or therapeutic procedures. Noise levels in the following industries frequently approach or exceed 90 dB(A):

- metal foundries (grinding, cleaning, dressing or finishing of castings and ingots);
- ship building or ship repairing industries (use of pneumatic percussive tools on metal);
- quarries and mining (drilling);
- drop-forging plants (shaping metal);
- textile manufacture (weaving fibres or bulking up of fibres);
- woodworking machinery (operation of band saws, circular saws, planers, tenoning machines);
- forestry (use of chain saws);
- printing industry.

Impulse noise can cause direct trauma, perforation of the ear drum, disruption of the auditory ossicles (causing conductive hearing loss) and high-frequency sensorineural hearing loss (Touma 1992). Industrial sources of impact noise include drop forging, hammering, riveting and the use of compressed airlines.

Physiological and psychological symptoms, such as headaches, dizziness and nausea, have been associated with high levels of infrasound (frequencies below 20 Hz) and ultrasound, with no evidence of hearing loss. Infrasound (Acton 1983) can be generated in ships' engine rooms, compressor rooms and some motor vehicles. Ultrasonic cleaning baths and mixers are commonly used in industry.

Vibration is oscillatory motion (i.e. motion to and fro between two points), the direction of which varies with time. The magnitude of vibration is expressed as the acceleration in metres per second squared ($m\,s^{-2}$), and the frequency is expressed in hertz (Hz). Increasing industrial use of mechanical tools has resulted in vibration at critical frequencies and acceleration becoming important causes of injury. The types of vibration important in the area of occupational health are whole body vibration (WBV), which may affect vehicle operators, and hand-transmitted vibration (HTV), affecting users of tools vibrating with a frequency in the range 20–1000 Hz.

The effects of vibration on the human body will vary according to the frequency, direction (vertical or lateral), point of entry, acceleration and duration. WBV can produce discomfort, interfere with the performance of activities and cause pathological and physiological changes in the body. WBV may affect drivers of heavy vehicles, such as tractors, trucks and earthmovers. The most significant frequency bands are 0.1–1.0 Hz and 1–20 Hz. The whole body has a resonance frequency at 5 Hz in the head to toe axis, but 1–2 Hz in the horizontal axis. Disorders of the spine have been reported in subjects exposed to long-term WBV in tractors, haulage vehicles and earthmovers. The first survey in the USA (Milby & Spear 1974) found an excess of musculoskeletal conditions, including disc protrusions, degenerative spinal changes and lumbar scoliosis.

Hand–arm vibration syndrome (HAVS) is a chronic progressive disorder which may be caused by vibration in the frequency range 2–1000 Hz; the most damaging frequencies are thought to be between 5 and 20 Hz. HAVS is characterized by vascular changes, such as whitening of the finger ends, and neurological effects, including numbness and tingling of the fingers, reduced grip strength and impaired dexterity. Tools associated with hand–arm vibration are listed in Table 5.4.

Extremes of *temperature* present another important physical hazard. Workers at risk from high heat load include smelters, steel workers, firefighters, blast furnace operators and glassblowers. The extent of heat stress in an individual is determined by environmental factors (heat gain and loss by conduction, convection, radiation and evaporation), the metabolic rate, the extent of protective clothing worn by the individual

Table 5.4 Tools potentially associated with vibration injuries. (After Griffin 1990.)

Type of tool	Example of tool type
Percussive metal working tools	Riveting tools Caulking tools Chipping tools Chipping hammers Fettling tools Hammer drills Clinching and flanging tools Impact wrenches Swaging Needle guns
Grinders and other rotary tools	Pedestal grinders Hand-held grinders Hand-held sanders Hand-held polishers Flex-driven grinders/polishers Rotary burring tools
Percussive hammers and drills used in mining, demolition and road construction	Hammers Rock drills Road drills
Forest and garden machinery	Chain saws Anti-vibration chain saws Brush saws Mowers and shears Barking machines
Others	Nut runners Shoe pounding-up machines Concrete vibro-thickeners Concrete levelling vibro-tables Motorcycle handlebars

and the exposure duration. The rate at which body moisture (sweat) evaporates is dependent on the relative humidity (RH) of the air, being slowest when RH is high. RH is given as:

$$\mathrm{RH} = \frac{\text{Partial pressure of water vapour}}{\text{Vapour pressure of water at the same temperature}} \times 100\% \qquad (5.7)$$

It is generally accepted that RH should be between 30 and 70%. If RH is below 30%, a feeling of discomfort is produced; conversely, high RH (>70%) produces a feeling of stuffiness. Increased environmental temperature can lead to heat cramps, heat exhaustion and heat stroke, as well as impaired performance and an increased risk of accidents. In contrast, cold stress is an occupational hazard for cold room workers, dry-ice workers, liquefied gas workers and divers. Cold injuries include freezing injuries (frostbite), non-freezing injuries (due to poor circulation, e.g. trench foot) and hypothermia.

The increased *pressure* experienced in diving and the decreased pressure experienced in aviation may present hazards due to rapid pressure changes. The effects of increased pressure amongst divers may include barotrauma and decompression sickness. In addition to these physical hazards, divers also encounter problems due to gas toxicity. The main components of air, oxygen and nitrogen, are both toxic at depths greater than about 50 m. Gaseous nitrogen induces narcosis and oxygen inhalation can cause a toxic reaction. At high altitudes, the decreased pressure will reduce oxygen blood absorption, and hypoxia may occur at altitudes greater than 3000 m.

It is important that workplace *lighting* is maintained at an acceptable standard. Lighting levels must be sufficiently high to enable workers to clearly see their tasks, but not so high as to cause glare. Glare occurs whenever one part of the visual field is much brighter than the average brightness to which the visual system is adapted. Where there is direct interference with vision, the condition is known as disability glare. Where vision is not directly impaired, but there is some discomfort, irritability, distraction or annoyance, the condition is called discomfort glare. Poor workplace lighting not only creates eye strain, but can also cause fatigue. Fatigue may lead to errors in the work and an increased likelihood of accidents brought about by the worker's failing or incorrect perception. Very intense light may lead to tissue damage or damaged sight. The amount of light falling on a surface (light level) is termed the illuminance, expressed in lux. The required illuminance in working areas depends largely on two factors: the type of work being performed and the hazard associated with it. Table 5.5 shows the recommended average illuminance and minimum measured illuminance for different types of work. As well as determining the required illuminance and avoiding glare, it is also important to consider the illuminance in adjacent areas and the plane (vertical or horizontal) on which it is provided. A large difference in illuminance between adjacent areas may cause visual discomfort or even affect safety in places where there is frequent movement.

Ergonomics

The basic approach of ergonomics is that of fitting the person to the task. The task in this context includes the totality of those aspects of the working environment which may influence the individual's effectiveness and comfort. A crucial point of concern is the interaction of the worker with the machinery and equipment with which he/she works, i.e. the worker–machine interface. By conducting task analysis (see Chapter 6) and making measurements of human characteristics (anthropometry), the ergonomist is able to design or improve the workplace, equipment and work procedures to ensure a safe, healthy and efficient performance.

Table 5.5 Average illuminances and minimum measured illuminances for different types of work. (After HSE 1989.)

General activity	Typical locations/ types of work	Average illuminance (lx)	Minimum measured illuminance (lx)
Movement of people, machines and vehicles*	Lorry parks, corridors, circulation routes	20	5
Movement of people, machines and vehicles in hazardous, areas; rough work not requiring any perception of detail*	Construction site clearance, excavation and soil work, docks, loading bays, bottling and cleaning plants	50	20
Work requiring limited perception of detail†	Kitchens, factories assembling large components, potteries	100	50
Work requiring perception of detail†	Offices, sheet metal working, bookbinding	200	100
Work requiring perception of fine detail†	Drawing offices, factories assembling electronic components, textile production	500	200

*Only safety has been considered, because no perception of detail is needed and visual fatigue is unlikely. However, where it is necessary to see detail to recognize a hazard or where error in performing the task could put someone at risk, for safety purposes as well as visual fatigue the figure should be increased to that for work requiring the perception of detail.
†The purpose is to avoid visual fatigue; the illuminances will be adequate for safety purposes.

One of the main reasons for physical stress on the job is the mismatch in size between the worker and the workplace, equipment or machinery. Overexertion and repetitive trauma injuries, such as low back pain, strains, sprains and tendonitis, are caused by jobs that involve excessive physical effort or highly repetitive patterns of localized muscle and joint usage. Awkward work posture is frequently an aggravating factor in these injuries. These injuries frequently occur on jobs that involve manual handling of materials (lifting, pushing, pulling or carrying of objects) or highly repetitive hand motions, such as working on an assembly line. Examples of workers at risk of work-related cumulative trauma disorders of the hand and arm include:

- plasterers;
- carpet layers;
- typists;
- cleaners;
- data processors;
- polishers;
- packagers;
- equipment assemblers.

Mechanical hazards

Machine operators may be injured as a result of movement of the machine, being trapped between the machine and materials or being struck by materials ejected from the machine. In identifying machinery hazards, it is useful to consider three factors: (i) the different phases of a machine's life (construction, installation, commissioning, operation, cleaning, maintenance and decommissioning); (ii) the circumstances giving rise to the injury; and (iii) the hazards that can cause the injury. For the different types and ranges of machines used, the hazards can be summarized as follows.

- *Traps.* There are three different types of trap: reciprocating traps (due to vertical or horizontal motion of machines), shearing traps (produced by a moving part traversing a fixed part) and in-running nips where limbs are drawn into a trap (e.g. where a moving belt or chain meets a roller or a tooth wheel).
- *Impact.* Machinery parts can cause injuries by their speed or movement if a person gets in the way.
- *Contact.* Burns, lacerations or other injuries may be caused due to sharp, abrasive, hot, cold or electrically live machine components.
- *Entanglement.* Limbs, hair or clothing may become entangled with unguarded moving parts.
- *Ejection.* Machines may eject particles, metals or actual parts of machines, e.g. grinding machines.

Psychosocial hazards

Psychosocial or organizational hazards are those which relate to the interaction between job content, work organization, management systems and environmental conditions, on the one hand, and workers' competence and needs on the other. Certain psychosocial and organizational characteristics of work are associated with stress, job dissatisfaction and ill health. Table 5.6 outlines nine different work characteristics of jobs, work environments and organizations which, under certain conditions of work, may result in stress and/or ill health. Stress-related situations may result from work demands which are not well matched to the knowledge and skills of the workers or their needs, especially where the workers have little control over the work and receive little support. It is important to note that stress-related problems may result as much from conditions of non-demanding, monotonous work as from high demands conventionally associated with occupational stress. Possible effects of stress include absenteeism, poor concentration, poor quality of work and increase in unsafe behaviour and accident rates.

All organizations present the potential for workers to be exposed to psychosocial hazards. Attempts have been made to rank broad occupational groups in terms of stress levels (Cooper *et al.* 1988), i.e.

Table 5.6 Psychosocial and organizational hazards of work. (After World Health Organization (WHO) 1993.)

Work characteristic	Hazard conditions
Organizational function and culture	Poor communication Organization as poor task environment Poor problem solving environment Poor development environment
Participation	Low participation in decision making
Career development and job status	Career uncertainty or career stagnation
Role in organization	Role ambiguity or role conflict Responsibility for others or continual contact with other people
Job content	Ill-defined work or high uncertainty Lack of variety Fragmental or meaningless work Underutilization of skill Physical constraint
Workload and workplace	Quantitative work overload or underload Qualitative work overload or underload High levels of pacing Lack of control over pacing Time pressure
Work organization	Inflexible work schedule Unpredictable hours Long or unsociable hours Shift working
Interpersonal relationships at work	Social or physical isolation Lack of social support Interpersonal conflict and violence Poor relationships with supervisors
Home–work interface	Conflicting demands of work and home Low social or practical support from home Dual career problems

'extremely stressful', 'very stressful' and 'above average stress levels'. Those falling into the 'extremely stressful' category include organizations dealing with accident and emergency situations or violent incidents, notably the police, fire, ambulance and prison services. Occupations ranked as 'very stressful' include civil aviation pilots, broadcasters, journalists, musicians, actors, doctors, dentists, nurses, teachers, social workers and those working in the mining and construction industry. Groups ranked as having 'above average stress levels' include workers employed in marketing and publishing, printing, the retail trade, catering and public transport.

Biological hazards

In the UK, the COSHH Regulations 1994 define a biological agent as any 'microorganism, cell-culture or human endoparasite, including any which have been genetically modified, which may cause any infection, allergy, toxicity or otherwise create a risk to human health'. Microorganisms can be classified according to the hazard they present and the precautions required when handling them. An example of a microorganism hazard group classification system is shown in Table 5.7, ranging from those that are unlikely to cause disease (Group 1) to those that may cause very serious diseases (Group 4).

Microorganisms include viruses, bacteria, fungi and protozoa. Occupational infections can occur following contact with infected persons, as in the case of health care workers, with infected animals or human tissue, secretions or excretions, as in laboratory workers, or with infected animals, as in agriculture. Occupational diseases transmitted from animals to humans are called 'zoonoses', and include anthrax, leptospirosis, orf, Q fever, ornithosis, glanders fever and brucellosis. A good review of biological agents and exposed groups is given in Collins *et al.* (1997) (Table 5.8).

Hepatitis (viral hepatitis) is an inflammatory condition of the liver. It is usually caused by infections or exposure to toxic substances, such as organic solvents. Of the blood-borne types of hepatitis, the most common is hepatitis B. People at risk of acquiring hepatitis B are those who come into contact with infected blood and other body fluids. These include health care workers, especially those working in dialysis units, blood banks, clinical laboratories, operating rooms, dental practices and washing areas for glassware and other equipment. Other occupational groups at risk include police officers, prison officers and clinical waste handlers.

Occupational respiratory conditions include extrinsic allergic alveolitis (farmer's lung, malt worker's lung, bagassosis, dry rot lung, sewage sludge disease, mushroom picker's lung, metal worker's lung) and asthma. Occupational asthma has been associated with a number of pro-

Table 5.7 Classification of microorganisms into groups on the basis of hazard. (Adapted from HSE 1997.)

Group 1	Agents that are most unlikely to cause human disease
Group 2	Agents that can cause human disease and might be a hazard to workers; they are unlikely to spread in the community; effective prophylaxis and/or treatment is usually available
Group 3	Agents that can cause severe human disease and which present a serious hazard to workers; there may be a risk of spread in the community; effective prophylaxis and/or treatment is usually available
Group 4	Agents that cause severe human disease and present a serious hazard to workers; there may be a high risk of spread in the community; effective prophylaxis and treatment are not available

Table 5.8 Classical biological agent-induced infectious occupational diseases.

Group	Disease	Source	Occupations at risk
Viruses	Rabies	Cats, dogs, wild animals	Vets, spelunkers, farmers, ranchers
	Orf	Sheep, goats	Shepherds, shearers, vets, stockyard workers
	Milker's nodule	Cattle	Dairy operators, vets, ranchers
	Newcastle disease	Birds	Poultry handlers, vets
	Hepatitis	Humans	Health-care workers
	AIDS	Humans	Health-care workers
Rickettsia	Rocky Mountain Spotted fever	Ticks	Outdoor workers in wooded areas
	Q fever	Ticks	Placental tissue of domestic animal handlers
	Psittacosis	Birds	Pet shop owners, poultry handlers, vets, taxidermists, zookeepers
Bacteria	Tetanus	Various	Those with risk of skin-breaking injury by contaminated objects
	Anthrax	Livestock	Goat hair, wool and hide handlers
	Brucellosis	Mainly livestock	Packing house employees, livestock handlers
	Leptospirosis	Rodents, livestock, dogs	Farm workers, livestock handlers, troops, sewer workers
	Plague	Rodents, lagomorphs	Western US—shepherds, ranchers, farmers, field scientists
	Tuberculosis	Humans	Health-care workers
	Mycobacteriosis	Soil, milk, water	Gulf Coast fishermen, pet store owners, health-care workers
	Erysipeloid	Surfaces	Animal, meat, poultry, fish handlers
	Tularemia	Ticks, wild and some domestic animals	Deer, rabbit, animal handlers, forestry workers
	Lyme disease	Ticks, wild animals	Workers in certain localized wooded areas
Fungi	Candidiasis	Humans	Dishwashers, cooks, bartenders, bakers, meat handlers
	Aspergillosis	Composting vegetation	Farmers, grain handlers, hemp workers
	Coccidiomycosis	Soil	Farmers, excavators, troops, textile workers
	Histoplasmosis	Bird-dropping enriched soil	Farmers, spelunkers, pigeon handlers
	Mycetoma	Soil, composting vegetation	Farmers
	Sporotrichosis	Sphagnum moss	Gardeners, farmers
	Chromomycosis	Soil, composting vegetation	Farmers—Southern US
	Dermatophytoses	Humans, sometimes animals	Pet hide and animal handlers, farmers, athletes, lifeguards

From Perkins (1997).

cesses, including flour handling, food protein manufacture, cheese making, cereal and grains and enzyme manufacture. Legionnaire's disease is a type of pneumonia caused by the inhalation of aerosols containing a specific bacterium, *Legionella pneumophila. Legionella* is frequently found in many recirculating and hot water systems, particularly in large, complex systems, such as in multistorey office blocks, factories and hospitals. Particular sites for bacterial growth are air conditioning systems, cooling towers, water standing in condensation trays, humidifiers and hot and cold water storage tanks. Microbial allergies mostly affect the respiratory tract, and result from the inhalation of spores of fungi, actinomycetes and other bacteria or their constituents or metabolites.

References

Acton, W.I. (1983) Exposure to industrial ultrasound hazards, appraisal and control. *Journal of the Society of Occupational Medicine* 33, 107–113.

Collins, C.H., Aw, T.C. & Grange, J.M. (1997) *Microbial Diseases of Occupations, Sports and Recreation*. Butterworth Heinemann, Oxford.

Cooper, C.L., Cooper, R.D. & Eaker, L.H. (1988) *Living with Stress*, 1st edn. Penguin Books.

Griffin, M.J. (1990) *Handbook of Human Vibration*. Academic Press, London.

Harrington, J.M. & Gardiner, K. (eds) (1995) *Occupational Hygiene*, 2nd edn. Blackwell Science, Oxford.

HSE (1989) *Lighting at Work. Health and Safety: Guidance Booklet No. HS(G)38*. HMSO, London.

HSE (1995) *Chemical (Hazard Information and Packaging for Supply) Regulations 1994 (CHIP 2)*. HMSO, London.

HSE (1996) *A Guide to the Reporting of Injuries, Diseases and Dangerous Occurrences Regulations 1995*. HSE Books, Sudbury, Suffolk.

HSE (1997) *General Control of Substances Hazardous to Health (COSHH) Approved Code of Practice, COSHH Regulations 1994*. HMSO, London.

International Electrotechnical Commission (1993) *Safety of Laser Products, Equipment Classification, Requirements and User's Guide*. IEC 825-1. IEC, Geneva.

Lide, D.R. (1996) *CRC Handbook of Chemistry and Physics*, 77th edn. CRC, Boca Raton, FL.

Milby, T.H. & Spear, R.C. (1974) *Relationship Between Whole-body Vibration and Morbidity Patterns Among Heavy Equipment Operators*. DHEW/NIOSH Publication No. 74-131. NIOSH, Cincinnati.

Moore, J.E. & Hautala, E. (1983) Odor as an aid to chemical safety: Odor thresholds compared with threshold limit values and volatilities for 214 industrial chemicals in air and water dilution. *Journal of Applied Toxicology* 3, 272–290.

Ness, S.A. (1991) *Air Monitoring for Toxic Exposure*. Van Nostrand Reinhold, New York.

Perkins, J.L. (1997) *Modern Industrial Hygiene, Vol. 1. Recognition and Evaluation of Chemical Agents*. Van Nostrand Reinhold, New York.

Riggins, R.M. & Petersen, B.A. (1985) Sampling and analysis methodology for semivolatile and nonvolatile organic compounds in air. In: *Indoor Air and Human Health, Major Indoor Air Pollutants and Their Health Implications* (eds. R.B. Gammage & S.V. Kaye), pp. 351–359. Lewis Publishers, Chelsea, MI.

Touma, J. (1992) Controversies in noise-induced hearing loss (NIHL). *Annals of Occupational Hygiene* **36** (2), 199–209.

Vincent, J.H. (1990) The fate of inhaled aerosols: a review of observed trends and some generalisations. *Annals of Occupational Hygiene* **34**, 623–637.

WHO (1993) *Psychosocial and Organisation Hazards at Work. Control of Monitoring*. European Occupational Health Series No. 5. WHO Regional Office for Europe, Copenhagen.

Chapter 6 Hazard identification techniques

Steven S. Sadhra

Introduction

This chapter aims to provide a brief review of the different techniques used to identify hazards from the concept of plant/processes/machines to their operation in the workplace. Practical guidance on workplace inspections is provided, with a proposed format for the systematic identification of occupational hazards. Different hazard types and their characteristics, as well as specific hazards arising from different industrial processes, are discussed in Chapter 5.

The need for hazard identification

A *hazard* is defined as a source of potential harm, and can include substances or machinery, methods of work and other aspects of work organization. Harm includes death, injury, physical or mental ill health, damage to property, loss of production, or any combination of these. In the context of occupational health, ill health includes acute and chronic effects caused by physical, chemical or biological agents, as well as adverse effects on mental health. *Hazard identification* is defined as the process of recognizing that a hazard exists and defining its characteristics.

It could be argued that the identification of hazards is the most important step in any risk assessment. Only the identified hazards can be assessed, and risk assessments will rarely reveal unidentified hazards. Once the potential hazards have been identified, and perhaps ranked according to their possible effects, the risk can be assessed by estimating the frequency and likelihood of their occurrence (see Chapter 10). Ideally, hazard identification techniques should be applied as early as possible in the development of a process, i.e. the concept stage (and especially at the process design stage), when it is generally possible to make changes which are less expensive, rather than having to enter into costly modifications once the process is up and running. The hazard identification process must then continue in different forms throughout the life of the process to ensure that the procedures developed are correctly followed and that process modifications, variations and faults are identified. In the process industries, hazard identification has received more attention at the initial design stage than at any other point during the rest of the project. Furthermore, regulations in a number of

European countries, as well as the USA, now require the application of hazard identification to existing plant presenting major hazards (discussed below).

Both continuous and non-continuous hazards need to be identified. *Continuous hazards* are those which are inherent in the work activity or equipment under normal conditions, e.g. noisy/unguarded machinery or toxic/flammable substances. *Non-continuous hazards* are hazards which arise from system failures (machine breakdown) non-routine operations (handling spillages, emergency procedures) or human errors. Various qualitative approaches to hazard identification are available; the selection of the most appropriate procedure will depend largely on the type of process and hazards involved. Procedures range from the use of a simple checklist by a single person to the more complex and detailed, open-ended, hazard and operability (HAZOP) studies carried out by multidisciplinary teams. In every case, it is essential to ensure that the reviewers are properly qualified and adequately experienced in the technique to be used and in the process being reviewed.

Hazard causes (awareness)

Before discussing the different techniques used to identify hazards, it is worth considering the factors relevant to the existence and development of hazards in the workplace. Once the causes of hazards have been identified, it is possible to establish the interventions required to prevent or minimize their potential (see Chapter 11).

Hazards are caused by unsafe acts and omissions or by unsafe conditions (Fig. 6.1). *Unsafe acts* are acts that deviate from a specified or accepted system of performance of a task, e.g. using a defective machine, taking up unsafe positions, unauthorized use of machinery, etc. *Unsafe acts of omission* are failures to conform to the requirements of the activity, e.g. failure to use personal protective equipment, unsafe use of equipment, failure to follow procedures and work methods, etc. As shown in Fig. 6.1, unsafe acts and omissions can be summarized as follows:

- inappropriate attitudes;
- inappropriate knowledge;
- inadequate skill;
- inadequate supervision;
- failure to do 'something'.

Unsafe conditions are inadequacies in either the situation or the system of work, and can include the inherent hazards of the materials used, hazardous work procedures, inadequacies in the layout of the plant and equipment, etc. The relationship between health effects or accidents and unsafe acts and conditions (Fig. 6.1) suggests that a hypothetical threshold must be crossed before an accident or effect can occur. This may be true, as hazards can exist for long periods of time without an accident or apparent effect on health.

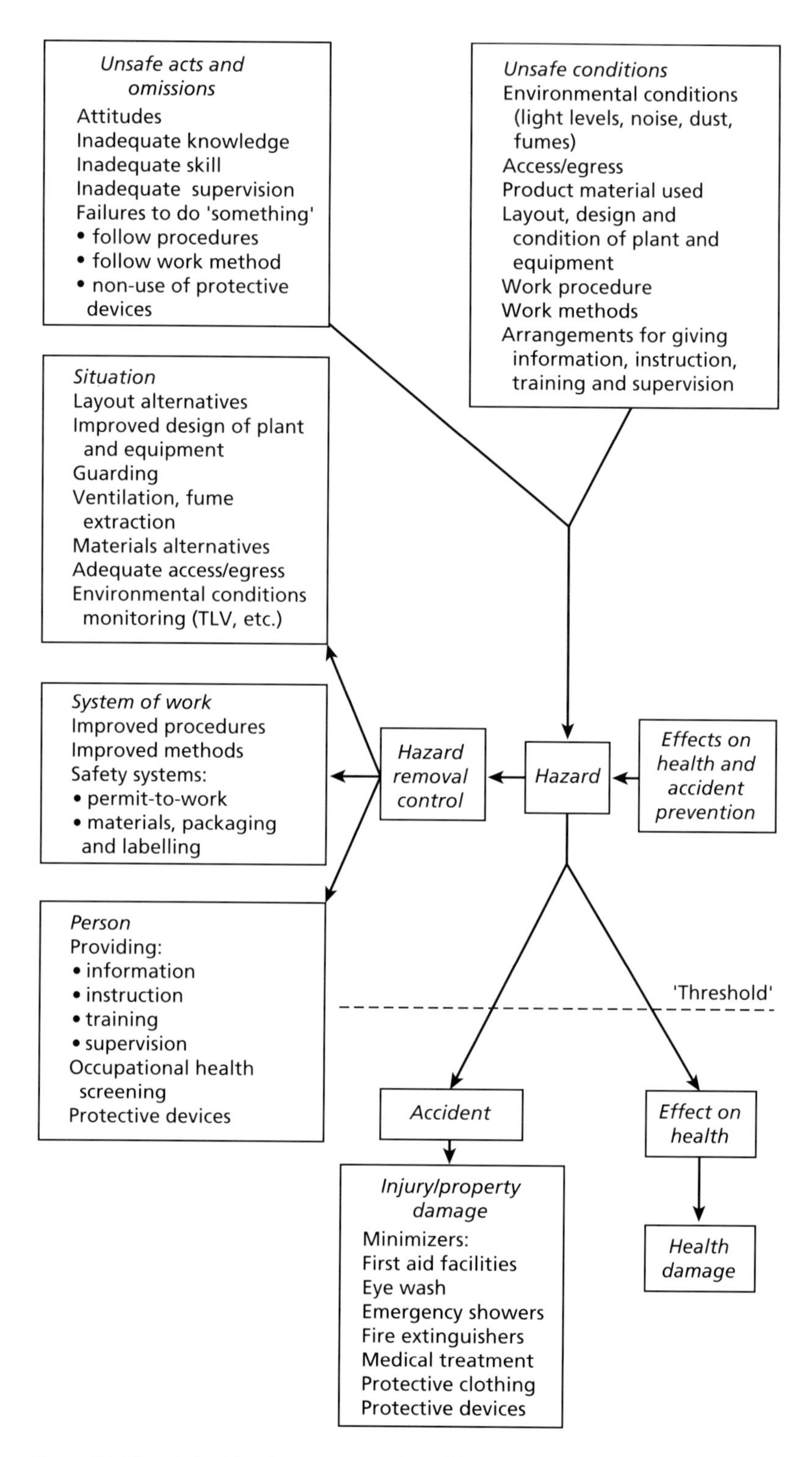

Figure 6.1 The relationship of unsafe acts and conditions to accidents. (After Wallace 1995.)

Major hazards

Following the Seveso accident in Italy (1976), in which a runaway reaction at a chemical works resulted in a release of a toxic chemical, the European Commission (EC) issued the so-called 'Seveso Directive' on the 'Control of Major Accident Hazards of Certain Industrial Activities'. This was adopted in the UK in the form of the Control of Industrial Major Accident and Hazard (CIMAH) Regulations 1984 (HSE 1991). The CIMAH Regulations cover industrial premises which, by virtue of the quantity of 'dangerous substances' on the premises, present a major accident hazard. The manufacturing processes covered are listed in a schedule to the regulations, but in effect apply to any chemical manufacturing process involving flammable or toxic materials that are likely to constitute a hazard. The primary objective of these regulations is the prevention of major accidents from industrial activities, and the limitation of the effects of such accidents on humans and the environment. Major accident hazard sites are, through these regulations, required to prepare a safety case assessing the nature and degree of the hazard and an evaluation of the types and consequences of major accidents. The preparation of safety cases is discussed in Lees and Ang (1989). The CIMAH Regulations are currently being updated, and will be replaced with the Control of Major Accident and Hazard (COMAH) Regulations which are based on quantitative risk assessment (QRA).

Hazard identification methods

Within an organization, there are several ways in which hazards may be identified. These may include the following.

1 *Specialized techniques used to identify hazards in the planning and design stages.*
   - Hazard and operability (HAZOP) studies: a qualitative technique used to identify hazards from hardware failures and human errors.
   - Failure mode and effect analysis (FMEA): an inductive technique used to identify hardware failures.
   - Task analysis: an inductive technique used to identify likely sources of human error.

2 *Methods used to identify workplace hazards.*
   - Accident and ill health statistics.
   - Investigation of accidents, ill health effects and complaints.
   - Audits.
   - Checklists.
   - Workplace inspections, including discussions and use of basic occupational hygiene instrumentation.

Hazard identification in the planning stage

With the development of the process from the planning to the operation stage, the flexibility to eliminate certain hazards is much reduced. For this reason, it is recommended that hazard identification should start at the planning stage, which will enable the areas where more information or research is needed to be identified. This section provides an introduction to the application and limitations of the common hazard indices and specialized structured methods used in the identification of hazards in the process planning and design stages.

Hazard indices—fire and explosions

The hazard classification guide developed by the Dow Chemical Company provides a method of evaluation of the potential hazards and potential loss from a process (Dow Chemical Company 1994). The *Dow Index* is aimed primarily at identifying the fire, explosion and chemical reactivity hazards during plant design. A number of material factors (flammability, reactivity, etc.) and process hazards (process temperature, pressure levels, potential for corrosion/erosion and how near the process operates to the flammable range, etc.) are considered in deriving a Fire and Explosion Index (F&EI). The larger the value of F&EI, the more hazardous the process. The F&EI values can then be used to determine what preventive and protection measures are needed, or to assess the potential loss taking into account the prevention and control measures incorporated into the plant design.

The *Mond Index* (Mond fire, explosion and toxicity index) expands on the Dow Index by providing a value for F&EI based on a more extensive evaluation of the material factors, including acute health hazards and process layout. A manual setting out the calculation procedure for the Mond Index has recently been revised (Imperial Chemical

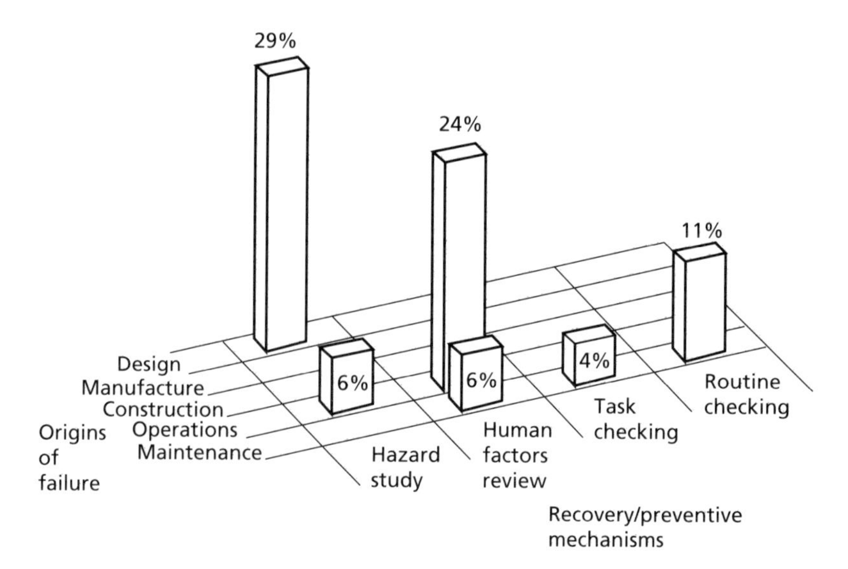

Figure 6.2 Prevention and recovery mechanisms for different origins of failure/failure types. (After Pitblado & Turney 1996.)

Industries (ICI) 1993). Both the Dow and Mond Indices are employed mainly in the chemical and petrochemical industries, and their use at an early stage in process design may reveal a hazard potential which is relatively easy to alleviate before design is advanced. Detailed guides for both indices should be studied before applying the technique; however, a good brief guide for both indices, with worked examples, is presented in Sinnott (1996).

Hazard and operability (HAZOP) method

A HAZOP study is a systematic, qualitative technique for hazard identification, which was developed by ICI. Although the technique can be applied at every phase of project development, including its operation, it is particularly effective when applied at the design stage. This is exemplified in Fig. 6.2, which shows that the use of the HAZOP method, by itself, may prevent 29% of design incidents and 6% of operational incidents, a higher proportion than any other single technique. A brief description of the HAZOP technique is given below, and further information on HAZOP studies and examples may be found in the Chemical Industries Association (CIA) publications on the subject (CIA 1979). The method and its applications are also fully explained by Kletz (1992).

Essentially, a HAZOP study takes a full description of the process and systematically questions every part of it to discover how deviations from the intentions of the design can occur, and decides whether these deviations can give rise to hazards. Each part of the design is subjected to a number of guide words asking 'what if?' questions. Each of the theoretical deviations is then considered to decide how it could be caused and what would be the consequences. A HAZOP study is normally carried out by a small, multidisciplinary team of experienced people, who have complementary skills and knowledge, led by a team leader experienced in the technique. A typical HAZOP team will consist of safety, process, instrumentation, operation, electrical and mechanical engineers. Other disciplines may be added to the team to suit the particular requirements of specific plant.

The study is based on a set of key words which stimulate thought. The set of key words contains two subsets, i.e. guide words which are applied to property words. The property words, such as flow, pressure, concentration, temperature, etc., focus attention on the design conditions and the design intentions, whilst the guide words (see Table 6.1) focus on possible deviations from the design intentions. If, for example, the flow of a chemical is under study (see Table 6.1), the team will define the *intention* of the system and then assess the possible *deviations*, *causes* and *consequences* of each of the following: 'no' flow, 'more' flow, 'less' flow, 'as well as' flow, 'reverse' flow and 'other than' flow, i.e. different chemicals.

The success of a HAZOP study depends on a number of factors: the accuracy of drawings and relevant data, the technical skill of the

Table 6.1 HAZOP guide words.

Guide words	Meaning	Comments
No or not	The complete negation of the intention, e.g. flow	No part of the intention is achieved, but nothing else happens
More or less	A quantitative increase or decrease, e.g. temperature	These refer to quantities and properties, such as flow rates and temperatures, as well as activities, e.g. 'heat' and 'react'
As well as or part of	A qualitative increase (e.g. purity) or decrease (e.g. wrong concentration)	All design and operating intentions are achieved with some additional activity, or only some of the intentions are achieved
Reverse	The opposite of the intention, e.g. reverse flow	This is mostly applicable to activities, e.g. reverse flow or chemical reaction
Other than	Complete substitution, e.g. flow of wrong materials	No part of the original intention is achieved. Something else quite different happens

multidisciplinary team and the ability of the team to assess the relative importance of the hazards identified. Furthermore, the team approach encourages creative thinking and generates good understanding of plant/process health and safety issues.

Failure mode and effect analysis (FMEA)

An FMEA (American Institute of Chemical Engineers (AIChE) 1992) is an inductive hazard identification technique which explores the effects of failures or malfunctions of individual components within a system. This approach answers the question: 'if this part fails in this manner, what will be the result?'. An FMEA can be applied to a number of situations (engineering products, chemical processes, manufacturing operations, human tasks), where the health and safety of employees may be put into jeopardy by a component failure.

An FMEA starts with the selection of a system, which should be clearly defined and broken down to its lowest level, i.e. the component parts. The following basic questions are asked about the system.

- How can each component fail?
- What mechanisms might produce these modes of failure?
- What effects will these failures have on other components in the system or on the whole system?
- How serious are these failure modes?

- How is each failure mode detected?
- Are there any compensating features in the design?

After completing the evaluation of the individual component failure modes, an FMEA summary sheet is prepared. On this sheet, the mode of failure, the cause(s) and the recommended remedial action(s) can be recorded on a standard table. The corrective actions may include design, procedural or organizational changes. This qualitative analysis can be enhanced by making a semiquantitative evaluation of each failure mode (using failure probability values), which will assist in the ranking of the severity of the failure modes. Overall, FMEA is most suited to specific equipment, and supplements HAZOP analysis which is best applied to whole processes.

Task analysis

Task analysis is used to analyse the human characteristics of systems, operations and procedures to identify likely sources of error (Kirwan & Ainsworth 1992). The data for such analysis comes partly from the analysis of what should happen and partly from observations of what does happen. For example, for a given system, all functions are defined and, for each function, all actions performed by the operator are listed. Each task and subtask is then described, indicating the nature of the action being performed by the operator (monitor, check, read, etc.). The error-likely situations for each task are then identified and ranked in order of severity. This type of analysis enables the development of training schemes for skill-based behaviour and design of controls, displays, buildings, environmental conditions and communications. The use of task analysis is generally limited to situations in which other techniques, such as HAZOP studies, have shown that human errors could lead to high risk. The main limitation of task analysis is the lack of reliable data on operator behaviour in error-likely situations. This may be explained by the number and range of factors (e.g. emotional state, training, experience, working environment and its interface) which influence human performance.

Identification of workplace hazards

More often, health and safety professionals are required to identify hazards in the workplace, and have limited involvement in the planning and design of processes. Hazards in the workplace can be identified by a number of methods, including accident and ill health statistics, investigations of accidents and incidences, audits, workplace inspections, checklists, etc. Workplace inspections, including inspection preparation, organization, information collection and records, are discussed later.

Accident and ill health statistics

The health and safety department should analyse data on injuries, accidents, near-misses and occupational ill health. The analysis of these data should compare the actual number of each type of incident against the set goals, which can be based on past experience. This comparison may reveal a pattern of injuries or accident types, unsatisfactory trends in operating procedures, unsafe systems of work, particular hazards and poor environmental conditions in the workplace. In addition, the frequency rates (see Chapter 4), e.g. fatality, major injury, reportable injury (discussed below), minor injury, sickness absence and damage, should be compared with previous years, other parts of the company, similar industrial sectors and the overall industry average. This comparison:

- enables the identification of areas or processes for further investigation;
- helps to justify expenditure;
- assists in the setting of future targets;
- helps to meet statutory reporting requirements of accidents, occupational diseases and dangerous occurrences;
- provides a performance indicator which can be compared with the rest of the industry and the industry average;
- is useful for educational purposes.

Overall, accident and incident statistics are useful in identifying uncontrolled hazards; if properly analysed, they will help to identify areas where control action (both organizational and physical) should be taken to prevent recurrence. Accident statistics are also very useful in assessing the likelihood that a particular hazard will cause harm, i.e. risk evaluation.

In the UK, the Reporting of Injuries, Diseases and Dangerous Occurrences Regulations (RIDDOR) 1995 cover the requirements to report certain categories of injuries and diseases (see Appendix 2) sustained at work to the relevant enforcing bodies, i.e. the Health and Safety Executive (HSE) or, in some cases, the local authority. The RIDDOR Regulations require the 'responsible person' to notify by the quickest practicable means:

- the death of any person, whether or not at work, as a result of an accident arising out of or in connection with work;
- any person suffering a specified major injury or condition as a result of an accident arising out of or in connection with work; and
- a scheduled dangerous occurrence (as outlined in Schedule 1 to the RIDDOR Regulations).

The 'responsible person' must also report, using the specified form, when:

- a person at work is incapacitated from his/her normal work for more than 3 days as a result of an injury (the injured person may not necessarily be away from work but, perhaps, undertaking light duties);
- the death of an employee, when death occurs within 1 year after a reportable injury which was directly responsible for that employee's death;
- a person being affected by a disease as specified in the RIDDOR

Regulations, provided that a doctor diagnoses the disease or condition, notifies the same in writing, e.g. by medical certificate, and the person's job involves a specified activity.

The RIDDOR data are compiled and published by the Health and Safety Commission (HSC) in the annual health and safety statistical report (HSC 1996). The occupational ill health statistics in this report are based on information from a number of sources, including death certificates, The Industrial Injuries Scheme (gives compensation for prescribed diseases), voluntary schemes for the reporting of occupational respiratory and skin diseases and household surveys, which yield estimates of the number of people who say that they have conditions which they believe have been caused by or made worse by work.

Investigations of accidents and incidents

Reports of accidents, symptoms or ill health effects should be analysed with regard to all the parameters available, including:

- department, type of operation and tasks performed;
- nature of injury, symptoms or illness;
- hazards exposed to and timing of symptoms or injuries;
- epidemiology of accidents, symptoms or illness among other workers;
- system of work and controls used.

The analysis of this type of information will help to identify the cause of the injuries or ill health effects, and will ultimately reveal the hazards at the root of the accidents or incidents. The identified hazard could be investigated further to determine the unsafe acts and unsafe conditions that allowed the harm associated with the hazard to be realized. Accident and incident investigations, on the whole, are useful in identifying information on hardware and software deficiencies, but provide limited information regarding human failures.

Audits

An audit is the systematic measurement and validation of an organization's health and safety programme against a series of specific and attainable standards. Audits may be conducted internally by employees or by external organizations, and usually involve a systematic examination of different aspects of the organization's activities (management policy, health and safety systems, attitudes, training, operating procedures, prevention and control procedures, emergency plans, accident records, etc.), with the object of identifying and rectifying hazards, as well as playing a major role in educating personnel at all levels in loss prevention. Independent audits may be conducted by a number of individuals or groups, including:

- engineering surveyors undertaking statutory inspections of, for example, boilers or pressure vessels;
- employers' liability surveyors;
- claims investigators, investigating accidents or damage claims under insurance policies;

- outside consultants conducting specific investigations;
- HSE or local authority inspectors undertaking investigations;
- insurance brokers' personnel undertaking inspections in connection with health and safety matters, such as fire.

The report of the audit team usually identifies major hazards and many minor hazards for the area audited. A list of actions should be drawn up to control the hazards identified. It is important to note that, for audits to be successful in the identification of hazards, they should be viewed as part of a 'learning' process rather than a 'police' action.

Checklists

An important tool in hazard identification is the checklist (example shown in Chapter 10). Like a standard or code of practice, a checklist is a means of passing on hard-won experience. It is difficult to envisage high standards in hazard control unless this experience is effectively utilized. As well as identifying hazards, checklists are also used to check compliance with good design and operating practices. An example of a checklist used for the assessment of manual handling operations is shown in Fig. 6.3.

Checklist questions for hazard identification can be derived from a number of sources, including industry codes, regulations, records of accidents, experience, knowledge of process and operating conditions, discussions, etc. The use of simple empirical checklists can be a valuable tool in the identification of hazards; however, the following points should be considered in the development and use of checklists:

- the analyst may ignore or overlook items not included in the list;
- items may be ticked without careful consideration;
- checklists are best organized using a list of words or phrases to stimulate questions concerning the subject rather than in a form which requires a simple yes/no response;
- checklists must be comprehensive, and the appropriateness of the questions must be reviewed regularly;
- checklists must be specific to the type of operation and process;
- checklists provide no quantitative measure, and hence do not allow the relative ranking of hazards;
- checklists may not be effective on their own to address new hazards or novel technology.

Untrained inspectors may characteristically miss hazards which are not detectable by the unaided eye, require active searching in, behind and under things or entail questioning about specific chemicals, process conditions or unplanned events such as machine breakdown. In summary, the use of checklists can help to make the identification of hazards systematic and can aid forgetfulness, but they should not be allowed to become a substitute for active thinking.

Workplace inspections

Many different individuals and groups within an organization will, at

Questions to consider: (If the answer to a question is 'Yes' place a tick against it and then consider the level of risk)	Yes	Level of risk: (Tick as appropriate) Low	Med	High	Possible remedial action: (Make rough notes in this column)
The tasks—do they involve: • holding loads away from body? • twisting? • stooping? • reaching upwards? • excessive vertical movement? • long carrying distances? • strenuous pushing and/or pulling? • unpredictable movement of loads? • repetitive handling? • insufficient rest or recovery? • a workrate imposed by a process? • team handling?					
The loads—are they: • heavy? • bulky/unwieldy? • difficult to grasp? • unstable/unpredictable? • intrinsically harmful (e.g. sharp/hot)?					
The working environment—are there: • constraints on posture? • poor floors? • variations in levels of work surfaces? • hot/cold/humid conditions? • strong air movements? • poor lighting conditions?					
Individual capability—does the job: • require unusual strength or stamina? • could the job be hazardous to pregnant workers or those with health problems? • does the job require special training or information?					
Other factors • Is movement or posture hindered by clothing or personal protective equipment? • Is there a risk to other employees and visitors?					

Figure 6.3 Manual handling assessment checklist. (Adapted from HSE 1992.)

some time, be involved in a workplace inspection: health and safety specialists, trade union safety representatives, inspectors of the enforcing authorities, insurance company surveyors and line managers. Inspections may be carried out for a number of reasons, including process familiarization, identification of breaches of the law, monitoring workplace controls, etc. However, the majority of workplace inspections are carried out to identify workplace hazards, and to ensure that

Part 1 Background information

Name of factory
Department(s) inspected

Date of inspection
Purpose of inspection
Inspection conducted by

Date of last inspection

(a)

Part 2 Inspection preparation checklist

1 **Plant, processes and materials**
Site plan
Processes and procedures, including typical operating conditions
Materials *(raw, intermediate, products, by-products, ancillary chemicals, process products, etc.)*
Control measures available *(engineering, administrative and personal protective equipment)*
Non-routine tasks and procedures *(machine breakdown, cleaning, maintenance etc.)*
Relevant legislation and codes of practice

2 **Personnel**
Number of workers and job titles
Age and sex and staff turnover
Working hours and shift systems
Sickness absence, accident rates and 'near-misses' history

3 **Services**
Welfare facilities *(canteen, changing rooms, showers etc.)*
Occupational health services *(staff, facilities, records and activities)*

(b)

Part 3 The inspection process

Department	Task	Materials and equipment	Hazard type	Location	Number exposed

Follow process flow
(Include ancillary processes and other areas which may support production processes)
Based on
Observations *(continuous and non-continuous hazards, routine and non-routine tasks)*
Information sources *(personal experience, communications, records, literature)*
Basic occupational hygiene equipment *(Tyndall beam, smoke tube, etc.)* and camera

(c)

Part 4 Records and actions

Activities, potential hazards, location, number exposed
Significant hazards
Agreed list of actions *(immediate, short and long term)*
Action by *(named individuals, competent, responsibility understood and accepted)*
Resources *(time, costs, etc.)*
Deadlines *(reasonable and agreed)*

Signature and review data

(d)

specific health and safety procedures are being operated. Inspections tend to follow similar formats, but are given many different names, including walk-through survey, health and safety inspection, hazard survey and safety sampling.

Preparation for the inspection

As stated above, workplace inspections can be conducted by various individuals or by a team. There are no hard and fast rules for the composition of a workplace inspection team. Ideally, it should include individuals with a knowledge of the process, production methods and materials, as well as health and safety specialists and engineers. The knowledge base for hazard identification is vital to a good inspection, which can be acquired in the following ways: personal experience of the hazard, consulting others, reviewing the literature and examining historical data on accidents, ill health effects and near-misses. A variety of checklists and survey record styles are used in conducting workplace inspections. Whatever format is adopted, the following aspects are vital to a good inspection:

- the exercise should be co-ordinated by one individual;
- the purpose of the inspection should be clearly defined and conveyed to team members;
- the inspection method should be agreed;
- actions should be recorded and monitored;
- those at risk must be informed of actions to be taken.

An example of a workplace inspection form is shown in Fig. 6.4. Parts 1 and 2 of the form provide the necessary background information for the inspection, which needs to be compiled and reviewed before proceeding on to the actual workplace inspection (Part 3). This should be followed up by a brief report of the findings and recommendations, as listed in Part 4. Part 1 of the form is fairly self-explanatory; however, it is worthwhile considering, in some detail, the information sources listed in Part 2 of the form (Fig. 6.4b).

Plant, process and material data (see Fig. 6.4b). Site plans and production flow charts are useful sources in planning and conducting the workplace inspection. The site plan ensures that any workplace visited is placed in the context of the rest of the work site, and that all relevant areas are eventually visited and evaluated.

The identification of potential hazards requires information on both the materials being processed and the equipment used in the process. A useful starting point is to create an inventory which may be organized by process, department or geographical area. The information recorded on the inventory should, as a minimum, include a list of all areas in the

Figure 6.4 (*Opposite.*) Workplace survey—hazard identification. (a) Part 1: background information. (b) Part 2: inspection preparation checklist. (c) Part 3: the inspection process. (d) Part 4: records and actions.

organization, the tasks performed, the substances and materials used and the place where the activity is carried out. When compiling material inventories, in addition to the raw materials purchased or used on site, consideration should also be given to the following list of substances:

- contaminants of raw materials (e.g. arsenic with other metals);
- intermediates and byproducts;
- final products, which may be single substances or formulations (paints, adhesives);
- ancillary chemicals used in the process (e.g. catalysts, solvents, biocides, surfactants);
- waste products, e.g. residues, used engine oils, etc.;
- proprietary products, e.g. cleaning agents, lubricants, paints, degreasing agents, adhesives.
- chemical agents produced as a result of processing, e.g. welding fume, vehicle exhausts.

Once the substances have been identified, specific information on their physical, chemical, toxicological and biological properties needs to be collected and collated (Chapters 3 and 5). The relevant data should include the physical form of the substance (gas, vapour, mist, fibre, respirable, inspirable, etc.), potential route of uptake (inhalation, skin absorption, ingestion, etc.), thermal reactivity (exothermic and endothermic reactions), flammability and explosive limits, toxicological (animal and human data) and biological (biodegradation, etc.) properties and current occupational exposure limits (OELs). The majority of this information can be obtained from the materials safety data sheets. However, further information may be obtained by reviewing and evaluating human epidemiology and toxicological data derived from scientific studies.

Certain UK legislation (Provision and Use of Work Equipment Regulations 1992, Manual Handling Operations Regulations 1992, etc.) demands risk assessments of activities in which materials are used. In most circumstances, it is impractical to base such assessments on material inventories; instead, a process inventory provides a better foundation for the identification and assessment of risks. As for material inventories, the process inventory can be organized by department, flow of materials or geographical area. The inventory should include the process, materials involved, normal operating conditions and procedures, potential hazards and control systems. This type of inventory is particularly useful in the identification of physical (noise, thermal, radiation) and mechanical hazards.

Personnel (see Fig. 6.4b). Information on the number of staff, working hours, shift patterns, job titles, age and gender is necessary for a number of reasons, including the assessment of exposure duration, the development of occupational hygiene sampling strategies and as a means of classifying exposure groups in epidemiological studies. Furthermore, this information may help to identify the more vulnerable individuals who may be 'especially at risk' as required by the UK Management of Health and Safety at Work Regulations (MHSWR) 1992. The individual characteristics relevant in this respect include gender, age, disability, shift work, pre-existing health conditions and other miscellaneous characteristics, such as personal/social habits of lifestyle choice, e.g. smoking.

Workers at high risk and processes with a relatively high hazard potential may be identified or highlighted by screening the accident and sickness absence data. Accident statistics (frequency, incidence, severity rates) are useful in identifying uncontrolled risks, as they will present data indicative of where control actions should be taken to prevent recurrence. Ideally, an analysis of injury, damage and near-miss accidents should be recorded. However, for the accidents and ill health statistics to be of use, the limitations of the indices measured should be fully understood. Recently, Amis and Booth (1992) questioned the significance and relevance of accident statistics as a measure of health and safety performance.

Occupational health service (see Fig. 6.4b). The services provided for the workforce enable an assessment to be made of the health, safety and welfare provisions in relation to any workplace hazards which may be identified. It is useful to know the composition of the occupational health team (physicians, occupational hygienists, first aiders, nursing staff, safety officers), and the facilities and equipment that are available for the assessment and management of individuals at risk. Ongoing activities, such as health surveillance (data on symptoms, inspections, biological and clinical data, audiometry, etc.), workplace inspections and audits and special services (counselling on health-related matters, immunization programmes, etc.), may provide further evidence for the existence of particular workplace hazards. The occupational health service may also collate and analyse data on injuries, ill health and sickness absenteeism.

The inspection

The workplace inspection must be systematic and comprehensive, examining all conditions affecting heath, safety and welfare in all parts of employment. It may be helpful to plan such a general inspection in one of three ways: (i) by following a geographical course through the site; (ii) by tracing a hazard; or (iii) by tracing tasks by process flow. Clearly, one approach will suit one particular workplace or one set of circumstances better than another.

The inspection process (see Fig. 6.4c). In the geographical approach, using the site plan, the inspector progresses through the plant area by area, department by department. The *geographical approach* is economical in terms of time, avoiding recrossing familiar ground. It is especially suitable for production units with simple processes, or where a number of processes are carried out on the same site. This approach, however, is not appropriate where the process is complex and difficult to understand, or where it must be followed through in order to identify the hazards.

The inspection by *hazard approach* ensures that full attention is given to a known or suspected hazard. The idea is to trace right through the plant all aspects of one problem, and to ignore other hazards. This may therefore result in a more consistent approach to a particular hazard across all activities. This approach is particularly relevant when trying to identify hazards in order to comply with requirements of specific health and safety legislation. The main disadvantage of this approach is that a particular hazard can be overemphasized or overlooked in the case of new or developing hazards.

The *task approach* to hazard identification relies on the identification of all activities carried out within the organization and a good understanding of the processes, their interactions and inter-relations. This pattern of inspection has the advantage of accurately describing the tasks performed by individuals, i.e. it is relevant to employees and is also cost effective in terms of time. The tasks carried out can be systematically identified by following the process flow, typically from goods in to the dispatch of products. The *process flow approach* is particularly useful, if not a necessity, in large manufacturing plants which may involve a number of complex stages, a large number of chemicals and numerous production lines. In order to identify all tasks, it is useful to supplement the process flow approach with the inspection of ancillary processes (cleaning, maintenance, etc.) and other areas (laboratories, boiler house, etc.) which may support the production process, and thus may be overlooked when using this approach.

When identifying hazards, it is important to distinguish between hazards arising from planned and unplanned events, sometimes referred to as continuous and non-continuous hazards (described earlier). Human error is also an important factor in events leading to an unwanted occurrence. Human error usually occurs because of an inadequacy of motivation, skill, training or capacity. It is possible to describe human error using a number of dimensions, e.g. the type of error, its cause, the probability of its occurrence within a specified time and its consequences. Thus, the identification of the role played by human error can, in itself, provide insight into the failure process.

During the inspection, it is important to communicate with individuals who operate, maintain or control the use of a particular machine/process. The purpose of the inspection should be explained to such individuals; furthermore, they should be encouraged to raise any questions regarding the health and safety aspect of the process, previous incidents, control systems and undesirable practices. By asking operators and others involved in a task for their view on the health and safety aspects of the task performed, information may be obtained on certain conditions, incidences and 'near-misses' experienced by the operators which may not be apparent during the inspection. This source of information is invaluable for the identification of hazards, particularly those of a non-continuous nature. In conducting the inspection, it is also useful to consider future tasks or situations that may affect the existing premises or process, such as the installation or modification of plant, new processes, proposed changes to the materials used and the demolition of buildings.

Use of occupational hygiene instrumentation. The majority of hazards may be identified from a knowledge of the process and materials safety data sheets, observation and understanding of the process, previous experience, records and the literature. However, in some situations, the hazard may not be obvious, or may require confirmation before proceeding to the risk assessment. Furthermore, as part of the workplace inspection, an initial assessment of ventilation systems and an understanding of how the contaminated volume of air moves may also be helpful. In such cases, the use of basic occupational hygiene instrumentation (smoke tubes, Tyndall beam dust lamp), photography techniques and numerous direct reading instruments can play an important role.

A smoke tube consists of a glass tube containing concentrated sulphuric acid absorbed into inert granules. A continuous stream of smoke is produced by coupling the smoke tube to a hand-held positive pressure pump (aspirator). The smoke may be released at different points in the workplace to trace air flow patterns. The technique is particularly useful for the rapid assessment of the suction inlets of local exhaust ventilation (LEV) systems, i.e. a smoke cloud can be released at the source of the contaminant to show whether air is drawn from the source into the LEV system. The 'dust lamp' employs the Tyndall effect to reveal the presence and direction of movement of respirable particles, which are normally invisible to the naked eye in normal lighting. The lamp produces a horizontal beam of light. When the beam passes through a cloud of dust, forward scattering of the light occurs, which is visible to an observer looking along the beam of light in the direction of the lamp. The lamp can also be used to evaluate the performance of LEV systems associated with dust-emitting processes, and the design can be modified if required to improve the capture efficiency. It is useful to photograph or video record the results from the use of smoke tubes and the Tyndall beam.

Other qualitative techniques used to visualize the flow of certain pollutants include infrared and schlieren photography. Infrared photography is based on the fact that the majority of gases and vapours have dipole moments in their molecular structure which cause them to exhibit strong absorption peaks in the infrared region. Schlieren photography is based on the visualization of small differences in density, which cause changes in the refractive index of the gas that can be made visible. It is also possible to integrate a pollutant sensor (e.g. a monitor for measuring particulate concentrations) with a video recorder so that a concentration marker can be displayed on the recording, enabling a direct correlation to be made between work activity and exposure profile.

Direct reading instruments play an important role in the identification or confirmation of suspicious hazards in the workplace. Instruments are available for measuring toxic gases, combustible gases, oxygen, flammable substances, aerosols, noise levels, lighting levels, radiation intensity, vibration, heat stress, etc. The instruments range from the simple, easy to use colorimetric detector tubes (for gases and vapours) to multispecific gas detectors (portable gas chromatographs, infrared analysers, photo-ionization detectors). The main advantages of such instruments are as follows:

- generally specific with a good sensitivity, and available for a large number of workplace contaminants;
- provide measurement results instantaneously;
- confirm suspicions regarding the type of hazard present and rule out other potential hazards;
- enable the identification of leaks and the spread of contaminants, including emergency response;
- enable sampling in confined spaces;
- enable the plotting of exposure profiles which can be related to work practices;
- can be linked to alarm systems which can be set at a percentage of the OEL or flammable limit;
- enable the identification and measurement of short-term peak exposures;
- can be used to assess the efficiency of control measures.

When using direct reading instruments, it is important that they are calibrated frequently to ensure accuracy and reliability. When properly calibrated and operated, they are capable of measuring atmospheric contaminants to an accuracy and reliability that are well within the requirements for the detection of occupational hazards.

Records and actions. After completing the inspection, it is important to discuss the findings and to list specific actions to be taken (Fig. 6.4d). The inspection will identify the hazard types and their characteristics, hazard location, number of individuals exposed, time of exposure and the control systems used. This information can also be used to carry out a qualitative exposure assessment by developing exposure rating groups and matching these to categories of likely health effects (Hawkins *et al.* 1991). The use of qualitative risk assessment based on the subjective ranking of exposure and health effects is discussed in Chapter 10. In some cases, the hazard can be eliminated or the working methods can be modified to minimize the hazard. More often, a detailed quantitative assessment may be required to assess the level of risk.

Individuals assigned to implement the actions must understand and accept their responsibilities, and must have the necessary time, resources, knowledge and experience to carry out the actions. In some cases, external assistance may be required, e.g. for exposure assessment, health surveillance, examination and design of control systems, development of health and safety procedures, etc. Deadlines must be agreed between the individuals concerned, and progress must be reviewed at suitable times. Records of all inspections, agreed actions and reviews must be kept in a suitable form and, if conducted properly, will provide a valuable information source for workplace risk assessments.

References

AIChE (1992) *Guidelines for Hazard Evaluation Procedures*, 2nd edn. Centre for Chemical Process Safety, AIChE, New York.

Amis, R.M. & Booth, R.T. (1992) Monitoring health and safety management. *Safety and Health Practitioner* 10, 43–46.

CIA (1979) *A Guide to Hazard and Operability Studies*. Chemical Industries Association, London.

DOW Chemical Company (1994) *DOW's Fire and Explosion Index Hazard Classification Guide and Chemical Exposure Guide*. AIChE Technical Manual, 2 vols., LC 80-29237. AIChE, New York.

Hawkins, N.C., Norwood, S.K. & Rock, J.C. (1991) *A Strategy for Occupational Exposure Assessment*. American Industrial Hygiene Association, Fairfax, VA.

HSC (1996) *Health and Safety Statistics 1995/6*. HSE Books, Sudbury, Suffolk.

HSE (1991) *A Guide to the Control of Industrial Major Accident and Hazard Regulations 1984; Guidance on Regulations*. HS(R) 21. HMSO, London.

HSE (1992) *HSE Guidelines on Manual Handling Operations Regulations 1992*. HMSO, London.

ICI (1993) *Mond Index: How to Identify, Assess and Minimise Potential Hazards on Chemical Plant Units for New and Existing Processes*, 2nd edn. ICI, Northwich.

Kirwan, B. & Ainsworth, L.K. (1992) *A Guide to Task Analysis*. Taylor & Francis, London.

Kletz, T.A. (1992) *Identifying and Assessing Process Industry Hazards*, 3rd edn. Institution of Chemical Engineers, London.

Lees, F.P. & Ang, M.L. (eds.) (1989) *Safety Cases Within the Control of Industrial Major Accident and Hazard (CIMAH) Regulations 1984*. Butterworth Scientific, London.

Pitblado, R. & Turney, R. (1996) *Risk Assessment in the Process Industries*, 2nd edn. Institute of Chemical Engineers, Rugby, Warwickshire.

Sinnott, R.K. (ed.) (1996) *Coulson & Richardson's Chemical Engineering*, 2nd edn., Vol. 6. Butterworth, Oxford.

Wallace, I. (ed.) (1995) *Developing Effective Safety Systems*. Institute of Chemical Engineers, Rugby, Warwickshire.

Chapter 7 Standard setting in occupational health

Leonard S. Levy

Introduction

Standards developed in occupations tend to be viewed like speed limits—above them danger exists, below them it is safe. In addition, practitioners of health and safety rules may simply turn to the figure in a table or list, and never consider the development or deeper purpose of the standard. The reality is that the standard, whether an air level for a chemical substance or a noise level, is set within a philosophical framework in a socioeconomic system within which the philosophy operates. This framework takes into account the purpose of the standard itself in terms of health protection (all people, some people, 'average' people), the way in which the scientific and medical data can be dealt with, the way in which uncertainties are dealt with (safety factor, default positions), the likely level of compliance by firms, the possibility of effective enforcement by regulatory authorities, the actual practicability of compliance with the standard and, lastly, the cost of achieving the standard. As can be seen, standard setting is a pragmatic process, and the standard itself cannot be divorced from the process by which it is set. It is thus not surprising that different bodies worldwide set different standards for the same substance or physical hazard, because not only may the science be interpreted in different ways, but the whole philosophy may vary. Even the composition of a standard setting committee may influence the way in which a standard is set. As an example, in a market economy country, a committee made up of industrially funded occupational health specialists may well suggest a very different level for a standard than a committee composed of trade union-funded occupational health specialists. For this reason, many occupational standards are set or agreed by the social partners as well as the government. This not only makes a reasonable compromise, but also means that the standard may achieve a much better chance of acceptance by all sides of industry. For these reasons, standards that are now set must be scientifically credible, defensible and receive broad acceptance by employers, employees and trade unions. In addition, the last decade has seen the inclusion of cost–benefit analysis in many standard setting processes. The methodology for this is not yet a precise science, but, broadly, the benefits from the introduction of a new standard or the reduction of an existing standard must be justified by comparing the benefits of the standard to the costs (financial, resources, person power, etc.) involved in achieving and maintaining the standard.

As an example of this procedure, if the Health and Safety Commission (HSC) in the UK wishes to set a new maximum exposure limit (a rigidly enforced air standard) for a chemical substance, the Health and Safety Executive (HSE, the competent national governmental authority) must make out a transparent and logical case showing where the chemical substance is used throughout all sectors of industry, where exposure is likely, how many people are exposed and at what levels, what means of control are available in different settings and what would be the practical means and the financial consequences of reducing exposure to particular levels right across all sectors of industry. This information is then set against estimates of what the potential health benefits would be from such exposure reduction. This could be in terms of the number of cancers prevented in the case of a carcinogen, or the number of cases of occupational asthma prevented in the case of an asthmagen. Such a standard setting exercise is a major undertaking, expensive in terms of both skilled person power and finance, and may take several years. For such reasons, this kind of rigidly enforced standard is not set for every chemical substance in use (there are many hundreds of thousands), but only for relatively few that are considered to be worthy of 'serious concern'.

Thus, at each stage of the standard setting process, questions must be asked regarding the philosophy of the overall procedure and what each stage is intended to achieve. Only then can one understand the true purpose of the standard and the level of protection/safety it is intended to achieve. This chapter explores how occupational standards are set, and how they can best be employed as a useful tool in the risk assessment, risk management process.

Types of standard

Probably the most abundant and widely known are the airborne standards, called occupational exposure limits (OELs); however, it should be borne in mind that, for many chemicals which can readily pass through the skin, relying on an airborne standard, which assumes that exposure (in the breathing zone) equals uptake (amount in the body), may seriously underestimate the total uptake. In this case, biological monitoring and biological effect monitoring can give a truer representation of the risk. For such substances, biological exposure indices (BEIs) (American Conference of Governmental Industrial Hygienists (ACGIH) 1996) have evolved in the USA and biological tolerance values (BATs) (DFG 1994) in Germany. Interestingly, both have a different scientific philosophical basis, which would not be recognized if one used the numerical figures from the tables; these will be described later. Although these two countries are the most advanced in setting such biological limits, other countries are now beginning to set their own, such as the UK, where biological monitoring guidance values (BMGVs) (HSE 1997) have been set, but with no regulatory status. Of course, most countries employ various forms of biological monitoring control for lead. In the case of physical agents, a number of countries have developed standards for various forms of industrially encountered radiation. These include lasers, microwaves and, of course, ionizing radiation. Other standards and guidance values exist for a wide range of physical agents, and may be set to provide protection to health, e.g. noise, heat, cold or manual handling, or where comfort is the chief target, e.g. workplace illumination or visual display unit (VDU) work. Again, as will be seen later, the philosophy is based on the protection of people from both short- and long-term exposure and the working schedule. Interestingly, all standards are built around the idea of a typical working week—some 40 h—and the standard is said to be adjusted for longer working hours. The most important thing for all standards is that they should be seen as an aid to risk management—they should not replace good professional judgement.

The evaluation of standards for occupational chemical exposure

The most highly refined and misunderstood standards are those controlling chemical exposure in the workplace. Generically, they are known as occupational exposure limits (OELs), and have now been produced for around 1000 of the most commonly used industrial substances. Different countries have different proprietary names for their exposure limits—some are similar, but some are quite different in terms of setting and applicability. The earliest OELs were set in the 1880s within the rapidly growing German chemical industry, but were usually concerned with short-term limits set to protect people from acute effects, usually in fairly dangerous conditions. From this time through to the 1920s and 1930s, few countries employed more than a handful of OELs. This was partly due to a lack of suitable, usable, analytical techniques—after all, it is no use having a standard if one cannot measure it.

The real leap forward in the development of OELs came in the USA in the 1940s, with the setting up of the ACGIH and their development of the threshold limit value (TLV) system (ACGIH 1996). Their innovations led to the concept of 'time-weighted averages' (TWAs) and a stated underlying philosophy of protecting 'nearly all workers'. Much of the philosophy of the TLV system, which still remains in OELs today, owes itself to the scientific paradigms that were accepted by the occupational health professionals of the 1940s and early 1950s. The most important scientific assumption made was that, for the standard setting process, there would be some form of dose–response relationship for any harmful effect in a population. Thus, there would be a variation in response corresponding to some form of normality, and some people would be more 'sensitive' (show an effect at a low level), whilst others would be more 'resistant' (show an effect at a high level). Even more important was the assumption made that, below a certain level, a 'threshold', no one would be affected. As can be seen, the concept of threshold became incorporated into the ACGIH's registered trademark, 'TLV'. Although both of these assumptions now seem to be naive in terms of our current knowledge of allergenicity (hypersensitive populations) and genotoxic carcinogens (no demonstrable safe levels), at the time they appeared to be justifiable as they appealed to what seemed reasonable in the real world of chemical exposure. All people do not respond in the same way to either good or bad effects at the same exposure levels, and the concept of thresholds fits in well with many harmful effects from chemical exposure, such as irritation and prenarcosis. In addition, much of the early experimental toxicological work showed that, for many common chemicals and harmful effects, there were thresholds.

What really accelerated the promulgation of the use of OELs was the development of portable, battery-operated sampling pumps in the 1960s, which enabled personal (breathing zone) measurements to be made. From this time onwards, OELs were set as personal sampling limits. This meant that OELs could be set on personal measurements.

One of the most difficult acts of faith to accept is that an OEL can protect workers from a whole range of potential toxic effects, both acute and chronic. Clearly, a massive amount of oversimplification needs to take place in the process of standard setting, but the most basic is that all chronic effects can be controlled by the use of the ACGIH TWA concept, employing 8 h as a surrogate for a 40-h week, a 40-h week as a surrogate for 52 weeks and 1 year as a surrogate for 40 years (a lifetime's exposure). In other words, the OELs set as 8-h TWAs should protect the average worker from a lifetime's exposure with no chronic effect. In the case of acute effects (harmful effects which occur rapidly, such as inflammations or narcosis), these can be protected against by the use of a short-term exposure limit (STEL), which is usually set for 10 or 15 min. 'Instant' would be better, but the time reflects the reality of the time required for sampling. Table 7.1 describes the conditions required.

Table 7.1 Standard setting options for protecting against acute or chronic toxic effects.

Acute effects	Chronic effects
1 Usually caused by single, high overexposure over seconds to hours	1 Usually related to low, repeated exposures over months or years (acute effects are not seen)
2 Condition develops rapidly (minutes to days) with signs and symptoms	2 Condition develops slowly over months or years. Usually, incremental tissue damage with early stages undetected
3 Usually, damage completely reversible (unless fatal)	3 Damage usually irreversible. Cessation of exposure may arrest damage, or condition may become progressive
4 Protected by STELs (usually 15 min)	4 Protected by 8-h TWA

The standard setting process

As stated in the 'Introduction', any standard setting body needs to state its purpose, in modern parlance, in a 'mission statement'. That employed by the ACGIH in the USA (ACGIH 1996), developed in 1953, succinctly defines the reality of most market force countries in setting standards.

> Threshold limit values refer to airborne concentrations of substances and represent conditions under which it is believed that nearly all workers may be repeatedly exposed day after day without adverse effect. Because of wide variation in individual susceptibility, however, a small percentage of workers may experience discomfort from some substances at concentrations at or below the threshold limit: a smaller percentage may be affected more seriously by aggravation of a pre-existing condition or by development of an occupational disease.

This has been the wording of the TLV preface since 1953 and, initially, they did not include 'nearly all' in their definition, so strong was their initial belief in the protection offered by the threshold concept. Recently, they added the sentence: 'Smoking of tobacco may act synergistically with airborne chemicals encountered in the workplace, e.g. asbestos'.

Information that can be used in the standard setting process tends to be highly variable, but usually falls into one of three groups.

1 Industrial experience: these are typical exposure levels that may be found in the range of industries using the substance.

2 Human evidence: this will take the form of any case reports, volunteer studies or epidemiological investigations on workers exposed to the substance.

3 Animal and other experimental investigations: these data include a whole range of acute and chronic studies in animals, looking for a range of acute and chronic effects (hazards) as well as any dose–response relationships; data may also include cell culture studies, such as bacterial mutation tests.

In many cases, human evidence is often minimal or even missing, and OELs may have to be based on animal studies. In such cases, uncertainty factors may be employed, using the 'no observable adverse effect level' (NOAEL) from the animal study, for an interspecies comparison.

As can be seen from the ACGIH philosophy, the levels set may not be absolutely protective for all people for all effects. However, other philosophies represent other beliefs. For example, the Occupational Safety and Health Administration (OSHA) in the USA states that (cited in Calabrese 1978):

> No employee will suffer material impairment to health or functional capacity even if such employee has regular exposure.

In the former USSR (also cited in Calabrese 1978):

> No detectable change of any kind in a test organization.

The contrast between the Russian approach in the 1970s compared with the approach in the USA is shown in Table 7.2.

It is quite easy to see why the Russian standards are far lower for many substances than the levels in the USA. The Russian standards are entirely health based, whilst the standards in the USA are based on health plus other factors—a cost–benefit approach. This is not to say that one is better than the other. Remember, what determines worker protection is how the standards, whatever they are, are complied with and enforced in workplaces. Since the break-up of the USSR and the collapse of communism in the countries of Central and Eastern Europe, there has been a move in standard setting to more market force-based standards. Harmonization will thus increase across Europe and internationally, and this will be aided by the use of agreed databases and the interchange of scientific ideas.

Developments in the UK and European Union (EU)

The developments in the UK act as a good model of what has happened in most of the rest of the world as they have developed their own approaches to incorporating standards into their own health and safety legislation. Many countries simply 'borrowed' the US ACGIH figures, and in this case the UK was no different. The then UK Factory Inspectorate published the ACGIH TLV list in 1960 in the form of a booklet entitled: *Toxic Substances in the Atmosphere*. Following the set-up of the HSE in 1974, a new set of Guidance Notes included one, *EH15*, which was the previous year's TLVs (HSE 1975). This continued until 1980 (at which time only 11 true UK standards were set). In 1984, the

Table 7.2 Contrasts in approaches to standard setting in the USA and the USSR in the 1970s. (Adapted from Calabrese 1978.)

USA	USSR
1 Minor physiological adaptive changes are permitted	1 Maximum allowable concentration will not permit the development of any disease or deviation from normal
2 Economic and technological feasibility are important considerations in the development of standards	2 The principle is that standards should be based entirely on health and not on technological and economic feasibility
3 Values are time-weighted averages	3 Concentrations are maximum values
4 Research emphasis is on pathology	4 Research emphasis is on nervous system testing
5 Except for carcinogens, goals of near-zero exposure are not widely adopted	5 The goal is a level of exposure that does not strain the adaptive and compensatory mechanisms of the body

HSE published its own philosophy of two forms of exposure limit, control limits (CLs) and recommended limits (RLs), as *Guidance Note EH40*/year (an annual update) (HSE 1995). Although this contained much of the US ACGIH philosophy in terms of STELs, 8-h TWAs and protecting 'nearly all workers', the two forms varied in their level of enforceability. In general, CLs were set for substances of serious health concern (usually carcinogens) and where no safe level (threshold) could be agreed. For these, the legal requirement was to be as low as reasonably practicable, but never above the CL value. For RLs, where a threshold of effect could usually be established with some level of assurance, they were used as guidelines for good practice and not so rigorously enforced.

The system for setting OELs in the UK is interesting, as it represents a model system in which the social partners' views are taken into account as well as those of the HSE. Initially, a tripartite subgroup, called the Working Group on the Assessment of Toxic Chemicals (WATCH), which is an essentially technical group of toxicologists, hygienists and occupational physicians, form an opinion. This is then considered by another committee, the Advisory Committee on Toxic Substances (ACTS), which takes socioeconomic as well as technical issues into account. Over the last decade, with the change of regulations in the UK and the interpretation of these OELs into a broader chemical control framework (the Control of Substances Hazardous to Health (COSHH) Regulations 1994) (Worksafe Australia 1990), the CLs and RLs have become transmuted into maximum exposure limits (MELs) and occupational exposure standards (OESs), with the following definitions for the purpose of compliance. MELs:

> Where there is exposure to a substance for which a maximum exposure limit is specified in Schedule 1, the control of exposure shall, so far as the inhalation of that substance is concerned, only be treated as being adequate if the level of exposure is reduced so far as is reasonably practicable and in any case below the maximum exposure limit.

As can be seen, there is no basic difference between this definition and that for CLs, and so no anomaly has been created.

The situation for OESs is somewhat different in that a novel definition was produced that did not match up to any previous UK definition, nor one elsewhere in the world. The definition set out in the COSHH Regulations reads:

> Without prejudice to the generality of paragraph (1), where there is exposure to a substance for which an occupational exposure standard has been approved, the control of exposure shall, so far as inhalation of that standard is concerned, be treated as being adequate if:
> (a) that occupational exposure standard is not exceeded, or
> (b) where that occupational exposure standard is exceeded, the employer identifies the reasons for the standard being exceeded

and takes appropriate action to remedy the situation as seen, as is reasonably practicable.
(Paragraph 1. Every employer shall ensure that the exposure of his employees to substances hazardous to health is either prevented or, where this is not reasonably practicable, adequately controlled.)

As stated earlier, other countries have different approaches to setting standards. In Germany, the MAK Commission initially recommends standards; this Commission consists entirely of academics and toxicologists sitting apart from government (DFG 1994). The value must then be considered by the government for adoption. In Australia, 'Worksafe Australia' has approved a list of exposure limits which is essentially the TLV list (Levy & Lunau 1990). This is still common in many countries.

However, great caution is needed when importing standards from one country to another. As has been demonstrated in this chapter, standards do not stand alone, but are usually part of a regulatory/control framework within the socioeconomic and political system of the country in which they are set. They may also take into account local environmental conditions and reflect the composition of the standard setting committees (academics alone, government scientists alone, a mixture of representatives of all the social partners, etc.). Thus, if a standard is imported from another country, the whole paraphernalia surrounding the intended setting, compliance and enforcement of that standard is also imported. This may be no bad thing in itself, but it should be clearly understood by those who adopt the standards. Ideally, each country should 'set' its own standards to take into account its own situation, but this does not mean that it necessarily has to set up teams of scientists to write critical scientific reviews based on hundreds of scientific papers. Harmonization of standards at a global level, as will be illustrated later, may be a more appropriate use of resources, but individual countries will still need ultimate decision-making powers.

What is important is the transparency of the process: not just the way the data are handled, but the setting out of the operating system and guidelines under which the standard setters operate. Again, to illustrate this point, the HSE in the UK has produced a set of 'indicative criteria' which are meant to assist, but not constrain, both WATCH and ACTS in their deliberations. For OESs, these are as follows.

1 The available scientific evidence allows for the identification, with reasonable certainty, of a concentration averaged over a reference period at which there is no indication that the substance is likely to be injurious to employees if they are exposed by inhalation day after day to that concentration; and

2 Exposures to concentrations higher than that derived under Criterion 1, and which could reasonably occur in practice, are unlikely to produce serious short- or long-term effects on health over the period of time it might reasonably be expected to identify and remedy the cause of excessive exposure; and

3 The available evidence indicates that compliance with the OES, as derived under Criterion 1, is reasonably practicable.

For MELs:

1 The available evidence on the substance does not satisfy Criterion 1 and/or 2 for an OES; a numerically higher value is necessary if the controls associated with certain uses are to be regarded as reasonably practicable.

As can be seen, there is quite a lot of room for discussion within each of the criteria, and so this is not simply a checklist approach to arriving at a figure—good judgement and consensus are paramount.

Within the EU, the Single European Act of 1992 has led to the need to harmonize health and safety standards in the workplace. The reasons are twofold. Firstly, the economic cost of health and safety should be equal between member states and, secondly, the level of protection for a worker moving from one job in one member state to another member state should also be the same when doing the same job. This applies to OELs and, for this reason, Directorate General V (DGV) set up a Scientific Expert Group on Exposure Limits (SEG), made up of nominees from member states, to advise them on setting EU OELs. Recently, the SEG has become more formalized as the Scientific Committee on Occupational Exposure Limits (SCOEL), and has produced a number of OELs. These are known as indicative limit values (ILVs), and must be taken into account when individual member states establish their own national values. At present, the system is slowly bedding into the health and safety activities of the EU member states, but points the way to the harmonization of standards.

Application of OELs and standards

The application of any standard to any given working situation relies entirely on good professional judgement. All standards will have imperfections in their setting, either through incomplete data or socioeconomic compromise, causing some people to be at risk. For this reason, the limitations of the standards must be appreciated, and their application must be used intelligently by the trained health and safety specialist. There are many examples of where allowances have to be made in the interpretation of air standards. A simple one would be that, if a worker is involved in a 12-h shift, the OEL for any substance he/she works with should be reduced on a *pro rata* basis so that the spirit of not overloading the system with the substance is adhered to. The model of risk assessment being divided into a number of discrete phases is useful in this context. The first two components of risk assessment—hazard assessment (toxicity) and dose–effect relationships (how much to cause the hazard)—are those which go into setting the standard. However, it is the third stage, exposure characterization, together with the previous two stages, that will provide the risk assessment by characterizing the risk and allowing effective risk management to be used. Another problem that occurs within the interpretation of chemical exposures is that of *complex mixtures*. Although most OELs are for single substances, the commonest situation that arises in the workplace is where people are exposed to a cocktail of mixtures, often of varying proportions. Several different types of interaction may occur between chemical constituents present in a mixture. Chemicals may act independently of each other or may interact in an additive manner. Alternatively, chemicals may interact synergistically, i.e. when the overall effect on health is significantly greater than the sum of the individual effects. Clearly, synergistic interactions present the most serious outcome and, where toxicological data indicate synergistic interactions, strict control is required. In most situations, information on the type of interaction which may be expected is not available, and to predict harm is impossible. However, the sensible use of OELs can lead to very practical, although pragmatic, control. For this reason, bodies such as the HSE and ACGIH are able to give advice which, although scientifically difficult to justify, seems to work in producing protection. Quite simply, the assumption is made that if two or more substances are present, and they are not known to be toxicologically independent of each other, they should be treated as additive and a 'combined OEL' can be made which should not exceed unity. For example, if chemical A with an OEL of 50 ppm is measured as X ppm and chemical B with an OEL of 100 ppm is measured as Y ppm, for a mixture of A and B, $X/50\,\text{ppm} + Y/100\,\text{ppm}$ should be less than unity.

In the case of organic solvents, where health effects may be very similar, such as mucous membrane irritation and prenarcosis, it is easier to justify the additive approach on toxicological grounds (Scheffers *et al.* 1985). In many other cases where mixtures are involved, the toxicology of all substances is either incompletely characterized or there are many potential divergent health end-points. Thus, although this approach may defy deep scrutiny, it is simple and workable, and probably affords a good deal of protection (Holmberg & Lundberg 1985; Levy & Lunau 1990). In the UK, OELs exist for some commonly encountered mixtures, such as foundry fume, where airborne particulate acts as a surrogate for overall exposure, or rubber fume, where exposure is assessed by measuring total particulate and cyclohexane-soluble material. With another commonly encountered mixture, welding fume, overall exposure is controlled by an OES, although for some welding fumes which contain substances with specific OELs, these OELs will need to be applied. A more complex scientific and regulatory problem exists for handling the issues surrounding the risk assessment and control of carcinogens. Because the outcome is so serious, risk reduction measures invariably need to be shown to be stringent; thus, if a carcinogenic substance cannot be banned, standards must be set and complied with. Many carcinogens act by genotoxic mechanisms and thus, in theory at least, there is no safe level; consequently, there is a need to have exposure levels which continuously put pressure on exposure reduction measures. When it comes to standard setting, three broad approaches have emerged to derive numerical values. One favours the use of mathematical modelling based on quantitative linear extrapolation and makes many assumptions; the second tries to use a 'no observable adverse effect level' approach, but then uses safety factors of perhaps 100 or 1000; the third approach uses a 'lowest technically achievable' approach, but takes into account the presumed risk levels (Vainio & Tomatis 1985).

Conclusions

The importance of standards is not the figures themselves, but the fact that they exist, can be agreed upon and that organizations will attempt to use them to control or limit the exposure of working people. Harmonization worldwide would be a laudable achievement, and there are moves to share data, experience and approaches. This is particularly important for chemical substances, where probably over 50 000 are used in workplaces, but standards exist for only around 800–1000 of these.

References

ACGIH (1996) *Documentation of the Threshold Limit Values and Biological Exposure Indices*, 6th edn. ACGIH Inc., Cincinnati, OH.
Calabrese, E.J. (1978) *Methodological Approaches to Deriving Environmental and Occupational Health Standards.* Wiley, New York.
DFG (1994) *Biological Exposure Values for Occupational Toxicants and Carcinogens*, Vol. 1. VCH Verlagsgesellschaft, Weinheim and New York.
Holmberg, B.O. & Lundberg, P. (1985) Exposure limits for mixtures. *Annals of the American Conference of Governmental Industrial Hygienists* **12**, 111–118.
HSE (1975) *Threshold Limit Values for 1975, Guidance Note EH15.* HMSO, London.
HSE (1995) *General COSHH ACoP (Control of Substances Hazardous to Health), Carcinogens ACoP (Control of Carcinogenic Substances) and Biological ACoP (Control of Biological Agents). Control of Substances Hazardous to Health Regulations 1994. Approved Code of Practice.* HSE Books, London.
HSE (1997) *EH40/97 Occupational Exposure Limits 1997.* HSE Books, Suffolk.
Levy, L.S. & Lunau, F.W. (1990) Occupational exposure limits for mixtures. In: *Indoor Air Quality and Ventilation* (eds. F. Lunau & G.L. Reynolds), pp. 15–22. Selpher Ltd, London.
Scheffers, T.M.L., Jongeneelen, F.J. & Bragt, P.C. (1985) Development of effect-specific limit values (ESLVs) for solvent mixtures in painting. *Annals of Occupational Hygiene* **29**, 191–199.
Vainio, H. & Tomatis, L. (1985) Exposure to carcinogens: scientific and regulatory aspects. *Annals of the American Conference of Governmental Industrial Hygienists* **12**, 135–143.
Worksafe Australia (1990) *Exposure Standards for Atmospheric Contaminants in the Occupational Environment.* National Occupational Health and Safety Commission, Canberra.

Chapter 8 Requirements of monitoring exposure to workplace contaminants

Steven S. Sadhra and Kerry Gardiner

Introduction

Exposure monitoring in occupational health is an important tool that can be used to provide a reliable estimate of exposure to workplace contaminants. The most common reason for such monitoring is to compare the data obtained with legal or recommended standards or recognized guidelines to yield a crude determination of risk. Two common techniques used to evaluate individual exposure are atmospheric monitoring and biological monitoring. Atmospheric monitoring is used to evaluate exposure when the main route of uptake is inhalation. Biological monitoring of blood, urine or exhaled air may be most appropriate for the evaluation of exposure in certain occupations where skin absorption and ingestion are the most important routes of entry into the body. It could be argued that biological monitoring is the best way to determine the actual or integrated exposure to the body; however, atmospheric monitoring may enable the exposure to be identified and quantified more rapidly without ethical difficulties before it can manifest harm. The role of biological monitoring in the evaluation of individual exposure is discussed in Chapter 16.

This chapter provides an overview of exposure monitoring, with emphasis on the principles of monitoring and the use and limitations of exposure data in the context of workplace risk assessment. Specific sampling and analysis techniques for different hazards are not covered; however, the importance of the development of a suitable sampling programme, which is applicable to the design of employee monitoring for all hazard types, is discussed in detail. Details of specific sampling and analysis methods for different occupational hazards can be found in other textbooks (Ashton & Gill 1992; Bisesi & Kohn 1995; Harrington & Gardiner 1995). The use of modelling techniques to predict exposure to hazardous agents in the workplace is discussed in Chapter 9.

Atmospheric monitoring methods

Atmospheric monitoring can be defined as the measurement and assessment of agents (physical, chemical, biological) in the workplace to evaluate inhalation exposure levels and health risks compared with an appropriate standard. Air monitoring often involves two stages, i.e. sampling of the agent, followed by analysis. Sampling and analysis techniques can be divided into several categories (listed below) on the basis of factors such as time, location and methods of collection and analysis.

- Instantaneous or real time monitoring.
- Integrated or continuous sampling.
- Personal monitoring.
- Static (area) monitoring.
- Active or passive (diffusion) flow monitoring.
- Bulk sampling.

Instantaneous monitoring

Instantaneous monitoring (direct reading) refers to the collection of a sample for a relatively short period, ranging from a few seconds to typically several minutes. The main categories of instantaneous instrument are:

- instruments designed to sample a single contaminant, e.g. carbon monoxide analyser;
- instruments which can be adjusted to sample for several individual contaminants, e.g. infrared analysers for the identification and quantification of different gases and vapours;
- instruments which respond to a number of contaminants at once and cannot differentiate between them, e.g. flame ionization detector (FID) used to measure total volatile organic compounds (VOCs).

The main advantage of these instruments is that both collection and analysis are provided immediately. The data represent the concentrations of contaminants at specific times of monitoring. Instantaneous monitors may also be used to detect explosive concentrations, oxygen deficiency and asphyxiant concentrations and, in many cases, can be linked to an alarm device which sounds when a particular concentration of a contaminant reaches a predetermined level. Other applications include hazard detection, leaks, spread of contaminants and the investigation of exposure variability with time and process. In many cases, direct reading instruments, which are usually physically small and portable, qualify as personal sampling devices, thus reducing labour and analytical costs. As a result of the increasing use of microprocessor technology in many direct reading instruments, equipment is available that will memorize and format the data to a computer for data storage and manipulation.

Integrated monitoring

Integrated monitoring refers to the collection of a sample continuously over a period of time. The need to collect a sufficient quantity of contaminant, in excess of the limit of detection of a laboratory method, means that integrated sampling must be conducted over a prolonged period, usually 15 min to several hours, including whole shift sampling. Integrated monitoring provides a single time-weighted average (TWA) concentration, which can be compared with occupational exposure limits (OELs) normally expressed over the reference periods of 15 min and 8 h. For most forms of integrated monitoring, part of the sampling device, or a medium held within it, must be submitted to a laboratory for analysis. The TWA concentrations may be determined by drawing air at a known flow rate over the reference period through the sampling instrument, or by arithmetic calculation from several results obtained during the reference period. The result is a sample representing the average concentration present in the air over the sampling period. The TWA is calculated as follows:

$$\text{TWA} = \frac{C_1(T_1) + C_2(T_2) + \cdots + C_n(T_n)}{\text{Length of working day}} \quad (8.1)$$

where C is the concentration of each sample and T is the sampling time for that sample.

For example, in a typical 8-h shift, a worker in a woodworking shop operates a band saw for 2 h, a circular saw for 1 h and a sander for 3 h. The remainder of the day is spent outdoors in the storage area. The average exposures in the woodworking shop during the three activities are measured to be 3.8, 4.4 and 6.8 mg m^{-3}, respectively. Assuming that there is no exposure to wood dust in the storage area, the 8-h TWA is given as:

$$\text{TWA} = \frac{(3.8 \times 2) + (4.4 \times 1) + (6.8 \times 3) + (0 \times 2)}{8} = 4.05\ \text{mg m}^{-3} \quad (8.1\text{a})$$

Personal and static sampling

Personal sampling involves the placement of an integrated monitor (or an instantaneous monitor, e.g. a noise dosimeter) onto an individual. The sampling device is usually located within the individual's breathing zone to sample the microenvironment from which the person is believed to breathe. Samples which are not taken on the individual are generally referred to as static (or area) samples. The two main benefits of static sampling are for the collection of a large sample volume when the air concentration is low, and for the determination of the concentration of a contaminant in a specific location over time, such as before and after the implementation of control techniques. Static sampling techniques are not always capable of measuring an individual's daily exposure accurately, especially when exposure sources are close to the breathing zone, during unplanned incidents, such as machine breakdown or spillages, or when the individual is very mobile in the workplace. Thus, personal sampling is preferred over static sampling when assessing the exposure of specific personnel conducting jobs/tasks of interest. Furthermore, almost all OELs are based on personal exposure levels, and thus require personal sampling of individuals within the breathing zone to determine the level of compliance. The use of personal and static sampling is discussed further under the heading: 'Where to collect the sample?'.

Passive and active sampling

Most monitoring techniques for the collection of airborne contaminants involve an active flow method, i.e. an air sampling pump is used to pull the air through the sampling medium or the instrument at a known flow rate. Passive sampling techniques are capable of taking samples of vapour pollutants from the atmosphere at a rate controlled by physical properties, such as diffusion, but do not involve the active movement of air through the sampling device. Most passive samplers have been designed for personal sampling, and may be incorporated into a badge or an instrument. For example, this method can be used for diffusible gases, vapours and ionizing radiation. Diffusive samplers are relatively inexpensive, light, robust and easy to use. Although there is a growing market of passive samplers, it is generally accepted that active samplers provide greater accuracy and precision. Regulatory authorities usually recommend the testing of passive samplers against active methods prior to their use.

Bulk sampling

In all situations, the nature of the contaminant needs to be identified before making any decision about air sampling or what actions need to be taken. In such cases, bulk sampling (large volume area sampling) of air, liquids or settled particulates may need to be performed for an in-depth qualitative and quantitative laboratory analysis. Different collection techniques are used, depending on the nature of the material. In the case of airborne particulates, a high-volume mechanical or electrical pump may be used with a suitable filter. The collected particulates could then be analysed for fibres, metals, non-metals, organics (polyaromatic hydrocarbons), particle size distribution, etc. Bulk samples of airborne gases and vapours can be collected in bags, evacuated containers or sorbent tubes, and then analysed to identify the hazardous constituents. Headspace vapour analysis of collected solid and liquid samples can also be performed using either a direct reading instrument (FID) or high-resolution laboratory instrumentation, e.g. gas chromatography–mass spectrometry (GC–MS).

In the case of liquid mixtures, it may be necessary to establish the relative concentrations of substances in the raw material. A good example of this is paint, which may contain a number of solvents (from materials safety data sheets), but it may not be certain which are present or in what proportions. In this case, a representative sample of the paint could be taken and analysed for organic solvents. The data could then be used to calculate an 'in-house' exposure limit for the paint. In this calculation, it is assumed that the atmospheric composition of the vapour above the mixture is similar to that of the mixture and the percentage composition (by weight) of the liquid mixture is known:

$$1/\mathrm{OEL}_{\mathrm{sol}} = \mathrm{FR}_{\mathrm{a}}/\mathrm{OEL}_{\mathrm{a}} + \mathrm{FR}_{\mathrm{b}}/\mathrm{OEL}_{\mathrm{b}} + \mathrm{FR}_{n}/\mathrm{OEL}_{n} \quad (8.2)$$

where $\mathrm{OEL}_{\mathrm{sol}}$ is the occupational exposure limit of the hydrocarbon solvent mixture ($mg\,m^{-3}$), OEL_a is the occupational exposure limit or guidance value of component 'a' ($mg\,m^{-3}$) and FR_a is the fraction (w/w) of component 'a' in the solvent mixture.

The use of the above formula requires an OEL for each component in a mixture of hydrocarbons. Some hydrocarbons may already be assigned OELs; however, other hydrocarbons can be divided into discrete groups and assigned guidance values based on structural similarity and critical health effects. For instance, in the case of white spirit, the following OELs and guidance values (approved by the Health and Safety Executive (HSE)) can be used to arrive at an OEL for white spirit.

White spirit typically contains the following percentages of hydrocarbons:

- alkanes $\geq C_7$, 52%; guidance value, 1200 $mg\,m^{-3}$;
- cycloalkanes $\geq C_7$, 27%; guidance value, 800 $mg\,m^{-3}$;
- aromatics (excluding xylene and trimethylbenzene), 10%; guidance value, 500 $mg\,m^{-3}$;
- C_8 aromatics (*o*-, *m*-, *p*-xylene or mixed isomers), 1%; occupational exposure standard (OES), 435 $mg\,m^{-3}$;
- trimethylbenzenes, 10%; OES, 123 $mg\,m^{-3}$.

Therefore

$$1/OEL_{sol} = 0.52/1200 + 0.27/800 + 0.1/500 + 0.01/435 + 0.1/123 = 1.807 \times 10^{-3}$$

$$OEL_{sol} = 553\ (550\ mg\,m^{-3}) \qquad (8.2a)$$

Preliminary considerations

Before discussing strategies for air monitoring, it is necessary to discuss briefly the main reasons for monitoring exposure and other considerations, such as the selection of appropriate sampling and analysis techniques, the prioritization of sampling needs, the importance of quality control and the factors which influence airborne concentrations.

Purpose of air sampling

Before deciding what, when and how to measure exposure, it is first necessary to consider the reasons for making the measurements and how they may affect the design of the sampling strategy.

The most common reason for sampling is to determine whether the exposure of an individual or a group of individuals exceeds an OEL. This usually requires the a priori selection of part of a workforce undertaking a certain task using certain contaminants, and is usually designed to be a 'worst case scenario'. If the exposure to these individuals is significantly less than the standard, it is believed, by default, that this will also apply to everyone else's exposure. When conducting a chemical risk assessment for compliance purposes, atmospheric monitoring may be legally required for certain substances, such as vinyl chloride monomer, chromic acid, lead and asbestos. In other cases, exposure monitoring may be considered to be required under the following conditions (Control of Substances Hazardous to Health (COSHH) Regulations 1994):

- when failure or deterioration of the control measures could result in serious health effects, either because of the toxicity of the contaminant or because of the extent of potential exposure;
- when measurements are necessary as an additional check of any control provided;
- when measurements are necessary so as to be sure that OELs are not exceeded.

A great deal of the legislation currently emanating from the European Union (EU) requires the 'assessment of risk'. This can be both quantitative and qualitative, thereby moving away from the prescriptive and limited comparison of exposure levels with exposure standards. No health risk assessment can take place without some form of qualitative evaluation. For instance, in the case of exposure to hazardous substances, the assessment process must relate to the biological phenomena which dictate the risks of disease, i.e. the rate of uptake (inhalation, skin absorption and ingestion), the rate of elimination, and therefore the burden (dose), and the rate of repair. Atmospheric monitoring alone cannot answer any of these aspects satisfactorily. Furthermore, different monitoring approaches are needed when the disease outcome manifests itself quickly (acute) or over a longer period (chronic). Some pollutants, such as noise or ionizing radiation, may produce both effects.

In addition to the assessment of health risks and the conformity or compliance with OELs, atmospheric monitoring may be carried out for a number of other reasons, each having its own requirements in terms of accuracy, type of sampling (personal or static), averaging time and methods to be used:

- the identification of hazards;
- epidemiological studies;
- the selection of control requirements;
- the assessment of the effectiveness of control measures;
- litigation.

Exposure monitoring can provide useful information on the location, identity or spread of a contaminant in the workplace. This information will be particularly useful as part of the workplace inspection in the identification of workplace hazards (Chapter 6). Atmospheric monitoring may be required as part of an epidemiological study, the main objective of which is to determine whether exposure to a contaminant affects the health status of a group of individuals. To be most useful for health effect studies, these assessments would ideally include the exposure of all employees to essentially all contaminants over the whole time period of the study. Thus, the requirements of the sampling strategies are more akin to those of health risk assessment than to those of compliance, as one is more interested in the precise estimation of the mean group exposure from low to highly exposed groups than to the measurement of specific individuals undertaking specific tasks. Clearly, the study design, whether it be prospective, cross-sectional or retrospective, will dictate the sampling strategy. Specifically, if sampling prospectively, an additional reason why epidemiological requirements are likely to be different from those of compliance testing is that one is likely to be concerned with contaminants believed to be harmless at the time and/or well below the current OELs.

If it has been decided that a contaminant and/or process is not under adequate control, it may be necessary to take measurements to determine by how much the exposure needs to be reduced. Unfortunately, actual measurements are often needed to justify capital expenditure. Examples include the choice of face velocities/hood design/volume flow rates, etc. for ventilation systems, respirator selection and octave band analysis for noise control. Once a contaminant and/or process is deemed to be under control, it may be necessary to ensure the continued performance of the system. This can be carried out either by the measurement of the contaminant or by the direct assessment of the process itself. These measurements may range from simple, instantaneous, non-specific leak detection, to part of a monitoring and maintenance programme, to the full examination and testing of local exhaust ventilation systems.

It is unfortunate that the exposure to contaminants may cause detrimental health effects, but in these litigious times some redress is being found. However, the measurement of the contaminant(s) of interest and the strategy for its collection may have an impact on both the plaintiff and defendant.

Prioritization of sampling needs

Having determined the reason for sampling, it is then necessary to make an a priori prioritization of which contaminants and/or processes are associated with the highest degree of risk (Corn 1985). Some risk determinants include: the number of potentially exposed individuals, the toxicity of the substance(s), the quantities used over some arbitrary reference period, the likely duration and concentration of exposure (plus exposure via routes other than inhalation), i.e. dose, the existence of and confidence in control measures, the likelihood and magnitude of change to the process and its control, and the presence of substances which may be potentiators or act synergistically or antagonistically.

Occupational hygiene surveys can be broken down into four levels related to the priority assigned: an initial assessment, a preliminary survey, a detailed survey and routine monitoring. The level of survey is obviously related to the nature and importance associated with the answer (as described on p.133) and the magnitude of the survey is related to the factors involved (numbers of people, variability, etc.). Figure 8.1 shows a self-explanatory flow diagram to aid in the visualization and under-standing of this process. Further details of the information needed/obtained by these various levels are available elsewhere

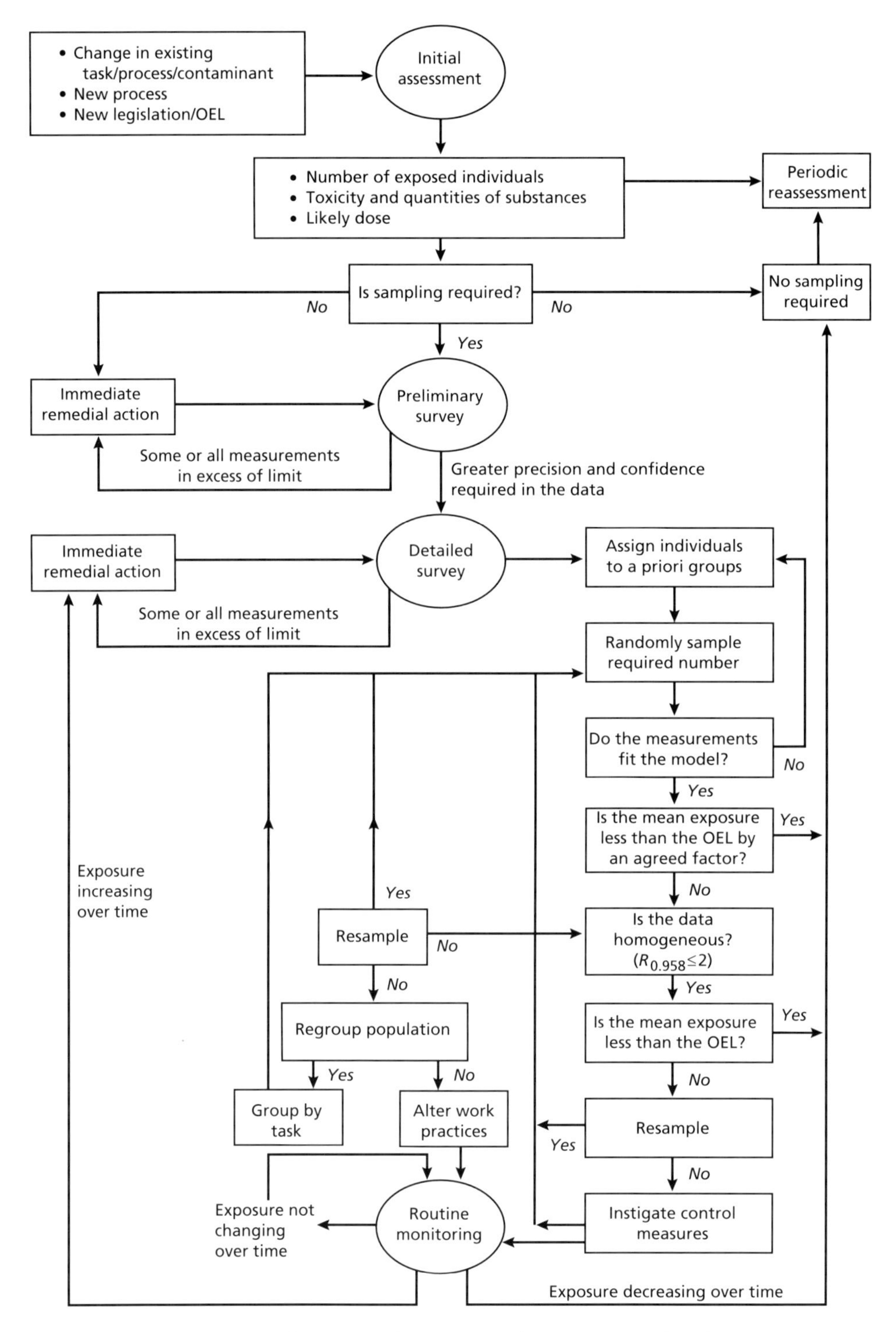

Figure 8.1 A decision logic flow diagram. (After Harrington and Gardiner 1995.)

(HSE 1989; British Occupational Hygiene Society (BOHS) 1993).

Selection of sampling and analysis methods

Frequently decisions are dependent upon measurements; therefore, it is essential that measurements are made using appropriate sampling and analysis methods with the inherent limitations fully understood. Depending on the survey objectives, very precise and accurate measurements may not always be necessary. However, the accuracy and precision of the method needs to be known. In selecting the most appropriate sampling and analysis methods, the following factors should be considered.

For sampling methods:

- the physical and chemical properties of the contaminant;
- the stability of the sampling medium;
- the compatibility of the sampling medium with the subsequent analysis method;
- the pump flow rate range and the ability to sample over periods relevant to the OEL;
- the capacity and the collection efficiency of the sampling medium;
- the type of analysis and information required;
- the intrinsic safety of the equipment;
- the portability, reliability and ease of equipment maintenance.

For analysis methods:

- specificity: the ability to measure the contaminant of interest in the presence of interferences;
- sensitivity: the ratio of the change of the instrument response (I) with the corresponding change in the concentration (C) of the substance analysed; thus, the slope of the calibration curve (dI/dC) can be used to determine the sensitivity value;
- accuracy: the difference between the mean of a set of measurements and the true or correct value for the quantity measured; accuracy includes both systematic errors (bias) and random errors (precision);
- precision: a measure of the method's variability when repeatedly applied to a homogeneous sample under controlled conditions, without regard to the magnitude of displacement from the true value; precision can be expressed by the standard deviation;
- limit of detection: the smallest amount of a contaminant which will produce a reliable instrument reading which is distinguishable from the background; quantitatively, it is often defined as three times the standard deviation of the blank signal above the blank signal.

Occupational hygienists are accustomed to comparing measured exposure data with relevant exposure limits. This approach may overlook the instrumental and analytical errors, as well as the normal, but larger, variations in workplace concentrations over space and time. When evaluating how well the measured exposure levels represent the working environment, it is important to recognize and distinguish between random (or random variation) and systematic (bias) errors. A random variation is a fluctuation of a quantity around its long-term average exposure value. If the instrument sometimes reads too high, sometimes too low, but on average gives the correct reading, it is exhibiting random error. On the other hand, if the instrument is calibrated incorrectly, i.e. the readings are constantly too high (or too low), it is exhibiting systematic error. Systematic error cannot be reduced or eliminated by repeating the measurements at the same point. Ideally, systematic errors should be eliminated or estimated by independently measuring the quantity in question with a different apparatus, preferably one which operates on a different principle from the original apparatus.

Another common source of error is contamination, both of the sampling device in the field and of the sample during laboratory analysis. The positive bias produced by various sources of contamination should be eliminated at the source and by the analysis of appropriate field blanks. Field blanks are defined as sampling devices which are treated exactly as samples, except that no air is drawn through them.

In addition to the above, when sampling for certain contaminants, such as organic solvents, the sampling efficiency of liquid absorbers (impingers) and the desorption efficiency of solid adsorbents (charcoal, silica gel, Tenax) may also need to be determined, so that the airborne concentrations of substances can be corrected accordingly. The desorption efficiency of a sorbent can be obtained by adding a known amount of the contaminant of interest to the adsorbent tube. This sample is then included unidentified in the analysis with field and blank samples, and is often referred to as a 'spiked' sample.

Fortunately, the concentrations of contaminants in the workplace are generally low. Thus, a sufficient quantity of sample must be collected to enable the analyst to determine the amount of contaminant accurately. Recommended minimum sampling volumes can be calculated using the following equation:

$$\text{Minimum volume (m}^3\text{)} = \frac{10 \times \text{Sensitivity of the analytical technique (mg)}}{\text{Atmospheric exposure limit (mg m}^{-3}\text{)}} \quad (8.3)$$

Furthermore, when comparing the measured airborne exposure levels with the OELs, it is important to ensure that the measurements and OELs are expressed at standard temperature and pressure. For example, as the exposure limits are based on a temperature of 20°C and a pressure of 760 mmHg, the concentrations of any pollutant not measured at these values should be corrected as follows:

$$C_{corr} = C(760/P)(T/293) \quad (8.4)$$

where C_{corr} is the corrected concentration, P is the actual pressure of the air sample (mmHg) and T is the absolute temperature of the air sampled (K).

Where available, standard methods of sampling and analysis should always be used. The International Standards Organization (ISO), the European Committee for Standardization (CEN) and various national bodies have published several methods for workplace measurements. Primary sources are the compendia of methods recommended by the regulatory bodies, i.e. the HSE in the UK or the National Institute for Occupational Safety and Health (NIOSH) and the Occupational Safety and Health Administration (OSHA) in the USA. The HSE has published *Methods for the Determination of Hazardous Substances* (MDHS) for over 80 specific substances (HSE 1981–1998); OSHA and NIOSH have published manuals with more than 500 and 100 sampling and analytical methods, respectively (OSHA 1985; NIOSH 1994). Secondary sources are published literature references in, for example, *Annals of Occupational Hygiene*, *The American Industrial Hygiene Association Journal*, *Applied Occupational and Environmental Hygiene* and *Analytical Chemistry*, and books such as *The Intersociety Committee's Methods for Air Sampling and Analysis* (Intersociety Committee 1988).

Exposure variation

Any air sampling exercise will be limited by a number of factors which influence the individual's exposure to a specific agent. The fluctuations in the concentrations of air contaminants are dependent on a number of factors (listed below). Exposure can also vary greatly, both within and between individuals, days, shifts, etc. (Fig. 8.2a–f). In order to obtain representative exposure data for risk assessment, these variables need to be understood and considered carefully in the design of appropriate sampling strategies (discussed later).

The main sources of variation which need to be considered include:

- variation in shift patterns and the average exposure of individuals;
- variation associated with the type and nature of processes;
- variation in the contaminant concentration in the breathing zone of operators over the duration of the shift;
- variation in individual exposure levels, even when working in the same place carrying out the same tasks on the same shift.

Fluctuations in exposure concentrations within and between shifts can be due to any combination of the following:

- variation in the number of emission sources;
- variation in the rate of release of the contaminant from a source;
- variation in the dispersion of a contaminant, i.e. the effect of air currents and turbulence in the workplace;
- variation in ambient conditions, such as air temperature and humidity.

Quality in exposure monitoring

Quality assurance (QA) refers to all steps which may be taken to

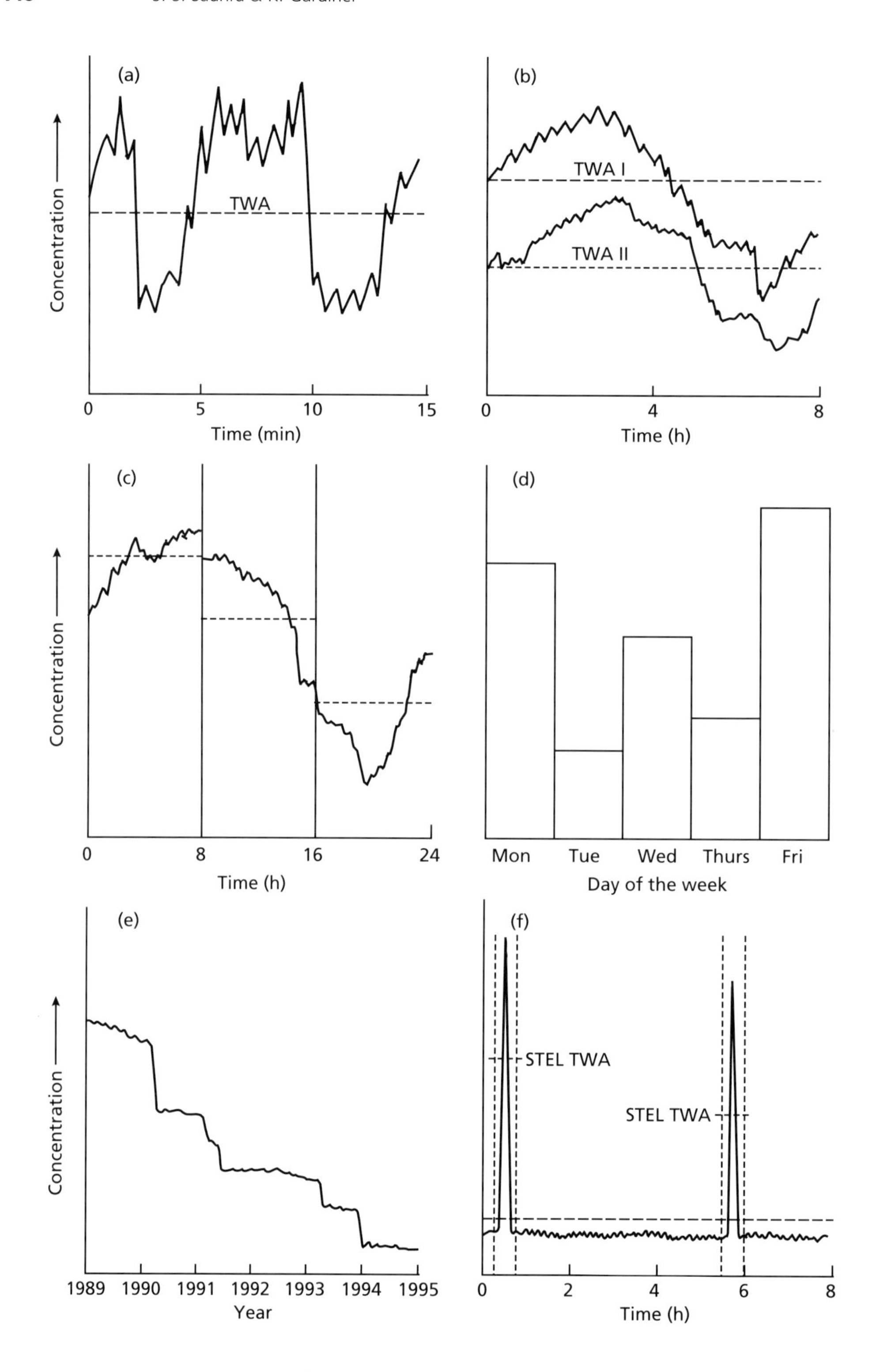
(a)
Concentration
TWA
0
5
10
15
Time (min)
(b)
TWA I
TWA II
0
4
8
Time (h)
(c)
Concentration
0
8
16
24
Time (h)
(d)
Mon
Tue
Wed
Thurs
Fri
Day of the week
(e)
Concentration
1989
1990
1991
1992
1993
1994
1995
Year
(f)
STEL TWA
STEL TWA
0
2
4
6
8
Time (h)

provide measurement data of a stated quality and reliability. As part of QA, quality control (QC) programmes are concerned with monitoring and controlling the precision and accuracy of sampling and laboratory analysis. In the USA, the Environmental Protection Agency (EPA) has developed an elaborate QA system for air monitoring (EPA 1986).

The factors which contribute to the measurement of the worker's personal exposure include the sampling strategy, sampling and analysis methodologies, internal and external quality control schemes, the measured concentration and its interpretation. Internal quality control is the set procedure undertaken by laboratory staff for the continuous monitoring of operations and results, in order to decide whether the results are reliable enough to be released. To do this, the results obtained are compared with predetermined limits of acceptability. External quality control (or proficiency testing) is a system for objectively checking laboratory results by means of an external agency. It includes the comparison of a laboratory's results with those of other laboratories, with the objective of interlaboratory comparison. Examples of external quality assessment schemes include the HSE Workplace Analysis Scheme for Proficiency (WASP) in the UK and the Proficiency Analytical Testing (PAT) of the American Industrial Hygiene Association (AIHA) in the USA.

All atmospheric sampling and laboratory analyses are subject to errors. The inherent random errors for both sampling and analysis methods are commonly described by the coefficient of variation (CV). The CV is also known as the relative standard deviation, and is a useful index of dispersion, as limits computed from the true mean of a set of data plus or minus twice the CV will contain about 95% of the data measurements. The CV value is often expressed as a percentage of the average value (X):

$$CV = (S/X) \times 100\% \tag{8.5}$$

where S is the standard deviation and X is the arithmetic mean of the measured values.

As most occupational hygiene measurements consist of both sampling and analysis stages, the CV of the measurement is given by:

$$CV_t = (CV_s^2 + CV_a^2)^{0.5} \tag{8.6}$$

where CV_t is the total coefficient of variation, CV_s is the coefficient of

Figure 8.2 (*Opposite.*) Examples of the variability of exposure: (a) hypothetical personal exposure as measured by continuous monitoring and the integrated 15-min TWA exposure; (b) hypothetical continuous trace and integrated TWA personal exposure for two individuals undertaking the same work over an 8-h period; (c) hypothetical continuous trace and integrated TWA personal exposure for three individuals undertaking the same work on different shifts over a 24-h period; (d) hypothetical 8-h TWA personal exposures for an individual undertaking the same work over a period of a week; (e) hypothetical trace of weekly TWA personal exposures for an individual undertaking the same work over a number of years; (f) hypothetical trace of personal exposure and 8-h and 15-min short-term exposure limit (STEL) TWAs of a contained process with occasional fugitive omissions. (After Harrington and Gardiner 1995.)

variation of the sampling error and CV_a is the coefficient of variation of the analytical error.

For example, if the CV of the sampling pump and the analysis are 0.05 and 0.08, respectively, CV_t is calculated as:

$$CV_t = (0.05^2 + 0.08^2)^{0.5} = 0.09 \quad (8.6a)$$

Sampling strategies

In general, the major purpose of a sampling strategy is that, by careful consideration of the issues involved (of which more later), the validity of the data generated will be maximized, thereby strengthening the inferences drawn. This should also ensure the most cost-effective approach. This section of the chapter will attempt to highlight and integrate the many issues which need to be considered before embarking on a sampling programme, whether one or thousands of samples are to be taken, but is not meant to be a definitive exposition of the mathematical derivation of the underlying statistics of sampling methodologies. These issues are applicable to the measurement of all workplace hazards including, for example, stress—where the questions below are equally relevant if a slightly broader interpretation is used. Safety issues, such as the assessment of flammability or the ability of an environment to sustain life, will not be covered.

Having determined the reason for monitoring employees, i.e. risk assessment, and having selected suitable sampling methods for the pollutant of interest, six fundamental questions need to be considered in formulating a monitoring programme.

1 Whose exposure should be measured?
2 Where to collect the sample?
3 When to measure?
4 How long to sample for?
5 How many samples?
6 How often to sample?

Whose exposure should be measured?

In a workplace with a limited number of staff doing similar jobs, the need to separate people into groups as the basis for individual selection is limited; however, in large workforces undertaking a multitude of different tasks, the need is greater. As discussed previously, the option of which of the worker groups to sample is dictated by the reason for sampling; however, first it is necessary to determine the means by which the groups are defined.

If the strict definition of homogeneity is that all the exposure distributions of all workers have the same means and standard deviations (which is almost unheard of), one is left with the contentious issue of how homogeneity can be defined/tested in a usable/achievable manner.

There are two main methods by which the population to be sampled can be grouped and assessed for homogeneity: prospective and retrospective employee grouping.

Prospective employee grouping

Prospective employee grouping relies on the ability of the occupational hygienist to assign individuals to a group or 'zone' before sampling on the basis of the following criteria: similarity of tasks, exposure to the same range of airborne contaminants and similarity of the environment (i.e. process equipment/exposure and controls) (Corn & Esmen 1979). Although this technique was developed for epidemiological purposes, it lends itself to the needs of compliance testing. The major benefit is that, when the measurement of personal exposure confirms the homogeneity of the group, this allows an assessment of risk to be made with greater confidence. The zones in a workplace can be redefined, but this should again be a prospective exercise.

Care needs to be taken in the selection of certain individuals, such as those involved in maintenance or non-routine tasks. These individuals are also likely to be at the higher end of the exposure profile and may need grouping separately. There is no rigid definition of homogeneity, but it clearly relates to the variability of the data, and therefore measures such as the standard deviation or geometric standard deviation (where lognormality is known or has been determined) are used for sizeable data sets, and non-parametric measures such as the interquartile range for small data sets. The HSE (1989) states a crude, but useful, rule: if an individual's exposure is less than half or greater than twice the group mean, they should be reassigned to another group.

Retrospective employee grouping

It has been proposed that, instead of prospectively allocating individuals into groups before sampling, the whole exposed population should be sampled randomly with groups created retrospectively (Rappaport 1991). It is felt that this technique is the most appropriate means of assessing chronic exposure/effect (i.e. health risk assessment and/or epidemiology), as it is not always possible to identify individuals by inspection. Unlike compliance testing, where the highest exposure is of interest, for health risk assessment/epidemiology, the precise estimation of the mean exposure and the within/between worker variability are of importance (Kromhout *et al.* 1993; Rappaport *et al.* 1993).

After the random sampling of the workforce, the data collected must then be grouped. (In the main, exposure data are lognormally distributed, but if possible the distributional form should be tested.) However, it is necessary to first identify the components of exposure variability. The exposure to an airborne contaminant of all workers on all days ('total distribution') has a geometric mean μ_c and geometric standard deviation $\sigma_{g,T}$. Each individual has their own personal distribution of day-to-day exposures ('within worker distribution') which can be characterized by individual geometric means $\mu_{c,W}$ and geometric standard deviations $\sigma_{g,W}$. To assess these, one would need to undertake repeat measurements over a period of time on the same individuals. In addition, there are differences in mean exposure between individuals ('between worker distribution'); this has the same geometric mean value (μ_c) as the distribution of all exposures, but the geometric standard deviation of the total distribution ($\sigma_{g,T}$) is larger than the between worker geometric standard deviation ($\sigma_{g,B}$), as it represents the combination of both the within and between worker components of exposure variability. It is these differences in individual practices which are difficult to observe, thereby limiting the validity of the prospective approach.

As mentioned previously, 'usable' homogeneity has no strict definition, but Rappaport (1991) has arbitrarily defined a 'monomorphic group' with reference to the between worker distribution. A 'monomorphic group' is one in which 95% of the individual mean exposures lie within a factor of two. This implies that the ratio of the 97.5th percentile to the 2.5th percentile ($R_{0.95B}$) is no greater than two, and will have a between worker geometric standard deviation ($\sigma_{g,B}$) of 1.2 or less. In practice, this arbitrary factor of two may be too restrictive, as intimated by the HSE in the UK (HSE 1989); it recommends that an individual's mean exposure should be within a range of 0.5–2 times the group mean.

Where to collect the sample?

As mentioned previously, the occupational hygienist has two main choices with regard to the location of the sampling device: to place the equipment on the individual (personal), or to fix it to a tripod so that it is static over the duration of sampling (area or static). If a health risk assessment is being undertaken, the preferred location is personal, as this is most likely to reflect the individual's exposure. In fact, for all but a few substances (e.g. cotton dust, the annual maximum exposure limit (MEL) for vinyl chloride monomer and subtilisins (proteolytic enzymes)), OELs are specific to personal exposure.

It is convention to call the microenvironment to which an individual will be exposed the 'breathing zone'; it is defined as approximately 20–30 cm from the nose/mouth (Fig. 8.3a). However, recent work has brought into question this locality and the reliance on the results from it. One study (Vaughan *et al.* 1990) showed that, when a dust sampler was placed at equal distances from the nose/mouth on each lapel, there was at least a twofold difference between the results in 5% of cases. It is also known that substances with a high degree of thermal buoyancy, such as welding fume and colophony (from rosin core pyrolysis or flow solder baths), generate a reasonably well-defined plume which rises sharply. A significant proportion of this may miss the lapel-located sampler, but, as a result of the nature of the work and therefore the

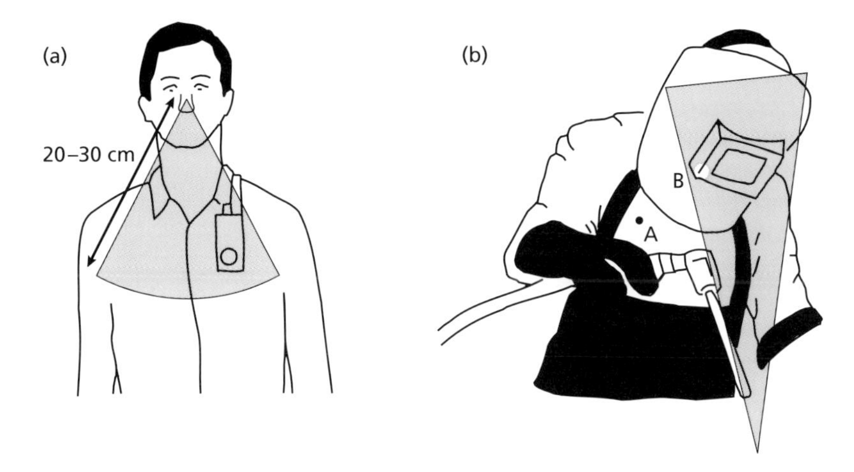

Figure 8.3 Location of sampler: (a) breathing zone highlighted with sampler located in its 'normal' lapel position; (b) well-defined plume missing the 'normal' lapel position; sampler located underneath welding helmet next to nose/mouth.

required body position, will generate significant exposure. The welding head sampler is therefore mounted on a cranial cap or on the inside of air stream welding helmets (Fig. 8.3b). Clearly, consideration of the work activity must be given before placement of the equipment, and discussion with the worker with regard to wearability may be fruitful.

As there is a poor relationship between static samples and real personal exposure, their use is less prevalent; however, they do have specific uses. The main one is in the assessment of the requirements and performance of control measures. The fixed location of the sampler strengthens the validity of comparison of the concentrations before and after control intervention, without the variability inherent with personal samples. Some measuring devices are large and barely portable, let alone suitable for personal sampling; this is especially true for continuous monitoring devices, or where very large volumes of air are needed to be sampled due to the low ambient concentrations. Occasionally, static samples can be used as a surrogate for personal exposure, especially where the nature of the work may make the wearing of additional sampling equipment more hazardous, or where a clear relationship between static measurements and personal exposure has been defined (e.g. lighting or, in certain environments, noise).

When to measure?

This question can relate to when to sample within a day/shift or on which day of the week/shift to sample. Processes can be split into three main types, continuous, cyclic or random, whether considered within a day or over a number of days. Indeed, most major processes will have elements of all three (i.e. in many chemical factories, the production part is continuous, the packaging of the material is cyclic and the maintenance work is random). A degree of familiarity with the process is necessary for this to be known, but should greatly improve the validity of the measurements.

Depending on the reason for taking the measurements, the sampling should reflect the nature of the process. For example, if the process is continuous, it will not matter greatly if the sampling is continuous, cyclic or random; however, if the process is cyclic, the time and/or day on which samples are taken is critical. This is because the period over which the measurement is taken could exactly match the duration of peaks or troughs; however, if the duration of the process cycles is much shorter than the duration of the sampling cycles, this is of less importance. Obviously, for health risk assessment and epidemiological purposes, the random choice of when to sample is more appropriate, provided that the frequency of sampling is great enough. This is to ensure that tasks rarely undertaken are likely to be included.

How long to sample for?

In the main, for the purposes of compliance testing, the duration over which the sample should be taken is dictated by the reference period of the OEL. In the UK, there are both long-term, 8-h, TWA exposure limits and short-term, 15-min, TWA exposure limits (STELs); however, for well-controlled, continuous processes with very little variability, periods shorter than the 8-h reference period may be sufficient as a surrogate for the whole working period. Also, it is not uncommon for two or more quite different tasks to be undertaken within one day, and therefore two or more separate samples are taken and the TWA is calculated relative to an 8-h reference period. Compliance testing against a STEL is difficult, due to the lack of sensitivity and precision of most techniques when the ambient concentration is low and the flow rate of the instrument is either limited (i.e. low flow pumps for adsorbent tubes) or set (cyclones used for measuring respirable dust). If the magnitude of the outcome of failure to control exposure to the STEL is great, it may be preferable to use continuous monitoring devices.

Chronic toxicants

The issue of how long to sample for with regard to health risk assessment and epidemiology is more complex. Rappaport (1991) has used the toxicokinetic properties of substances to produce a model which indicates that exposure variability must be transmitted through to body burden and, ultimately, damage if it is to affect the risk of disease. For those substances with a chronic effect, the transmission of the day-to-day variation in exposure diminishes rapidly if the biological half-life ($T_{1/2}$) is $10 < T_{1/2} < 100$ h, so that less than half of the variability is expected to reach the tissues when $T_{1/2} > 40$ h. This value of $T_{1/2}$ can be used as a strategic benchmark to identify contaminants for which the day-to-day variation in exposure is unlikely to be important (Rappaport 1988, 1991). This means that tissue damage, the very entity that we are trying to assess and ultimately prevent, will be related to the mean exposure and time. This presumes that linear kinetics prevail; however, issues such as synergism or antagonism (from concurrent exposure to other contaminants), allergic reactions to sensitizers and an upward curving burden–damage relationship (from periods of intense exposure saturating the normal clearance processes) may mean that the translation of exposure to damage is non-linear.

The major benefits for chronic toxicants are that, instead of taking five 8-h samples over the period of a week, fewer samples taken over a longer duration (e.g. a week) may be possible (depending on the ambient concentration and sampler overload). Clearly, however, information relating to compliance, task-specific, short-term fluctuations and control will be lost.

Acute toxicants

As discussed in Chapter 3, for substances with an acute effect, the rate constants for biological elimination and repair are in the range of seconds to hours, and therefore the transfer between exposure and tissue damage occurs within the time frame of a single shift. In addition, the transmission of exposure variability to the site of damage (the tissues) is likely to be efficient. Non-linearity, together with acute responses, means that short-term exposure variability cannot be ignored as it is likely to be the primary determinant of acute response.

As mentioned above, the sensitivity and precision of the measuring techniques are often not capable of characterizing exposure accurately, whether it be for compliance or the assessment of health risk, and therefore continuous monitoring may be more appropriate. However, it may be advantageous to differentiate between those acute responses that lead to potentially irreversible effects (phosgene—pulmonary oedema) and temporary effects, such as irritation or narcosis (sulphur dioxide, xylene), as well as the likely variability of the process/job. It is often thought that, instead of struggling to measure short-term exposure, it may be better to concentrate on the elimination or control of the problem.

How many samples?

Hopefully, it is becoming apparent that the variability of exposure data is such that taking one or two samples on one day is insufficient to reach any conclusions about the workplace, particularly the risk it poses to those working there. Therefore, in the main, the greater the number of samples taken the better. However, everyday constraints, such as time and money, mean that, in large workforces (i.e. greater than 10 people doing the same job), the exposure of only a proportion of the workers can be assessed. The number of samples taken is also dependent upon the pre-existing knowledge of within and between person exposure variability, as most methods rely upon group homogeneity already having been defined. For example, instead of having a workforce of 100 with the generic title of lathe operator, one may have 10 homogeneous subgroups of varying sizes. The following are some examples of the means by which the number of samples can be calculated.

General rules

If no information is available on the cohort of interest, then general guidance is required. The HSE (1989) suggests that at least 1 in 10 individuals should be sampled (perhaps suitable for a very large population), with Corn (1985) suggesting that at least three samples should be taken from the population of interest and, if the difference between them is greater than 25%, additional samples should be taken. It is often stated that an occupational hygienist can 'cope' with between 5 and 10 'sampling trains' at the same time; it would therefore be prudent to define the homogeneous group to be sampled in such a way that the 5–10 samples constitute as large a proportion as possible (i.e. if possible, sample everyone, but the greater the proportion the better).

Statistical methods

The number of samples to be collected can be determined on a statistical basis as described below, in which case sample numbers can be extremely large and resources may not be available for such an extensive exercise. However, these large samples result from the fact that workplace exposure is highly variable.

The NIOSH method. A method has been promulgated by NIOSH in which one measurement from the sampled population is chosen to be in the top $T\%$ with $C\%$ confidence (Leidel *et al.* 1977). This method for calculating the number of measurements can be used without a knowledge of the standard deviation and the data distribution form. The method was designed specifically as a compliance tool, but has been used in epidemiological studies (Gardiner *et al.* 1992). Tables exist wherein one specifies the upper fraction of exposure (e.g. top 10%) and the confidence with which one wants to find an exposure measurement in that fraction (e.g. 95% confidence). The total number of individuals in the defined homogeneous group is determined (group size), and the required number of samples to be taken in that day is read off from

Table 8.1 Size of partial sample for Top 10% and confidence 0.90 (NIOSH).

Group size N	8	9	10	11–12	13–14	15–17	18–20	21–24	25–29	30–37	38–49	50+
No. of samples n	7	8	9	10	11	12	13	14	15	16	17	18

Table 8.1. For example, suppose an equal expected exposure risk group of size $N = 26$ is considered. To be 90% confident that at least one of the three (i.e. 10% of 26) individuals with the highest of all exposures is included in a partial sample, 15 workers (see Table 8.1) should be randomly chosen for sampling from the total of 26.

Using the estimated mean and standard deviation. A knowledge of the geometric mean (GM) and geometric standard deviation (GSD) from previous surveys or experience can be used to calculate the required number of samples. If no data are available, mean exposures and their standard deviations can be either estimated or extracted from published data for comparable industries. A figure of approximately 2.0 can be used to provide an initial estimate of the GSD; however, it is preferable to overestimate (GSD > 2.0) rather than underestimate the GSD, as this will maximize the sample size. Therefore, the number of samples required (n) can be calculated from these data using the formula:

$$n = \left(\frac{t\text{CV}}{E}\right)^2 \qquad (8.7)$$

where CV is the coefficient of variation (standard deviation/mean), E is the acceptable or chosen level of error and t is the t-distribution value for the chosen confidence level ($n_o - 1$) degrees of freedom.

For example, normally distributed data for wood dust include an estimated (based on a preliminary survey) arithmetic mean of 10.0 mg m^{-3} and a standard deviation of 4.0 mg m^{-3}. With a chosen error limit of 10% and 95% confidence level, $t = 1.960$ (degrees of freedom, ∞). The number of samples can be calculated as:

$$n = \frac{(1.96 \times 4.0/10.0)^2}{(0.1)^2} = 57.76\ (58) \qquad (8.7a)$$

Therefore, to estimate the mean concentration of the population within 10% of the 'true' mean with 95% confidence, 58 full-shift samples from the same group would be needed! Clearly, the greater the homogeneity and acceptable/allowable error and the less the confidence required, the smaller the number of samples needed.

It is suggested that, if the data are known or suspected to be lognormally distributed, the same formula can be used. This is because the central limit theorem states that the distribution of means is approximately normal even for lognormally distributed data sets.

An alternative formula can be used if the population of interest is small, i.e. when $10n < N$ (where N is the population size):

$$n\frac{(N-1)}{(N-n)} = \left(\frac{t\text{CV}}{E}\right)^2 \qquad (8.8)$$

Using the figures quoted in the example above and a total population of 50:

$$n\frac{(50-1)}{(50-n)}=\frac{(1.96\times 4.0/10.0)^2}{(0.1)^2}=27.05\ (28) \quad (8.8a)$$

The figure for the number of samples should always be rounded up.

Comparing mean exposures with OELs

If compliance testing is being undertaken, it is possible to choose the number of samples relative to the required degree of compliance to the OEL. Rappaport and Selvin (1987) have promulgated an equation to test the arithmetic mean exposure against the OEL with a certain statistical significance and power, thereby providing the required sample size (Table 8.2). Again, it is clear that the greater the variability and the closer the mean value to the standard, the greater the number of samples required. For sample durations of less than the complete shift, it has been postulated that approximately 25% of the exposure duration should be sampled (with the proviso that there is no significant systematic variation in exposure).

It is important to note that the techniques mentioned above do not specify that each individual should be sampled at least twice (preferably the same number of repeats on each individual), thereby facilitating the calculation of within and between worker variances. If the number of samples and the resultant exposure indicate that the question of overexposure cannot be resolved, it is necessary to resample, choosing to take either the same number of repeat samples from extra people or to take repeat measurements on all of those already sampled and, by so doing, to ensure that the numbers of repeats on each individual remain balanced. If overexposure exists, a review of the within and between worker variances should indicate where control measures should be focused: engineering controls for high within worker variance (i.e. day-to-day) and administrative (behavioural) controls for high between worker variance (Gardiner 1995).

Epidemiological studies

In epidemiology (see Chapter 4), the determination of the number of

Table 8.2 Sample size requirements for testing the mean exposure from a lognormal distribution of 8-h TWAs (95% significance and 90% power).

	Sample size (n) at geometric standard deviation of				
Mean/OEL	1.5	2.0	2.5	3.0	3.5
0.1	2	6	13	21	30
0.25	3	10	19	30	43
0.5	7	21	41	67	96
0.75	25	82	164	266	384
1.25	25	82	164	266	384
1.50	7	21	41	67	96
2.00	2	6	11	17	24
3.00	1	2	3	5	6

samples required often relies on detailed information about the partitioning of the exposure variability before a study commences formally. Also related to the number of samples is the within group variance (homogeneity) and the between group variance (contrast) (Boleij *et al.* 1995; Kromhout & Heederick 1995). Obviously, an optimal grouping would be one in which the groups are homogeneous, great contrast exists between the groups and the mean exposure in each group is precise. Unfortunately, however, these are rarely compatible due to the practical realities of a limited number of samples, i.e. small, homogeneous groups have poor contrast and precision, with larger groups having greater precision and contrast, but less homogeneity.

How often to sample?

The question of 'how often to sample' within a day has been covered in the section: 'When to measure?'. However, there still remains the issue of the frequency of routine monitoring.

For some substances/processes, a long-term routine monitoring programme based over the period of a year or longer may be appropriate. The decision about whether periodic monitoring is required should be based on the results of the initial sampling exercise and the characteristics of the work environment and tasks performed. Factors which should be considered include:

- reliability of controls;
- exposure variability;
- closeness of exposure levels to limits;
- changes in work practices;
- changes in the working environment.

There are a number of schemes in which the frequency of monitoring can be related to the ratio of mean exposure to the OEL. It has been suggested by Roach (1977) that, the closer the measured exposures are to the OEL, the greater the frequency of sampling, and those values which are either significantly above or below the OEL need to be sampled less frequently. The frequencies of sampling, per 10 employees, are given in Table 8.3.

Specific monitoring strategies for compliance

Two methods used to develop sampling strategies for compliance with

Table 8.3 Minimum frequency of regular monitoring.

Shifts to be sampled (per 10 employees)	Exposure/OEL
1/month	1–2
1/quarter	0.5–1 or 2–4
1/annum	0.1–0.5 or 4–20
None	<0.1 or >20

exposure limits include the NIOSH method and the zoning method of occupational hygiene sampling, and are summarized below.

The first manual of an occupational exposure strategy for compliance testing was published by NIOSH (Leidel *et al.* 1977; Leidel & Busch 1994). In this method, a decision is made for each personal sample after a confidence interval has been calculated (based on analytical errors associated with the sampling technique) as to whether it is an overexposure, a possible overexposure or within compliance. The employees believed to have the highest exposure (worst case approach) are selected for personal sampling. These 'high-risk' employees are identified for every operation, and the factors considered in determining them include: distance from the source, worker's movement (mobility), ventilation patterns and differences in individual work habits. If the high-exposure workers cannot be identified for an operation with reasonable certainty, a random selection of employees is made from groups expected to have similar exposure. The sample size of the subgroup is chosen (see section: 'How many samples?') so that there is a high probability that the random sample will contain at least one worker from those with the highest exposure. Although the NIOSH method is used by OSHA to evaluate samples obtained during inspections, this single measurement technique does not take into account the environmental variability, which is considered to be far more important than the sampling and analytical variability.

Another approach, which is based on multiple measurements as opposed to single measurements (i.e. the NIOSH method), is presented by Corn (1985). This is known as the zoning method, and is used to determine the exposure for a group of workers based on job similarities and the similarities of the environment in which they work. Each zone must fulfil four basic requirements.

- *Work similarity*, i.e. employees in the zone must perform similar tasks.
- *Similarity with respect to the hazardous agent*, i.e. zone members must use the same agent, and the potential for exposure to the agent must be similar.
- *Environmental similarity*, i.e. ventilation, process equipment, etc. must be similar for all zone members.
- *Identifiability*, i.e. the same employees must not be classified in more than one zone.

Having classified the zones and the group size in each zone, an appropriate number of workers from each zone are then randomly (using a table of random numbers) selected and sampled. The analysis of the data collected is based on the lognormal distribution of the exposure measurements. The GM, the GSD and the arithmetic mean for each zone and agent combination are calculated. The means are compared with the exposure limit for that agent. If a mean is greater than the exposure limit, at least one of the workers in the zone is exposed at a level above the limit. If a mean is less than the exposure limit, the probability of finding workers with exposure in excess of the limit is determined. The expected number of workers with exposure in excess of the limit can also be calculated. Recently, the AIHA has published a sampling strategy similar to the zoning method for occupational exposure assessment (Hawkins *et al.* 1991).

Data interpretation

It is presumed that, because the reason for sampling in this case is the assessment of health risk, the reader will have a clear idea of the means by which the data collected will be used for this purpose. Unfortunately, however, this is not always the case, and one is reminded of the adage: 'Don't ask a question if you don't know what to do with the answer'. To assist in this process, a brief outline is given below of some of the ways in which the data can be treated.

Probability plots

Small data sets (typically less than 20 or so measurements) may sometimes present difficulties when trying to determine exposure patterns. In such cases, it is useful to summarize the data graphically so that any underlying trends can be seen and examined before making comparisons with exposure limits. An example of a graphical method used to summarize exposure data is the log-probability plot (cumulative frequency plot). This method is based on the fact that almost all air sampling data are best described by a lognormal distribution, i.e. the logarithms of the data are distributed normally. A log-probability plot is a plot of the individual data points as a cumulative frequency curve, where the percentage scale has been adjusted so that lognormally distributed exposure data will produce a straight line. The drawn line will summarize the characteristics of the population from which the samples were taken and will enable generalizations and predictions to be made (Fig. 8.4).

To draw a log-probability plot, the data should be ranked in ascending order, the number of results counted, the appropriate plotting points taken from Table 8.4 and the results plotted against the corresponding point on log-probability paper (Chartwell 5575). If it is possible to draw a straight line 'by eye', then this should be done, but it is preferable to calculate the correct line. A number of useful measures, such as the GM and GSD, can be estimated from the plot, the GM by reading up from the 50th percentile until intersecting the line and then reading the concentration from the y axis, and the GSD by dividing the value gained from the 84th percentile by that gained from the 50th percentile. The gradient or slope of the line is therefore indicative of the variability of the results; the steeper the gradient, the greater the variability (Fig. 8.4).

Other valuable information which is readily obtainable from these

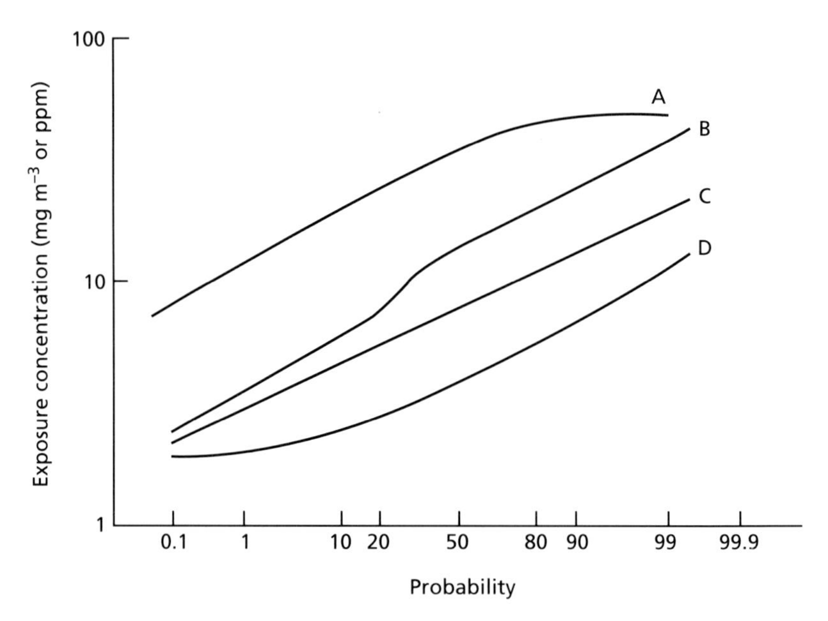

Figure 8.4 Four hypothetical probability plots: (A) probability plot of a right-truncated distribution; (B) probability plot of a mixture of two distributions; (C) probability plot of a lognormal distribution; (D) probability plot of a left-truncated distribution.

plots includes a simple guide to the proportion of the population above or below a certain level of exposure. For example, the proportion of exposure measurements likely to be above 10 (arbitrary units) in Fig. 8.4, line C is about 30%. In addition, if the line is right-truncated (i.e. flattened to horizontal at the top), it is suggestive of the measuring device reaching the point of saturation (line A); if the line is left-truncated (i.e. flattened to horizontal at the base), it is suggestive that the exposure is low and that the measuring device has reached its limit of detection due to insufficient sensitivity (line D). If there appear to be potentially two distinct line segments, this is suggestive that two separate populations have been measured (line B). Finally, two or more lines can be drawn on the same plot, perhaps to compare different systems of work or control techniques.

Comparison of results with standards

When comparing personal exposure data with exposure limits for compliance purposes, three basic conclusions can be reached.

1 Exposures are above the occupational exposure limit. There is a need to identify the reasons for the results and the steps required to control the exposure of the workers.

2 Exposures are well below the exposure limit; hence, controls need to be maintained.

3 There is insufficient information to decide whether exposures are

Table 8.4 Log-probability plotting points.

Rank order	Sample size *n*: 5	6	7	8	9	10	11	12	13	14	15	16	17	18	19	20	Rank order
1	12.9	10.9	9.4	8.3	7.4	6.7	6.1	5.6	5.2	4.8	4.5	4.2	4.0	3.8	3.6	3.4	1
2	31.5	26.6	23.0	20.2	18.1	16.3	14.9	13.7	12.7	11.8	11.0	10.3	9.8	9.2	8.7	8.3	2
3	50.0	42.2	36.5	32.1	28.7	25.9	23.7	21.8	20.1	18.7	17.5	16.4	15.5	14.7	13.9	13.2	3
4	68.5	57.8	50.0	44.0	39.4	35.6	32.4	29.8	27.6	25.7	24.0	22.5	21.3	20.1	19.1	18.1	4
5	87.1	73.5	63.5	56.0	50.0	45.2	41.2	37.8	35.1	32.6	30.5	28.7	27.0	25.5	24.2	23.0	5
6		89.1	77.1	67.9	60.7	54.8	50.0	46.0	42.5	39.6	37.0	34.8	32.8	31.0	29.4	27.9	6
7			90.6	79.8	71.3	64.4	58.8	54.0	50.0	46.5	43.5	40.9	38.5	36.4	34.5	32.8	7
8				91.7	81.9	74.1	67.6	62.1	57.5	53.4	50.0	47.0	44.3	41.8	39.7	37.7	8
9					92.6	83.7	76.3	70.2	64.9	60.4	56.5	53.1	50.0	47.3	44.8	42.6	9
10						93.3	85.1	78.3	72.4	67.4	63.0	59.2	55.8	52.7	50.0	47.6	10
11							93.9	86.3	79.9	74.3	69.5	65.3	61.5	58.2	55.2	52.5	11
12								94.4	87.3	81.3	76.0	71.4	67.3	63.6	60.3	57.4	12
13									94.8	88.2	82.5	77.5	73.0	69.1	65.0	62.3	13
14										95.2	89.0	83.6	78.8	74.5	70.6	67.2	14
15											95.5	89.7	84.5	79.9	75.8	72.1	15
16												95.8	90.3	85.4	81.0	77.0	16
17													96.0	90.8	86.1	81.9	17
18														96.2	91.3	86.8	18
19															96.4	91.7	19
20																96.6	20

For sample size > 20: plotting point = $\left(\frac{\text{rank order} - 0.3}{\text{sample size} + 0.4}\right) \times 100$.

above or below the limit. Either more information is necessary or prudent action should be taken to reduce the exposure of the workers.

When assessing for compliance, it is possible to take a pragmatic approach, and simply divide the measured concentration by the OEL and make decisions based on this dimensionless index of exposure. For example, if the value is 0.1 and the STEL conditions are fulfilled, compliance is assumed. However, when there is a high degree of variability in high-risk situations, incorrect conclusions may be drawn.

Another technique for the determination of compliance is to use the mean and variance of the exposure distribution to calculate the probability of a measurement exceeding the OEL. If the probability is $\leq 0.1\%$, then compliance is assumed; if the probability is $> 0.1\%$ but $\leq 5\%$, then the situation is probably compliant, but more measurements are needed; finally, if the probability is $> 5\%$, then the situation is not in compliance (Comité Européen de Normalisation 1992).

Period of work greater than 8 h

The ever-changing requirements of employers in terms of the duration of work or shifts may mean that potential difficulties arise when comparing exposures with OELs devised for five 8-h days per week. Clearly, the longer the day over which the contaminant is absorbed, the shorter the period of recovery before the next insult. For substances with very short half-lives, this may not be a problem, but for those whose half-lives approach or exceed 16 h (the period of recovery for an 8-h working day), the body burden may rise over the week/shift period. A number of sophisticated models utilizing pharmacokinetics have been put forward, but, unfortunately, they require a great deal of substance-specific information which is very rarely available. A more simplistic model by which OELs can be adjusted was postulated by Brief and Scala (1975) for longer working periods:

$$\text{OEL multiplication factor} = \frac{8}{H} \times \left(\frac{24-H}{16}\right) \tag{8.9}$$

where H is the number of hours worked per day.

Such a non-specific formula has limitations, but at least may afford the individual a degree of extra protection. However, the formula does not apply to continuous 24-h exposure, work periods of less than 7–8 h per day or 35 h per week or for concentration-dependent acute toxicants.

Record keeping

It is always necessary to record observations, both at the time of sampling and in any subsequent reports. It is also advisable to record more information than one would have thought necessary at first as, on enquiry, the memory may have rapidly faded and, if someone else is attempting to read and interpret the report, additional qualifying information is always of benefit.

Author and any assistants	Tel. no.	Date of sampling	Contaminant	1	2	3
Name of occupier			CAS no.			
Address of premises/location/identity			Product/trade name			
			Sampling/analysis details			
			MDHS/NIOSH/OSHA Ref.			
Total no. of people on site						
Total no. of people in area/process of interest						

	Ref. no.	Male/ Female (M/F)	Personal identifier	Sample type personal/ static (P/S)	Sample description (e.g. name/task /process/equipment)	Reason for sampling (compliance/ random, etc.)	Exposure modifier (e.g. other routes of absorption confounding factors, etc.)	Work period (i.e. shift)	Start/ stop times	Duration (min)	Result	TWA ppm or mg m^{-3}	Result	TWA ppm or mg m^{-3}	Result	TWA ppm or mg m^{-3}
1																
2																
3																
4																
5																
							Current occupational exposure limits	8 hour								
								15 minutes								

Figure 8.5 Sample record sheet.

Figure 8.5 shows an example of a sample record sheet which is useful for both on-site recordings and for formalizing the information provided in a report. It is essential to state clearly the reason for the measurement being taken, the person chosen, when the measurement was taken, etc., as retrospective reviews and exposure assessments of existing data are very difficult without this additional information.

Conclusions

It is hoped that a reasonable exposition of the various aspects of sampling atmospheric exposure in the workplace for the purpose of risk assessment has been made. The principles and factors affecting the choice of sampling method and analysis technique have been highlighted. The issues which need to be considered in the design of suitable sampling strategies and data interpretation methods have also been discussed.

In summary, atmospheric monitoring is an important tool in the estimation of airborne concentrations, and can be used in making decisions about the level of risk by comparing the measurements with suitable standards, or as part of a more sophisticated health risk assessment. However, in order to do this, the data must be representative and reliable and their limitations must be fully understood. It is also important to note that the evaluation of atmospheric exposures is only one phase in the overall effort to determine the extent of exposure. For instance, other routes of exposure, such as skin absorption and ingestion, may be equally or even more important in certain occupations, and individual breathing zone measurements may not reflect the true absorbed dose; hence, appropriate health surveillance methods, including biological monitoring, should also be considered.

References

Ashton, I. & Gill, F.S. (1992) *Monitoring for Health Hazards*, 2nd edn. Blackwell Scientific Publications, Oxford.

Bisesi, M.S. & Kohn, J.P. (1995) *Industrial Hygiene Evaluation Methods*. Lewis Publishers, London.

BOHS (1993) *Sampling Strategies for Airborne Contaminants in the Workplace*. BOHS Technical Guide No. 11. British Occupational Hygiene Society, H and H Scientific Consultants Ltd., Leeds.

Boleij, J.S.M., Buringh, E., Heederick, D. & Kromhout, H. (1995) *Occupational Hygiene of Chemicals and Biological Agents*. Elsevier, Amsterdam.

Brief, R.S. & Scala, R.A. (1975) Occupational exposure limits for novel work schedules. *American Industrial Hygiene Association Journal* 36, 467–469.

Comité Européen de Normalisation (1992) *Workplace Atmospheres—Guidance for the Assessment of Exposure to Chemical Agents for Comparison with Limit Values and Measurement Strategy*. prEN 689. CEN, Brussels.

Corn, M. & Esmen, N.A. (1979) Workplace exposure zones for classification of employee exposures to physical and chemical agents. *American Industrial Hygiene Association Journal* 40, 47–57.
Corn, N. (1985) Strategies of air sampling. *Scandinavian Journal of Work, Environment and Health* 11, 173–180.
EPA (1986) *Quality Assurance Handbook for Air Pollution Measurement Systems*. US Environmental Protection Agency, Research Triangle Park, NC.
Gardiner, K. (1995) Needs of occupational exposure sampling strategies for compliance and epidemiology. *Occupational and Environmental Medicine* 52, 705–708.
Gardiner, K., Trethowan, W.N., Harrington, J.M., Calvert, I.A. & Glass, D.C. (1992) Occupational exposure to carbon black in its manufacture. *Annals of Occupational Hygiene* 36 (5), 477–496.
Harrington, J.M. & Gardiner, K. (eds.) (1995) *Occupational Hygiene*. Blackwell Science, Oxford.
Hawkins, N.C., Norwood, S.K. & Rock, J.C. (eds.) (1991) *A Strategy for Occupational Exposure Assessment*. American Industrial Hygiene Association, Akron, OH.
HSE (1981–, in series). *Methods for the Determination of Hazardous Substances*. HSE Occupational Medicine and Hygiene Laboratory, Sheffield.
HSE (1989) *Monitoring Strategies for Toxic Substances. Guidance Note EH42*. HMSO, London.
Intersociety Committee (1988) *Methods of Air Sampling and Analysis*, 3rd edn. Lewis Publishers, Chelsea, MI.
Kromhout, H. & Heederick, D. (1995) Occupational epidemiology in the rubber industry: implications of exposure variability. *American Journal of Industrial Medicine* 27, 171–185.
Kromhout, H., Symanski, E. & Rappaport, S.M. (1993) A comprehensive evaluation of within and between-worker components of occupational exposure to chemical agents. *Annals of Occupational Hygiene* 37 (3), 253–270.
Leidel, N. & Busch, K. (1994) Statistical design and data analysis requirements. In: *Patty's Industrial Hygiene and Toxicology* (eds. R.L. Harris, L.J. Cralley & L.V. Cralley), 3rd edn., pp. 453–582. Wiley, New York.
Leidel, N., Busch, K. & Lynch, J. (1977) *Occupational Exposure Sampling Strategy Manual*. US DHEW (NIOSH) Publ. No. 77-173. NIOSH, Cincinnati, OH.
NIOSH (1994) *NIOSH Manual of Analytical Methods*, 4th edn. DHEW (NIOSH) Publ. No. 94-113. NIOSH, Cincinnati, OH.
OSHA (1985) *OSHA Analytical Methods Manual*. OSHA Analytical Laboratories, Salt Lake City, UT.
Rappaport, S.M. (1988) Biological considerations for designing sampling strategies. In: *Advances in Air Sampling* (ed. W. John), pp. 337–352. Lewis Publishers, Chelsea, MI.
Rappaport, S.M. (1991) Assessment of long-term exposures to toxic substances in air—review. *Annals of Occupational Hygiene* 35 (1), 61–121.
Rappaport, S.M. & Selvin, S. (1987) A method for evaluating the mean

exposure from a log normal distribution. *American Industrial Hygiene Association Journal* **48**, 374–379.
Rappaport, S.M., Kromhout, H. & Symanski, E. (1993) Variation of exposure between workers in homogeneous exposure groups. *American Industrial Hygiene Association Journal* **54** (11), 654–662.
Roach, S.A. (1977) A most rational basis for air sampling programmes. *Annals of Occupational Hygiene* **20**, 65–84.
Vaughan, N.P., Chalmers, C.P. & Botham, R.A. (1990) Field comparison of personal samplers for inhalable dust. *Annals of Occupational Hygiene* **34** (6), 553–573.

Chapter 9 Exposure modelling

Christopher N. Gray

Introduction

The term exposure modelling can be applied to a wide range of techniques used to predict exposures to chemical, physical or biological agents from limited data. Exposure models can be conceptual, qualitative or quantitative, and might involve simple algorithms, complex numerical techniques or, occasionally, scale models built of Perspex. Simple exposure models may be used to predict average exposures from the results of limited personal sampling; for example, if the typical exposure during the filling of a single road tanker with solvent was measured, the shift average exposure could be estimated from the number of tanker fills per shift. A more complex model might make use of a theoretically derived value for the solvent evaporation rate and calculations of vapour dispersal, together with assumptions about the workers' locations at different times, in order to predict the average exposures.

When no actual exposure data are available, it may be necessary to rely upon *ab initio* theoretical predictions, as in the second example above. This is generally the case when it is planned to introduce a new process, equipment or substance, and in certain other circumstances (Table 9.1). It may be possible to predict what exposures might result if a new process, equipment or substance is used in a certain way. For example, the manufacturers of industrial plant and equipment can often provide information on the sound power level, noise spectrum and noise directivity of their products, and this can be used to predict the sound field that would be obtained if the equipment was located in a given setting. By making assumptions about where and for how long workers will be located in this sound field, the expected noise exposures

Table 9.1 Examples of situations in which exposure modelling is valuable.

1. Prior to the introduction of new processes, equipment or substances
2. Prior to process modification
3. In the selection of substitutes for hazardous substances
4. To predict the potential exposures that could result from accidental releases of substances (spills, leaks, unplanned venting, etc.)
5. To help reconstruct exposures in the aftermath of an accident
6. To help reconstruct exposures in retrospective epidemiology

can be calculated. A similar approach is possible for other physical hazards, such as ionizing and non-ionizing radiation. For airborne chemical hazards, it is necessary to estimate the emission rate, the pattern of dispersal of the substance in the air and the location of the workers in the resulting concentration field.

Ab initio predictions of exposure are always subject to considerable uncertainty, and it is usually more reliable to use extrapolations from existing exposure data for analogous processes. In the absence of validation data, all predictions must be viewed with considerable caution. Nevertheless, they can often be of value in indicating the possible range of exposures, and in providing an understanding of the exposure process that can aid in risk control.

Types of exposure model

Exposure models consist essentially of a source, a transmission path and a receiver (the workers). They do not usually consider the dose or effect resulting from the exposure, although these may also be modelled as part of the overall risk assessment process (Fig. 9.1). However, if the exposure model is to provide the correct measure of exposure for risk assessment, it must take into account the key features of the dose and effect models. For example, in assessing the risk of acute central nervous system effects from organic solvents, the exposure model must deal with short-term high exposures and not just average exposures. It must also account for possible dermal contact, as this could be a significant route of uptake. As another example, models of respiratory exposure to dusts should take into account the aerodynamic size fraction relevant to the toxic effect under consideration: the respirable fraction in the case of crystalline silica and the inhalable fraction in the case of systemically poisonous substances.

The main components of exposure models, covering the source, the path and the receiver, can usually be considered separately. For example, the source can often be modelled as though it was independent of both the path and the receiver. This is not always a valid assumption;

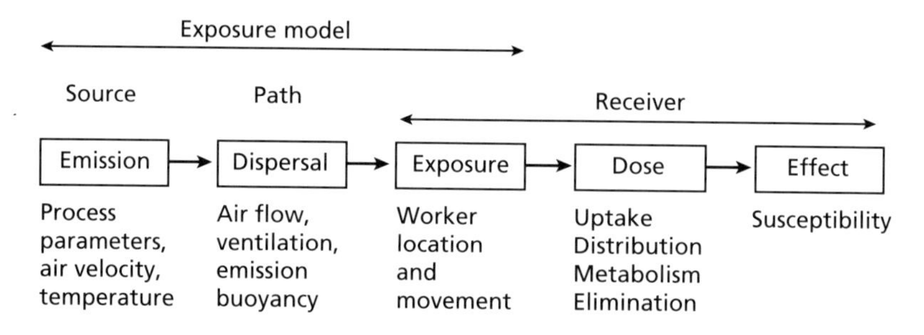

Figure 9.1 Outline of a simplified exposure model for an airborne substance showing the relationship to dose and effect and certain factors which influence each stage of the model.

for example, the location and activity of the workers may very well influence the emission rate of noise, chemicals and other hazardous agents. However, the assumption of independence is often a reasonable first approximation.

Modelling sources of emission

The first step in the sequence leading to exposure is the generation and release of the physical, chemical or biological hazardous agent. Emission rates from various sources can be estimated by measurement under controlled conditions or, in many cases, by calculation. Examples of sources and the basis for emission models in each case are given in Table 9.2.

Empirical emission rates

In many cases, exposure models can be based on empirical (measured) emission rates; if the source is available to be investigated, this is often the most reliable way of obtaining emission data. This is often the case for sources of noise, vibration, ionizing and non-ionizing radiation, bio-

Table 9.2 Examples of sources and emissions, and the corresponding basis for emission models.

Source	Emission	Basis of model
Sealed radioactive source	Ionizing radiation	Measurement or calculation of source activity
High-voltage apparatus	X-rays	Measurement of emission, wavelengths and directionality
Machinery	Noise	Measurement of sound power level, noise spectrum and directionality
Machinery	Vibration	Measurement of acceleration and frequency
Radio transmitter	Electromagnetic radiation	Calculation or measurement of power output, frequency and directionality
Paint, solvents and adhesives	Solvent vapours	Calculation or measurement of evaporation rate per unit area
Stacks (chimneys and other discharges)	Gases, fumes, etc.	Stack sampling or calculation based on materials used
Indoor materials and surfaces	Volatile organic compounds	Emission calculations or laboratory measurements
Glass fibre reinforced plastic resins	Styrene vapour	Calculation of evaporation rate or measurement of mass loss
Welding, brazing, soldering	Metal oxide fumes, flux components, gases	Calculation or measurement of metal fume composition, measurement of emission rates
Synthetic mineral wool insulation	Dust and fibres	Measurement of emissions under standard test conditions

aerosols and some chemicals. Empirical methods are used to evaluate a wide range of emissions, including solvents from resins, paints and adhesives, pyrolysis products from heated plastics, dust from insulation materials, gases from vehicle exhausts and fumes from factory chimneys. Emissions of hazardous substances are usually measured by sampling a known proportion of the emission, which is then analysed. For example, welding fume formation rates can be measured relatively easily in a ventilated box in which the fume is collected on a filter for weighing and analysis. A variant of this technique can be used to measure the formation rates of various gases, such as ozone, carbon monoxide and oxides of nitrogen.

Generally, the measurements are made under controlled or laboratory conditions, and the results must be adjusted to take into account different workplace conditions. For example, the evaporation rate of a solvent from a product, such as a paint or adhesive, could be measured under controlled conditions, and the evaporation rate at different temperatures and air speeds could be predicted by calculation using theoretical models as described below.

In some cases, rates of emission may be measured by a simple weight loss experiment, e.g. the rate of emission of styrene from polyester resins during curing. This simple procedure allows the emission characteristics of different resins to be compared, and low-emission resins can then be selected in order to reduce potential styrene exposures. Emission rates measured in this way cannot be used to predict accurately actual emission rates during the use of the resins, because these are dependent on temperature and air speed.

Theoretical emission rates

If it is not possible to obtain reliable empirical emission rate data, it may be possible to predict the emissions theoretically. For example, the emissions from radioactive sources can be predicted accurately from their isotopic composition and their size and shape (to account for self-absorption). Theoretical emission rates may also be derived for sources of non-ionizing radiation, and for some sources of chemicals, including hydrocarbon fuels, paints, resins, adhesives and some plastics. In a few cases, the theoretical average emission rate can be calculated simply from the rate at which a substance is used in a process. For example, in the use of adhesives, the daily average rate of emission of solvent is almost equal to the mass of solvent in the adhesive used each day, even though the emission rate may vary considerably over the course of the day. Usually, the theoretical calculation is more complicated than this, and requires a knowledge of the physical or chemical mechanism of the emission process.

Evaporation models

Many substances used in the workplace become airborne by a simple process of evaporation. This applies to the solvents in paint, adhesives, varnishes and resins, and to metals heated to high temperatures. Vapour compositions and evaporation rates can be predicted with reasonable accuracy from the vapour pressures and other physical properties of substances or mixtures. In welding, brazing and soldering, the fume compositions can be predicted from the vapour pressures of the metals in the alloy using semiempirical models (Gray *et al.* 1980; Thorne & Hewitt 1985). On the other hand, the theoretical prediction of the overall fume formation rate in welding has proved to be very difficult, and is the subject of continuing research, notably at Bradford University in the UK.

The vapour pressures (or saturated vapour pressures) of pure substances can be obtained from several sources, including materials safety data sheets (MSDSs), although these are often given for only one temperature. The temperature dependence of vapour pressure is given by the well-established Clausius–Clapeyron equation, details of which are given in most chemical reference books, such as the *CRC Handbook of Chemistry and Physics* (Lide 1996). Most commercial solvents are mixtures, and the vapour pressures of pure chemicals do not apply in such cases. For mixtures of similar types of chemical, such as petroleum, which consists of various hydrocarbons, the vapour pressures of the components are easily calculated. Such mixtures behave more or less 'ideally' and obey Raoult's law, i.e. the vapour pressure of each component is proportional to its molar fraction in the mixture. Simple ideal solution models have been used extensively in occupational hygiene calculations to predict vapour compositions, e.g. to predict the proportion of benzene in petroleum vapour. The composition of saturated vapour over a liquid mixture is proportional to the relative vapour pressures of the components of the mixture. This rule does not apply if the liquid totally evaporates, when, of course, the proportions by mass in the total vapour are the same as they were in the liquid before it evaporated.

Some solvent mixtures do not obey Raoult's law, that is to say the vapour pressures of the components in the mixture cannot be predicted easily from the vapour pressures of the individual components. This applies particularly to mixtures of chemically dissimilar compounds, such as organic compounds and water, as found in water-based paints, and ketones and hydrocarbons, as found in some adhesives. This often has the effect of significantly increasing the vapour pressures.

For such mixtures, it is necessary to know the thermodynamic 'activity' of each component, or its 'Henry's law' constant in the case of dilute mixtures. It is possible to find some values of activity coefficients and Henry's law constants in chemical data books, but these are limited, and it is often necessary to calculate them from theoretical considerations. These calculations are complex and beyond the scope of this book. However, several computer programs are now available which can perform them rapidly, and which can be used by non-specialists, e.g. the

SUBTEC package (Olsen *et al.* 1992). These only require the user to specify the ingredients and proportions of a mixture and to select a temperature, and all the calculations are performed automatically.

The saturated vapour pressure of a substance at a particular temperature represents the maximum concentration that it can attain in the vapour phase; higher concentrations can be obtained only if airborne droplets or solid particles are present. In an open workshop, or ventilated space, vapour concentrations rarely reach their saturated vapour pressures. Instead, the concentration is limited by the rate of evaporation, and the rate at which the vapour is removed by the natural and mechanical ventilation. Therefore, in order to predict the possible air concentration, we must estimate the evaporation rate.

For many organic solvents and commercial mixtures, the evaporation rates relative to *n*-butyl acetate are included in the MSDSs; a substance with a relative evaporation rate of 2.0 will have a vapour emission rate approximately twice as high as *n*-butyl acetate, used in the same way and under the same conditions of temperature and air speed. Various reference books have long been available which contain such data for a range of compounds (American Mutual Insurance Alliance (AMIA) 1966). Relative evaporation rates can be used to compare the theoretical emission rates of different volatile compounds when substitution is being considered, but they do not allow the actual values of the emission rates to be easily calculated. This requires more difficult calculations which are best achieved using commercially available computer programs, as will be described below.

The rate of evaporation of a substance is a function of its vapour pressure and its rate of diffusion in the air above the evaporating surface. In perfectly still air, the evaporation rate is limited by molecular diffusion according to Fick's law, but, in practical situations in the workplace, this is not an important mechanism. Instead, the rate of evaporation is determined by eddy diffusion caused by air movements. Air movements due to ventilation, draughts and the movement of the source, etc. rapidly carry vapour away from the evaporating surface (forced convection). Additionally, if the source is warmer than its surroundings, this causes the vapour to be buoyant so that it rises from the evaporating surface and again rapidly carries vapour away (free convection). In order to predict accurately the evaporation rate of a volatile compound, it is necessary to know its vapour pressure, its molecular diffusivity and the effect of free and forced convection.

There are several ways of dealing with these problems, which need not be discussed here, and the necessary calculations can be performed using a spreadsheet on a personal computer, provided that the necessary data can be found for the mixtures in question. Alternatively, several computer programs are available which can be used to predict evaporation rates.

Some early evaporation models were developed for outdoor situations, where air velocities can be relatively high (several metres per second) and the flow in the boundary layer over the evaporating surface can be turbulent. Such models tend to overestimate the predicted evaporation rate in indoor occupational settings, where air velocities are generally much less than $1\,m\,s^{-1}$ and boundary layer conditions are laminar. These include theoretical models proposed by Mackay and Matsugu (1973), Gray (1974) and Gmehling *et al.* (1989). The US Environmental Protection Agency (EPA 1987) also has a model of evaporation that was developed for outdoor conditions. This greatly underestimates evaporation rates in indoor laminar flow conditions. Evaporation models which are suitable for occupational risk assessment include the SUBTEC model (Olsen *et al.* 1992) and the isothermal model of Nielsen and Olsen (1995). The latter appears to give the most reliable prediction of indoor evaporation rates, but the SUBTEC model has the advantage of being available as a commercial computer program which allows occupational hygienists and other risk assessors to carry out reasonably reliable predictions for complex mixtures without a detailed knowledge of the underlying theory.

Modelling the path of an emission

Path models attempt to describe the process by which an emission becomes distributed in the workplace environment, and may be applied to any hazardous agent, including gases, vapours, dusts, mists, noise, vibration, radiation and biological agents.

In the case of noise, path models may take into account multiple sources, attenuation with distance, reflections, reverberation, sound absorption and insulation and structure-borne noise. It can be difficult to model a complete noise environment without the benefit of measurements, but the noise field of individual machines can often be predicted with reasonable accuracy provided that the characteristics of the noise source and proposed surroundings are known. Such calculations may be carried out before the purchase of a large piece of industrial plant, such as a pump or compressor. In the simplest cases, such models involve a calculation of the theoretical noise level at various distances from the equipment. This requires a knowledge of the sound power level and of any sound reflecting surfaces that will be near the source. More complex calculations are necessary if the equipment is a directional noise source or if reverberant conditions are possible, and in the case of multiple sources.

For airborne substances, the contaminant is dispersed from the source to the receiver by diffusion and air movements. These can be complex, and it is usually necessary to make certain simplifying assumptions. Use is sometimes made of physical scale models to deal with the complexity of the air flow in the real workplace; for example, scale models have been used to study the air flow and pollutant concentrations in coal mines (Vincent *et al.* 1991), and wind tunnels are used to examine contaminant dispersal in flowing air (Kim & Flynn 1991). Simple mathematical techniques that can be used include box models and diffusion models.

Box models

The simplest of all models of dispersal assumes that there is total and instantaneous mixing of the contaminant with the air in the work space. These are sometimes known as 'box' or 'stirred box' models. The contaminant enters the air at a rate equal to the emission rate of the source, and is removed by the natural or mechanical ventilation in the space. If the emission rate is $E\,\text{mg}\,\text{s}^{-1}$ and the total air flow into and out of the space is $Q\,\text{m}^3\,\text{s}^{-1}$, the average contaminant concentration in the space will build up to a steady state value of $E/Q\,\text{mg}\,\text{m}^{-3}$, independent of the volume of the space. If the air is initially clean, the concentration will build up exponentially towards the steady state value as long as the emission continues and, when the emission ceases, it will decay exponentially to zero (Fig. 9.2), the rate of build up and decay depending on the volume of the air space.

These calculations are simple, but the model has obvious limitations. Although it can provide a reasonable estimate of the average air concentration in the space, it totally ignores the inevitable variation of concentration from point to point and, in particular, the higher concentrations closer to the source. For localized sources, such as a gas leak or welding arc, this discrepancy can be so serious as to invalidate the model, particularly when workers are located close to the source. However, for multiple distributed or area sources, and where the workers are mobile throughout the space, a box model can provide a reasonable approximation of actual average exposures. A stirred box model has been used to predict the exposures of painters to organic vapours in a room during paint stripping with methylene chloride, painting with solvent-based paints and solvent cleaning (Bjerre 1989). Most of the measured exposures were within a factor of two of the predicted values. Box models are also used for predicting indoor air quality from the emission properties of the surfaces and furnishings, etc. and building ventilation rates (Mackay & Paterson 1983).

In more complicated box models, buildings or work areas are

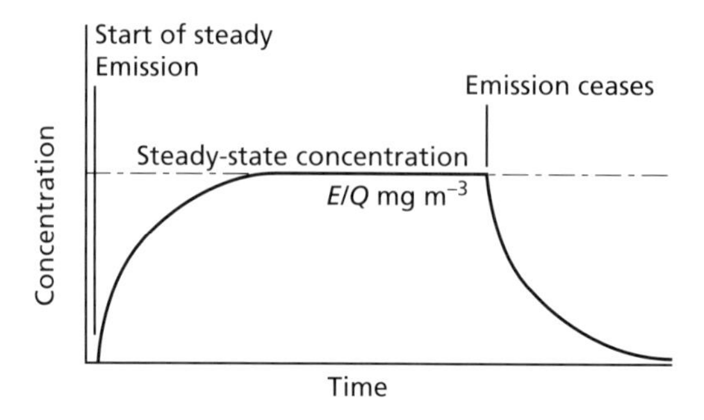

Figure 9.2 Build up and decay of the concentration of contaminant in a stirred box. When the emission rate is $E\,\text{mg}\,\text{s}^{-1}$ and the total ventilation rate is $Q\,\text{m}^3\text{s}^{-1}$, the steady state concentration is equal to $E/Q\,\text{mg}\,\text{m}^{-3}$.

notionally divided into separate zones, each of which is treated as a separate stirred box. For example, the local environments of several workstations in a large workshop might be treated as individual boxes, while the remainder of the air in the workshop might be treated as a separate single box. The air flows between the boxes and between each box and the outside environment must be taken into account, as well as the emissions in each. Such sequential box models have been found to be useful in studying the air flow and airborne contaminant concentrations in buildings, workrooms and enclosures (Zemba & Luis 1993), and in large tanks during the application of internal surface coatings (Haberlin & Heinsohn 1993).

Box models are also used in the design of general (dilution) ventilation for controlling less hazardous air contaminants, provided that the concentration is reasonably uniform. If the emission rate ($E\,mg\,s^{-1}$) is known and it is desired to reduce the air concentration to a particular value ($C\,mg\,m^{-3}$), a required minimum ventilation rate ($Q\,m^3\,s^{-1}$) can be calculated from $Q = E/C$. In practice, because the air flow is unlikely to be uniform throughout the room, a safety factor is usually introduced, and the required minimum ventilation rate is increased by a factor of several orders of magnitude (American Conference of Governmental Industrial Hygienists (ACGIH) 1995).

Diffusion models

Because box models are not reliable for localized sources, other types of model must be used in such cases. Airborne substances are transported from the source to the worker's breathing zone by diffusion and air movement. Molecular diffusion is insignificant in practice, and it is eddy diffusion (free and forced convection) that dominates the mass transfer process. Air movements in the room due to natural and mechanical ventilation may produce a more or less steady flow in one direction, but random air movements also occur due to draughts and the movement of people and equipment. In addition, there may be strong convection currents if the source is hot, e.g. in soldering, and weaker convection currents are produced by the body heat of the worker. This might suggest that modelling the dispersal of an emission is extremely difficult, but various simplifying assumptions can be made.

Dispersion models usually assume that, on average, the concentration profile about a point source follows a Gaussian statistical distribution, and the effect of a prevailing air movement is to skew the Gaussian distribution to one side. Similarly, a buoyant emission shifts the Gaussian distribution vertically upwards. It is beyond the scope of this book to explain these calculations in detail, but they are capable of being performed easily on a personal computer using a spreadsheet, provided that the required parameters can be selected. Often the greatest uncertainty involves the amount of eddy diffusion that may occur in the workplace, and sometimes a range of plausible values are used in order to calculate a range of possible concentrations.

Gaussian dispersion models have long been employed to calculate theoretical atmospheric pollution concentrations downwind of factory and power station chimneys, and the predicted ground level concentrations have been used in risk assessments and in planning decisions regarding chimney heights and factory locations. They are now being increasingly employed to model the dispersion of airborne contaminants in occupational settings. An early application of this technique was in modelling the effect of multiple leaks in chemical plants (Schroy 1981; Powell 1984). In research currently underway at Deakin University in Australia, Gaussian dispersion models have been used successfully to describe the concentration profiles of fume in the vicinity of a welding operation. In this case, the eddy diffusion coefficients were chosen to fit the empirical data and were not selected in advance, but further work might be able to provide values to use in predictive modelling.

Gaussian dispersion models have proved to be useful for describing the distribution of airborne contaminant concentrations around point sources. This can be useful in explaining the behaviour of emissions, and can help in the design of controls, including ventilation. However, their predictive capacity remains limited to situations in which there is a knowledge of air flows or where simple assumptions can be made.

Modelling the receiver

If it is possible to predict or to measure the distribution of a particular hazardous agent in a workplace, using the techniques described above, it is possible, in principle, to predict the exposures to that agent by making certain assumptions about the locations and movements of workers. If there are fixed workstations, this may be a relatively straightforward procedure. For example, if the noise field produced by a machine can be predicted, or measured, and the operator is to be located at one position, the noise exposure can also be predicted. Similarly, for hand-held tools where there is not much variation in the arm position, noise exposures may also be predicted with reasonable confidence. Where it is likely that a worker's tasks will vary over the work shift, it is necessary to make certain assumptions about the time spent in different locations and on different tasks. Often this cannot be done in great detail, but it may be possible to estimate that certain proportions of a worker's time will be spent in certain specified ways. For example, it might be estimated that, on a typical day, a furniture production worker will operate a circular saw for 90 min and a router for 120 min, in addition to being subjected to background noise of a certain level for 7 h. A similar approach can be taken for exposure to other agents, including radiation and airborne chemicals, and this permits the estimation of both short-term exposures and shift average exposures. Of course, there are considerable uncertainties in this procedure, and it is prudent to consider not just a single predicted value, but a range of possible exposures, as discussed later.

For workers in a fairly uniform exposure field, their actual location is less important, particularly if they are mobile throughout the exposure area. In the case of painters decorating a whole room, for example, the solvent vapour concentrations might not vary greatly, and their mobility would tend to average out their exposures. In such circumstances, sequential box models, which assume time-variable but spatially uniform concentrations within each notional box, are often satisfactory.

In the case of point sources of emission, the uncertainties can be considerable for any type of hazardous agent, but particularly for localized sources of airborne chemicals close to individual workers. Here, the concentration gradients can be very steep so that small movements of the worker or the source, or changes in air movement, can result in large fluctuations in exposure. In electric arc welding, where fume dispersal is dominated by the thermal buoyancy, the fume is highly localized, and the concentration can vary by an order of magnitude over a few centimetres. The precise position of welders with respect to the fume column varies considerably and cannot be predicted with any certainty; hence, fume exposures are also variable and rather unpredictable. It may be possible to predict approximately the average exposure for a group of welders using a particular welding process in a certain way, but this would have to be based, at least in part, on actual exposure measurements for similar work.

Modelling dermal and gastrointestinal exposure

The estimation of dermal exposure is a particular problem in occupational health risk assessment. In some circumstances, dermal uptake of chemicals may dominate over respiratory uptake, e.g. in the application of some pesticides and when there is routine skin contact with organic solvents. It is very difficult to measure dermal exposure and it is not often attempted, although biological monitoring can sometimes be used to measure the total uptake of a chemical by all routes, including the skin. For a few chemicals, the permeability of intact human skin to liquids and vapours has been measured, and there are some mathematical models of skin permeability that can be used to predict very approximately what rate of uptake would result if a certain area of skin was in contact with a particular chemical. Skin exposure models attempt to predict the extent and duration of skin contact with chemicals in a given situation. In modelling exposure to solvents and petroleum, some investigators have attempted to estimate the skin area and frequency and duration of dermal contact due to handling, spills and hand washing. Various models have been used to predict dermal exposure to pesticides (Van Hemmen 1993), but these are generally qualitative. The whole subject of dermal exposure and uptake is in need of further research. It is also recognized that accidental poisoning by ingestion occurs in some occupations. However, very little is known about occupational gastrointestinal exposure to chemicals, and modelling of such exposure is rarely attempted.

Effect of personal protective clothing and equipment

Exposure to all, or most, hazardous agents is influenced by personal protective clothing and equipment (PPE). Ear plugs reduce noise exposure, respirators reduce inhalation exposure and impervious gloves reduce dermal exposure to chemicals and some forms of radiation; if the influence of PPE is ignored; exposures will be overestimated. The results of manufacturers' or other performance tests can be used to estimate the possible effect of the protective clothing or equipment on exposure, but it must be realized that the performance achieved in the workplace may be considerably less than that achieved in controlled tests. For hearing protection, it is generally possible to obtain both the mean and standard deviation of the attenuation achieved in test conditions. This information could be used to calculate the distribution of theoretical protection factors, but, if the devices are not worn properly by all of the workers throughout the period of noise exposure, the actual protection may be very much less than predicted. Similarly, the performance of respirators may be severely compromised by improper and inconsistent use. In reality, the performance achieved will fall somewhere between the nominal or test performance and zero, often closer to the latter. If PPE is used routinely in a particular setting, it should be considered in the exposure model, but its influence can only be estimated by making various assumptions about how it is used in practice.

Dealing with the uncertainties

Every stage of exposure modelling is subject to some, sometimes considerable, uncertainty. This is inevitable, but it does not necessarily invalidate the approach; there are considerable uncertainties in the whole risk assessment process, but, if these are acknowledged, they can often be accommodated. One way of dealing with these uncertainties is to assume the worst case. This might involve choosing the data and assumptions that give the greatest emission rate for a source of an airborne chemical, choosing conditions that give the highest possible air concentration and, finally, assuming that the workers spend the maximum plausible time in the area of highest concentration without the benefit of effective PPE. It is also possible to carry out a 'best case' calculation in order to estimate a range of possible exposures. This may appear to be reasonable, but may be highly misleading, because the worst and best cases could be improbable, extreme values and the range could be unrealistically wide.

An alternative approach is to consider the natural ranges and uncertainties in all of the parameters of the model, and to use these to calculate a probability distribution for the exposure, rather than to calculate point estimates with unknown uncertainties. The most convenient way of doing this is often to carry out a 'Monte Carlo' simulation. This is a relatively simple computer technique in which, wherever appropriate, a range or distribution, rather than an individual value, is applied to the variables in the model. For example, we might not know the precise duration of a particular exposure, but we might know that it can be from 20 to 45 min. This range would be used in the model rather than an average or single estimated value. Similarly, ranges or distributions would be applied to the parameters of the emission rate, the dispersal, the location of the workers, etc. In calculating the exposure using the Monte Carlo technique, values are selected at random by the computer for each of the variables, from the appropriate range or distribution, and an exposure value is calculated. The process is then repeated (iterated) thousands of times in order to produce thousands of different estimates of the exposure. The important next step is to examine the distribution of these exposure estimates. Figure 9.3 shows the results of a Monte Carlo simulation, carried out by the author, of a simple model for exposure to a solvent during adhesive application. It is interesting to note that, although all the parameters of the model had simple range values, the distribution of the predicted exposure appears, at least superficially, to be lognormal. Additionally, the worst case estimate of exposure can be seen to be an extreme and very improbable value. A commercially available program called 'Crystal Ball' that can perform such simulations is available from the American company Decisioneering Incorporated. However, it is perfectly possible to carry out the calculations using a spreadsheet, such as Microsoft Excel, and this maintains the flexibility required for more complex modelling.

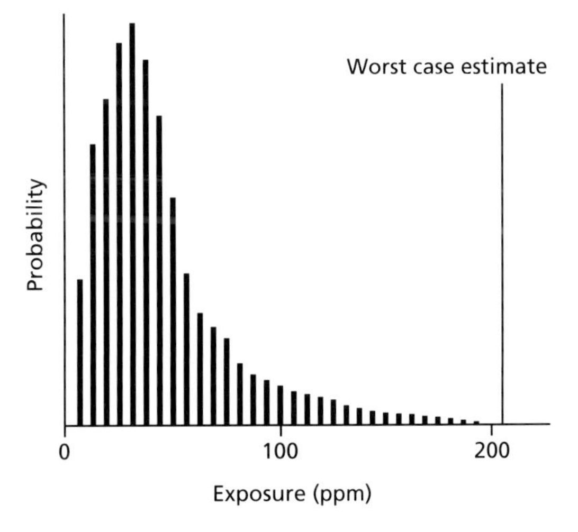

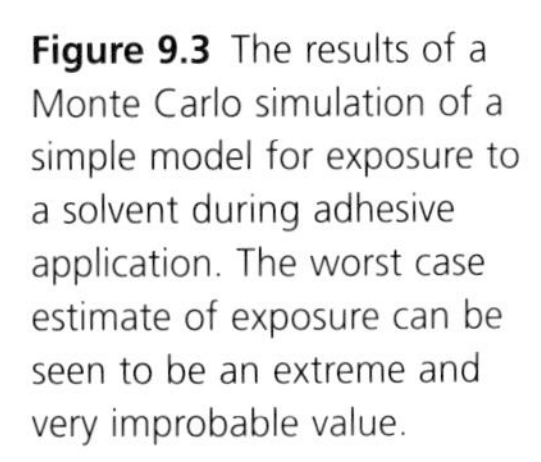

Figure 9.3 The results of a Monte Carlo simulation of a simple model for exposure to a solvent during adhesive application. The worst case estimate of exposure can be seen to be an extreme and very improbable value.

Conclusions

Exposure models are often useful for extrapolating from limited exposure data in order to predict exposures at other times and for circumstances different from those for which data are available. They may be applied to physical hazards, such as noise and radiation, to chemicals and to biological agents. Where there are no relevant exposure data, e.g. prior to introducing a new process, in planning for possible accidental releases and in reconstructing past exposures, *ab initio* modelling can sometimes provide an indication of the possible exposures. However, theoretically predicted values must be treated with caution, as it is difficult to be certain that the conditions and work practices are as expected; wherever possible, some exposure data should be obtained to attempt to validate the model. For most emissions, it is often possible to model the source, the path and the receiver (workers) independently. This simplifies the modelling process and allows empirical data to be introduced at various stages. Account should be taken of the possible effect of any personal protective clothing and equipment in use. This involves assessing not only its nominal performance, but also the way in which it is used in practice, as this often seriously compromises the protection achieved. Exposure models should consider all possible routes of exposure. Although inhalation exposure is usually dominant in the occupational setting, dermal and gastrointestinal exposure may sometimes be important, e.g. in pesticide application. It is difficult to model dermal exposure, and the skin permeability of many chemicals is not known. Little is known about occupational exposures involving ingestion, although accidental poisoning by this route is known to occur. These are areas requiring further research.

Exposure modelling is subject to considerable uncertainty, and it must be remembered that exposures are often highly variable for a given process. It is not valid therefore to predict a single value of exposure for a particular process. Instead, account should be taken of the natural variations in the parameters that determine exposure, and the uncertainty in these values. One way of doing this is to consider the best and worst case estimates as giving a possible exposure range, although this may be unrealistically wide. Another approach is to use a modelling technique that takes into account the ranges or distributions of the model parameters in order to calculate a probability distribution of predicted exposures.

References

ACGIH (1995) *Industrial Ventilation: A Manual of Recommended Practice*, 22nd edn. American Conference of Governmental Industrial Hygienists, Cincinnati, OH.

AMIA (1966) *Handbook of Organic Industrial Solvents*. Technical Guide No. 6. American Mutual Insurance Alliance, Chicago.

Bjerre, A. (1989) Assessing exposure to a solvent vapour during application of paints, etc.—model calculation vs. common sense. *Annals of Occupational Hygiene* 33 (4), 507–517.
EPA (1987) *Technical Guidance for Hazard Analysis: Emergency Planning for Extremely Hazardous Substances. Supplement to NRT-1, Hazardous Materials Emergency Planning Guide.* US Environmental Protection Agency, Washington.
Gmehling, J., Weidlich, V., Lehmann, E. & Frohlich, N. (1989) A method for calculating airborne concentrations of substances emitted from liquid product mixtures. *Staub-Reinhaltung der Luft* **49**, 227–230 (in German).
Gray, C.N., Hewitt, P.J. & Hicks, R. (1980) The prediction of fume compositions in stainless steel metal inert gas welding. In: *Weld Pool Chemistry and Metallurgy*. The Welding Institute, London.
Gray, D.C. (1974) Solvent evaporation rates. *American Industrial Hygiene Association Journal* **35**, 695–710.
Haberlin, G.M. & Heinsohn, R.J. (1993) Predicting solvent concentrations from coating the inside of bulk storage tanks. *American Industrial Hygiene Association Journal* **54** (11), 1–9.
Kim, T. & Flynn, M.R. (1991) Modelling a worker's exposure from a hand-held source in a uniform freestream. *American Industrial Hygiene Association Journal* **52** (11), 458–463.
Lide, D.R. (1996) *CRC Handbook of Chemistry and Physics*, 77th edn. CRC, Boca Raton, FL.
Mackay, D. & Paterson, S. (1983) Fugacity models of indoor exposure to volatile chemicals. *Chemosphere* **12** (2), 143–154.
Mackay, D. & Matsugu, R.S. (1973) Evaporation rates of liquid hydrocarbon spills on land and water. *Canadian Journal of Chemical Engineering* **51**, 434–439.
Neilsen, F. & Olsen, E. (1995) Prediction of isothermal evaporation rates of pure volatile organic compounds in occupational environments—a theoretical approach based on laminar boundary layer theory. *Annals of Occupational Hygiene* **39** (4), 497–511.
Olsen, E., Olsen, I., Wallstrom, E. & Rasmussen, E. (1992) On the substitution of chemicals—use of the SUBFAC-index for volatile substances. *Annals of Occupational Hygiene* **36** (6), 637–652.
Powell, R.W. (1984) Estimating worker exposure to gases and vapours leaking from pumps and valves. *American Industrial Hygiene Association Journal* **45** (11), A7–A15.
Schroy, J.M. (1981) Prediction of workplace contaminant levels. In: *Proceedings—Symposium on Control Technology in the Plastics and Resins Industry*, pp. 190–206. US Department of Health and Human Services, Publication 81-107. NIOSH, Cincinnati.
Thorne, B.D. & Hewitt, P.J. (1985) Generation of cadmium fume from alloy sources. *Annals of Occupational Hygiene* **29** (2), 181–189.
Van Hemmen, J.J. (1993) Predictive exposure modelling for pesticide registration purposes. *Annals of Occupational Hygiene* **37** (5), 541–564.
Vincent, J.H., Aitken, R.J., Mark, D. & Botham, R.A. (1991) Scale model studies of the transport of airborne pollutants on coalfaces. *Annals of Occupational Hygiene* **35** (4), 359–376.

Zemba, S.G. & Luis, S.J. (1993) *A User-Friendly Approach for Modelling Air Dispersion of Chemicals in Industrial Facilities*. Cambridge Environmental Inc., Cambridge, MA.

Chapter 10 Risk characterization

Hani Raafat and Steven S. Sadhra

Introduction

In addition to demonstrating compliance with relevant standards and regulations, risk assessment is a structured approach which aids in the consistency of decision making and the cost effectiveness of the allocation of resources. This approach has become the cornerstone of all harmonized health and safety legislation and standards.

Risk assessment may be defined as a structured and systematic procedure for the identification of hazards, evaluation of risks and prioritization of decisions in order to reduce risks to a tolerable level. As described in earlier chapters, risk assessment techniques are complementary to the more pragmatic ways of problem identification and assessment. They highlight systematically how hazards can occur and provide a clearer understanding of their nature and possible consequences, thereby improving the decision-making process for the most effective way to prevent injury and damage to health. The techniques of risk assessment range from relatively simple qualitative methods of hazard identification and analysis to the advanced quantitative methods for risk assessment in which numerical values of risk frequency or probability are derived.

The four principal elements of risk assessment for human health are: hazard identification, dose–response assessment, exposure assessment and risk characterization. *Risk characterization* can be defined as the process for estimating the incidence and severity of the adverse health effect likely to occur due to actual or predicted exposure to a workplace hazard. Thus, risk characterization is the product of the risk assessment process that can be used by the risk manager to develop and prioritize control strategies and to communicate risks.

As the final step in the risk assessment process, this chapter attempts to provide a summary of the previous chapters and describe ways in which the information presented can be combined to determine the level of risk and its tolerability/acceptability. Once the risk has been characterized, the risk manager has the responsibility to protect adequately the potentially exposed population. This responsibility will include socio-economic and political factors, as well as the consideration of societal concerns and the perception of risks (discussed in Chapters 12 and 14).

Risk assessment framework

As shown in Fig. 10.1, before commencing the risk assessment, its objectives and scope must be defined explicitly. The purpose of the study and the fundamental assumptions made must be clearly stated. In order to limit the analysis, the human–system boundaries must also be defined, as well as the intended design, use, operation and layout. The risk assessment procedure, shown in Fig. 10.1, contains two essential elements.

1 *Risk analysis*: hazards and hazardous situations are systematically identified and their consequences are analysed. The level of risk associated with each hazardous situation is estimated or measured.

2 *Risk evaluation*: a judgement is made as to whether the level of risk is acceptable/tolerable or whether some corrective/preventive actions are needed.

As discussed in Chapter 6, following any modification in the machine design or operation/maintenance procedures, there is a need to verify

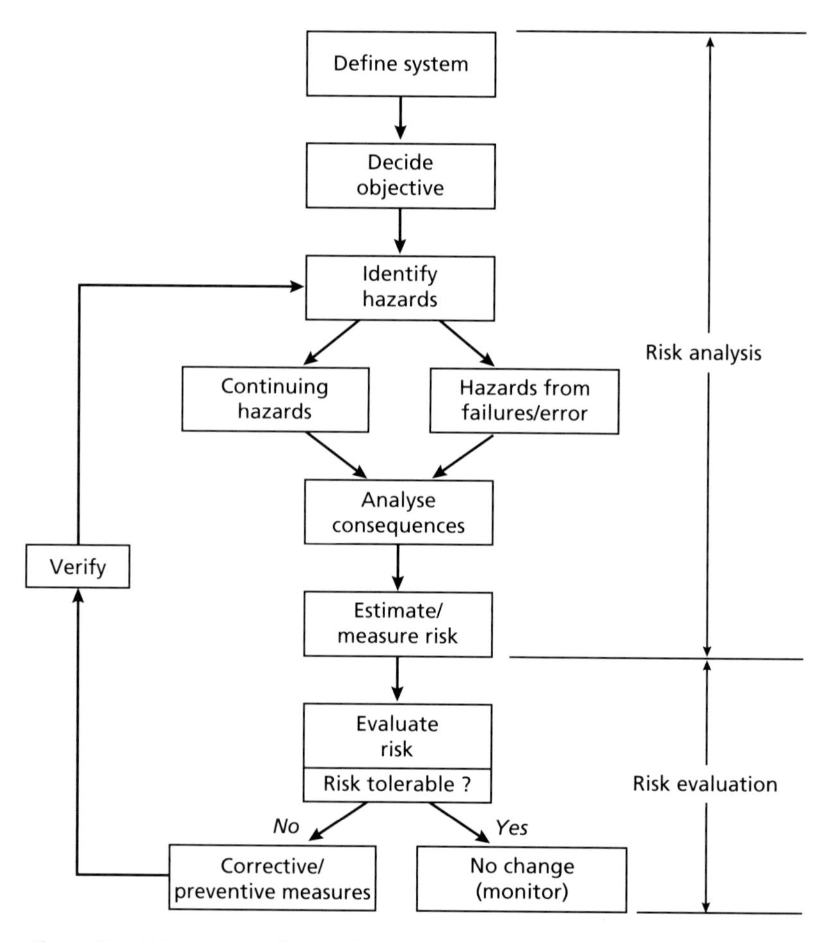

Figure 10.1 Risk assessment framework.

that the original hazards/hazardous situations are controlled, and that the risk assessment is updated as a result of design/procedural evolution. The risk assessment should be viewed as a living system, capable of learning from the experience of the individuals who run it, and should reflect what is actually taking place, and not what should happen.

Define the system/activity

The first step in any risk assessment is to provide a detailed description of the process/activity being studied. This description is needed at this stage in order to avoid confusion at a later stage, and to define the boundary and interfaces with other processes/activities. This step also involves the identification of the design objectives, material being handled/processed and exposure patterns for individuals involved in operation and maintenance.

Define the study objective

Because risk assessment is used as a means of demonstrating compliance with a number of regulations, it is important to limit the study to the range of hazards and potential consequences in relation to specific requirements, e.g. the Control of Substances Hazardous to Health (COSHH) Regulations, Noise at Work Regulations, Management of Health and Safety at Work Regulations, health and safety or economic risks.

Hazard identification

Having defined the scope and objectives, the identification of hazards is the third, but most important, step in any risk assessment study, because omitting any hazard at this stage will lead to the associated risk failing to be assessed. Hazard is defined as the potential to cause injury or damage to health. It is important in this respect to distinguish between continuing hazards (those inherent in the work activity/equipment under normal conditions) and those which can result from failures/error (e.g. hardware/software failures, as well as foreseeable human error). A brief summary of hazard identification techniques is provided below (for a more detailed discussion, see Chapter 6).

There are several qualitative approaches to hazard identification which provide a more formalized and structured procedure. The selection of the appropriate procedure will depend on the type of machine/process and the hazards involved. Procedures may range from simple checklists to a more open-ended approach. Checklists (Table 10.1) may be used to identify continuing hazards, while more open-ended techniques may be needed to identify and analyse failures and error. Hazards resulting from equipment failure and human error require the following:

1 A detailed hazard identification to be carried out for all stages of the

Table 10.1 Example of hazard identification checklist.

Type of hazards	Source	Task involved (who and when exposed?)
1 *Mechanical hazards*		
1.1 Crushing		
1.2 Shearing		
1.3 Cutting/severing		
1.4 Entanglement		
1.5 Drawing-in/trapping		
1.6 Impact		
1.7 Stabbing/puncture		
1.8 Friction/abrasion		
1.9 High pressure fluid injection		
1.10 Slips/trips/falls		
1.11 Falling/moving object		
1.12 Other mechanical hazards		
2 *Electrical hazards*		
2.1 Direct contact		
2.2 Indirect contact		
2.3 Electrostatic phenomena		
2.4 Short circuit/overload		
2.5 Source of ignition		
2.6 Other electrical hazards		
3 *Radiation hazards*		
3.1 Lasers		
3.2 Electromagnetic effects		
3.3 Ionizing/non-ionizing radiation		
3.4 Other radiation hazards		
4 *Hazardous substances*		
4.1 Toxic fluids		
4.2 Toxic gas/mist/fumes/dust		
4.3 Flammable fluids		
4.4 Flammable gas/mist/fumes/dust		
4.5 Explosive substances		
4.6 Biological substances		
4.7 Other hazardous substances		
5 *Work activity hazards*		
5.1 Highly repetitive actions		
5.2 Stressful posture		
5.3 Lifting/handling		
5.4 Mental overload/stress		
5.5 Visual fatigue		
5.6 Poor workplace design		
5.7 Other workplace hazards		

Continued

Table 10.1 *Continued.*

Type of hazards	Source	Task involved (who and when exposed?)
6 *Work environment hazards*		
6.1 Localized hot surfaces		
6.2 Localized cold surfaces		
6.3 Significant noise		
6.4 Significant vibration		
6.5 Poor lighting		
6.6 Hot/cold ambient temperature		
6.7 Other work environment hazards		

machine lifecycle. This ideally should include the identification of contributory causes for each hazard.

2 Analysis of systems of work and established procedures to identify who might be exposed to a hazard and when, e.g. operator under normal conditions, maintenance/tool fitter/cleaner, etc.

Following a review of the process or activity, a checklist may be used to identify the type of hazard, the source of the hazard, who may be exposed to the particular hazard (operator, maintenance, cleaner) and when.

Structured and systematic techniques which would assist in the identification of hazards might include the following, the procedures of which are discussed in Chapter 6.

- *Hazard and operability (HAZOP) study*: a qualitative technique to identify hazards resulting from hardware failures and human error (see example below).
- *Failure mode and effect analysis (FMEA)*: an inductive technique to identify and analyse hardware failures. A quantitative technique.
- *Task analysis*: an inductive technique to identify human error.

Analysis of the consequences

Consequence analysis is the process of describing and quantifying the relationship between the exposure to a hazard and the resulting adverse health effects, including fatalities, illness or injuries. The nature of the health effect can be minor and temporary, or severe and permanent. Health effects in an individual resulting from exposure to a given toxic substance will depend on a number of factors, including the level of exposure, frequency of exposure, exposure route(s), toxicity of substance (acute and chronic effects), metabolism, target organ(s) and control methods used to minimize exposure to the hazard. In addition, individual factors, such as age, sex, lifestyle, health status, diet and the individual's natural defence mechanisms, may also influence the effect of exposure. The health effect most frequently considered in consequence analysis is death; however, other health effects which are often estimated fall into one of four categories: cancer, reproductive effects, clinical effects and subclinical effects.

In the case of mechanical hazards, it is relatively easy to analyse their consequences in terms of injury severity. It is in situations in which a major fire or explosion may be identified as high risk that structured techniques may be needed to systematically follow the consequences in terms of whether people can escape in time or whether an overpressure can cause fatal injury. In such cases, an inductive technique, event tree analysis (ETA), may be used. However, for the vast majority of consequences relating to machinery hazards, HAZOP studies and FMEA are capable of providing such analysis.

Example. HAZOP study (feed supply system to a process reactor). A light hydrocarbon reagent is pumped from a nitrogen-blanketed storage tank into another nitrogen-blanketed buffer tank (T-1), which supplies the process reactor. A HAZOP study is conducted to identify the potential hazards and consequences of exposure.

A piping and instrument diagram (P&ID) is shown in Fig. 10.2. This is a typical HAZOP diagram as it shows the basic instrumentation of the process. These instruments include: pressure indicator (PI), pressure indicator controller (PIC) and flow indicator controller (FIC). To start the analysis, the process is divided into lines and vessels: storage tank (T-1), pumping line (L-1) and line (L-2). Starting with T-1, guide words such as 'more', 'less', etc. (explanation given in Chapter 6) are applied

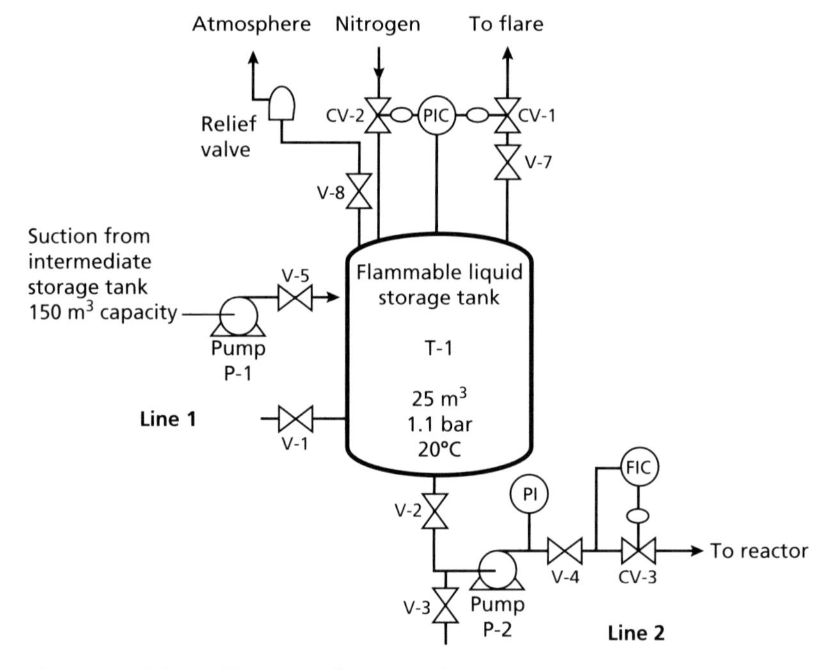

Figure 10.2 Piping and instrument diagram for the process.

as shown in Table 10.2. It should be noted that the guide words are not applied to all process intentions—only to level, composition and pressure in order to demonstrate the technique. A column headed 'action required' is included to list potential hazards, questions which need to be resolved as well as possible mitigating measures.

The notes on the worksheets can then be identified and classified into categories according to hazardous outcomes, and whether these relate to safety or operational problems. In some cases, more detailed design or process information may be required, whereas in others flammable release rates may have to be estimated. For example, deviations 3 (V-3 open or broken) and 4 (V-1 open or broken) would both result in similar reagent release rates. However, as V-3 could be isolated by closing V-2, the release time—and thus the total quantity released—could be minimized. On the other hand, if V-1 were broken, the entire tank

Table 10.2 Results of HAZOP study of proposed flammable reagent storage. HAZOP worksheet for storage tank T-1 (storing flammable reagent at 1.1 bar and 20°C).

Guide word	Deviation	Possible causes	Consequences	Action required
More	Level	1 Pump P-1 fails to stop	Reagent released	Incorporate high level alarm and trip
		2 Reverse from process	Reagent released	Consider check valve line 2
Less		3 Pump P-1 cavitates	Damage to P-1	Can reagent explode? If pump overheats?
		4 Rupture in line 2	Reagent released	Consider alarm and pump shutdown
		5 V-3 open	Reagent released	Consider alarm
		6 V-1 open	Same	Same
		7 Tank rupture	Same	What external events can cause rupture?
No		Same as less		
Other than	Composition	8 Wrong reagent	Possible reaction	Is reagent sampled before pumping?
As well as		9 Impurity in reagent	Possible overpressure, if volatile	What are the possible impurities?
Less	Pressure	10 Break in flare or nitrogen lines	Reagent released	Consider low pressure alarm
		11 Loss of nitrogen	Tank implodes	What is design vacuum of tank?
		12 CV-2 fails closed	Tank implodes	
		13 PIC fails	Tank implodes	
More		14 PIC fails	Reagent released via relief valve	What is capacity of CV-1?
		15 CV-1 fails closed	Reagent released via relief valve	
		16 V-7 closed	Same as 15	Is V-7 locked open?
		17 Overfill tank	See 6	Is V-8 locked open?

contents would be released. The information from the HAZOP study can then be used to prepare an action plan based on the proposed corrective measures. These measures should be primarily aimed at preventing the hazard occurring in the first place by design/technical changes. If this is not practicable, safe systems of work should be considered and developed. The last line of defence would be to mitigate the consequences should a hazard occur, e.g. to rely upon alarms, evacuation and personal protective equipment.

Although HAZOP studies and FMEA are valuable in identifying and analysing the consequences of exposure to hazards, in the majority of cases, the consequences of a hazard being realized may be straightforward, and may be classified broadly in terms of:

- injury or damage to health (employees, contractors);
- injury or damage to health (third party, e.g. public, contractors, visitors, others);
- economic consequences (damage to equipment/plant, interruption to production);
- public and media reaction to incidents/accidents on/off site;
- effects on the environment (e.g. temporary, widespread damage).

Estimation/measurement of risk

The estimation or measurement of risk is vital, if risk is to be evaluated. Risk is defined as the chance or probability of exposure to a hazard, combined with the consequences of such exposure. Risk estimates are sometimes formulated as a statement of frequency, i.e. an average number of events to be expected over a specified time; such measures of risk are most suitable where a large amount of evidence or data exists. Thus, we may express the probability of death in the oil and gas industry as 1 in 600 per person per year for offshore activities and 8 in 100 000 per person per year for onshore activities. This description is known as quantified risk.

When estimating or measuring risk, there will always be a certain degree of uncertainty associated with the determination. Uncertainty can be defined as the deficiency in knowledge relevant to the decision-making process, and is usually associated with either the volume or the quality of data collected or made available. One way of reducing the level of uncertainty is to develop and test appropriate models to evaluate hypotheses of what would happen under certain conditions. However, uncertainties will always be attached to any estimate of risk, as no model fully reflects reality. The models used to estimate workplace exposure (such as the Monte Carlo method) and the associated uncertainties are discussed in Chapter 9. A more detailed account of the methods used to estimate and analyse uncertainty is provided by Covello and Merkhofer (1993).

Risk may be defined in qualitative, semiquantitative or quantitative terms:

- *qualitative*: no figures; judgement is used to estimate the risk level;
- *semiquantitative*: risks may be ranked on a comparative scale or by using a risk matrix;
- *quantitative*: risks may be described as a frequency of death.

An example of a risk matrix is shown in Fig. 10.3. This risk matrix, intended to estimate risk on a semiquantitative basis, gives a clear definition of risk. If it is estimated that the chance of the operator being exposed to an explosion hazard is remote, but this exposure will result in a fatality, the matrix shows this risk level as 'B'. If, on the other hand, it was decided to quantify risk, it might be possible, for example, to describe the chance of individual risk as a result of exposure to a hazard resulting in a fatality. It is also possible to describe other forms of risk on the same basis. These include societal risk, environmental risk and economic risk.

Evaluation of risks

One of the most important steps in risk assessment is to evaluate risks, i.e. to determine whether the level of risk is tolerable, or unacceptably high and warrants some urgent attention. In order to define these levels, risk criteria (standards) need to be developed which may represent the view, usually of the regulator, of how much risk is acceptable/tolerable. Examples of such standards include occupational exposure limits, noise action levels, biological exposure indices and radiation dose. In other situations, it may be possible to compare the level of risk with existing codes of practice, or existing situations for similar activities, or indeed to set one's own risk target for acceptability.

The risk criteria usually fall into three categories: (i) *comparative or equity based*, where the standard is what is held to be usually acceptable in normal life, or refers to some other premise held to establish an expectation of protection; (ii) *cost–benefit analysis based*, where some

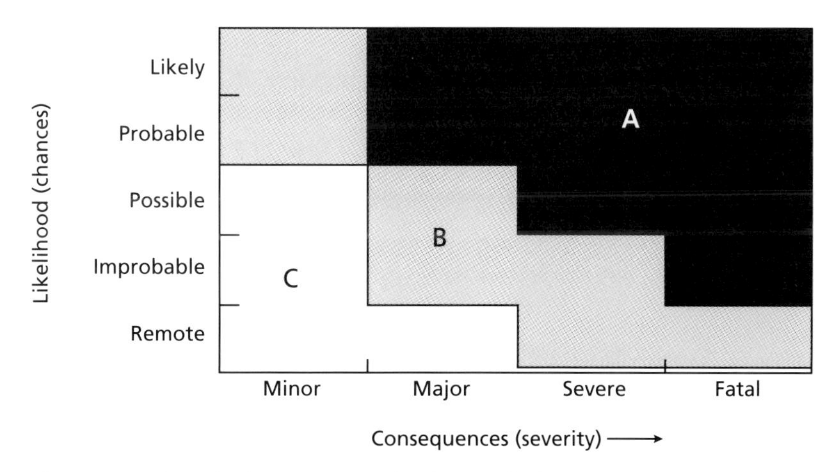

Figure 10.3 Criteria for the estimation and evaluation of risk.

direct comparison is made between a value placed on the risk of ill health and the cost of risk reduction/prevention measures; and (iii) *technology based*, which essentially reflects the idea that a satisfactory level of risk prevention is attained when relevant best or 'state-of-the-art' technology is employed.

The most widely used criteria for the evaluation of quantified risks in the UK are the risk criteria proposed by the Health and Safety Executive (HSE): *Tolerability of Risk from Nuclear Power Stations* (HSE 1992). Although the report concentrates on nuclear power, it has influenced the development of risk assessment in other fields. The report defines concepts (see Fig. 10.4) of:

- an 'intolerable' level of risk, at or above which immediate action to reduce the risk or terminate the activity is called for, irrespective of the cost;
- a broadly 'acceptable' level, at or below which further reduction measures are not required;
- a middle region, where additional risk reduction measures are necessary until the overall cost becomes grossly disproportionate to the risk reduction produced. This is classed as 'as low as reasonably practicable (ALARP)'.

As shown in Fig. 10.3, the three-tier framework sets the limit for the maximum tolerable risk of a fatal accident to a worker in a hazardous industry at 1 in 1000 per person per year, and the maximum tolerable level of risk for killing one member of the public as 1 in 10 000 per

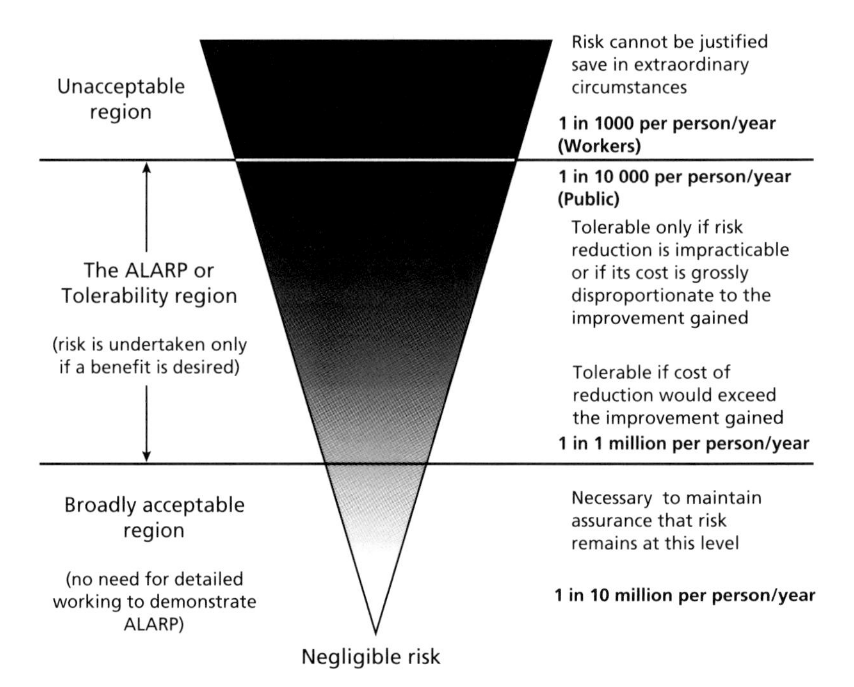

Figure 10.4 UK criteria for the tolerability of risk.

person per year. The level of acceptable risk is 1 in a million or below per person per year, when no further action is necessary.

The HSE criteria deal largely with fatal accidents, but stipulate that all risks should be reduced to a level ALARP. The ALARP principle may be taken for all practicable purposes as indistinguishable from 'ALARA' (as low as reasonably achievable, which still applies in radiation protection) and from the injunction 'so far as is reasonably practicable' (SFAIRP). All these injunctions are taken for purposes of regulations to mean that the cost of each incremental opportunity should be set against the presumed benefit in terms of the avoidance of injury (HSE 1995).

The evaluation of risk will depend on the method used to estimate the risk. Risk evaluation can be carried out qualitatively, semiquantitatively or quantitatively:

- *qualitative*: judgement is used, difficult to prioritize;
- *semiquantitative*: decide which area of the risk matrix represents intolerable risk;
- *quantitative*: use a target for the tolerability of risk if a fatal accident can result from exposure to the hazard.

The risk matrix shown in Fig. 10.3 is an example of a tool used to estimate as well as evaluate risks on a semiquantitative basis. The level of risk will determine the urgency of corrective and preventive measures.

- Risk level 'A' is regarded as 'intolerable'. The relevant activity cannot be justified on any grounds.
- Risk level 'B' is a region of uncertainty. Risk assessment is needed to ensure that risks in this region are ALARP.
- Risk level 'C' is 'broadly tolerable'. No further action is necessary.

The risk calculator

There are several drawbacks with the criteria described so far for the estimation and evaluation of risks, as they either focus attention on potential fatal accidents or they miss out a vital component in the measurement of risk. This is the proportion of time a person(s) is exposed to the hazard.

The risk calculator (Fig. 10.5) was developed to provide a semiquantitative tool for the rapid screening of risks, in order to focus attention on risk levels which are intolerable. The calculator also has the ability to compare several types of risk, including individual, societal, economic and environmental, on the same scale. It is important to note that the risk calculator does not pretend to be entirely accurate, and it must be borne in mind that the main objective of its development is the ranking of risks rather than to provide criteria for risk tolerability.

The risk calculator (Raafat 1995) is a tool developed for the screening of risks resulting from work machinery and equipment. It is intended as a rapid guide to the evaluation of the level of risks, or to decide which risks warrant more detailed risk assessment. One of the main

Consequences	I	II	III	IV	V	VI
Personnel	Insignificant	Minor	Major	Severe	Fatality	Multiple fatalities
Economic	< £1000	< £10 000	< £100 000	< £1 million	> £1 million	Total loss
Environment	Minor	Short-term damage	Major	Severe	Widespread damage	Catastrophe

Analysis of the consequences

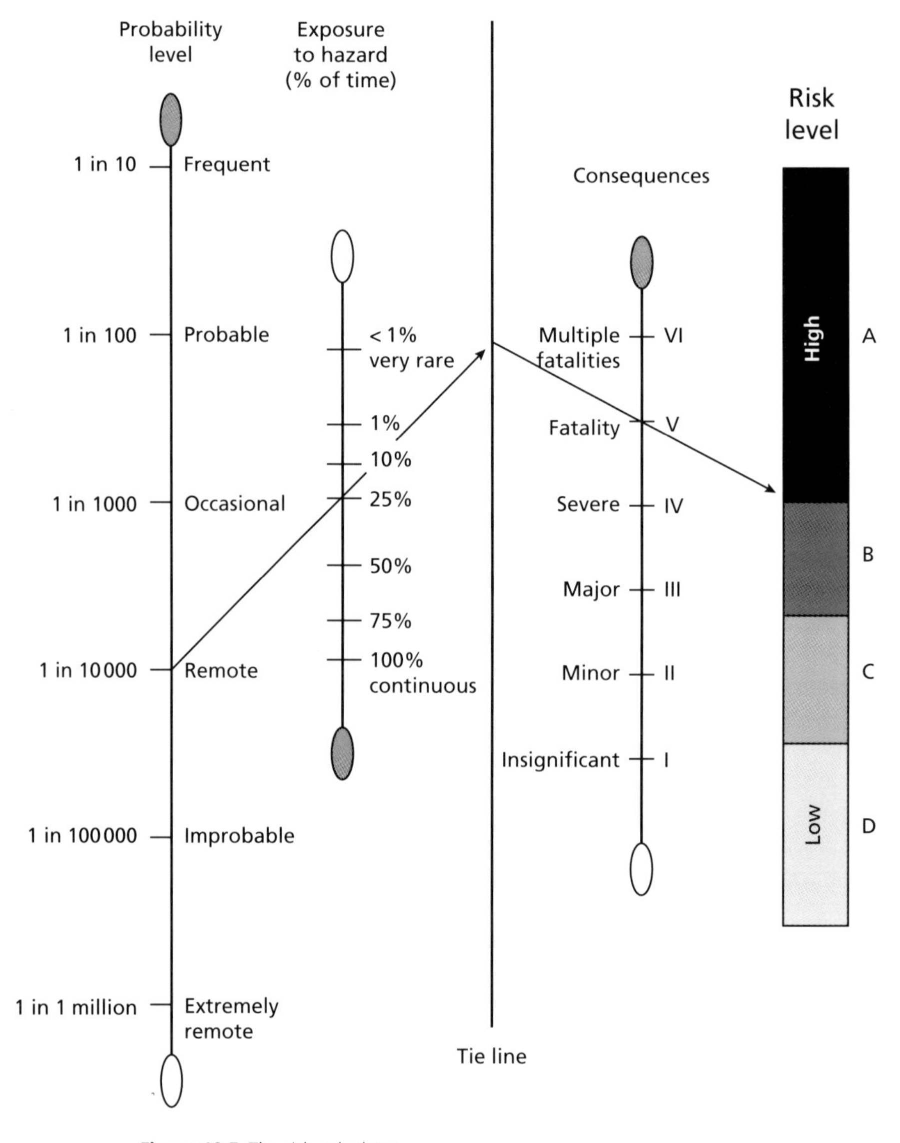

Figure 10.5 The risk calculator.

differences between the risk calculator and other risk matrices is that the calculator takes into account the frequency and duration of exposure to a hazard. The risk calculator is primarily based on a normogram introduced in the British Standard (BS) 5304 (Safeguarding of Machinery) (British Standards Institution (BSI) 1988).

The basic elements in calculating the order of magnitude of risk are (see Fig. 10.5):

- the likelihood of occurrence of a hazard ('probability level')—this ranges from frequent, or 1 in 10, to extremely remote, or 1 in a million; the probabilities are used to describe the order of magnitude of probable, remote, etc.;
- the frequency and duration of exposure to the hazard—this is measured on a scale ranging from very rare, or less than 1%, to continuous exposure, i.e. 100% of the time;
- the consequences or potential severity of injury/damage, measured on a scale ranging from category I, i.e. minor loss/first aid, to category VI, i.e. multiple fatalities/total loss, etc.

By connecting the appropriate points on each scale and using the tie line in the middle of the calculator, it is possible to determine the level of risk involved. The risk level is divided into four general categories:

- high risk (A), which indicates that the level of risk is unacceptable and cannot be justified on any grounds;
- substantial risk (B), which indicates that the level of risk should be reduced to a level as low as reasonably practicable: 'ALARP';
- moderate risk (C), which indicates that the risk is tolerable if the cost of reduction would exceed the improvement gained;
- low risk (D), which indicates that the level of risk is broadly acceptable and no further precautions should be necessary.

If the level of risk falls between high and low, it must be reduced to the lowest practicable level, bearing in mind the benefits flowing from its acceptance and the cost of any further reduction. As mentioned previously, the injunction laid down in general safety law is that any risk must be reduced as far as reasonably practicable, or to a level that is 'ALARP'. The area between the levels A and D represents the 'ALARP' region.

The HSE criteria for the tolerability of risk relate to individual risk (IR), which can be obtained using the following formula:

$$\mathrm{IR} = C \times T \times P \qquad (10.1)$$

where C is the chance of exposure to a hazard, T is the proportion of time exposed to the hazard and P is the probability that the exposure will result in death. The risk calculator is calibrated using HSE's ALARP criteria in relation to IR as follows:

1 If the hazard is present 100% of the time at work, and if an employee works 8 hours a day and 5 days a week, the proportion of time exposed to the hazard is approximately 25%.

2 If the annual chance of the hazard being realized is 1 in 1000 per year

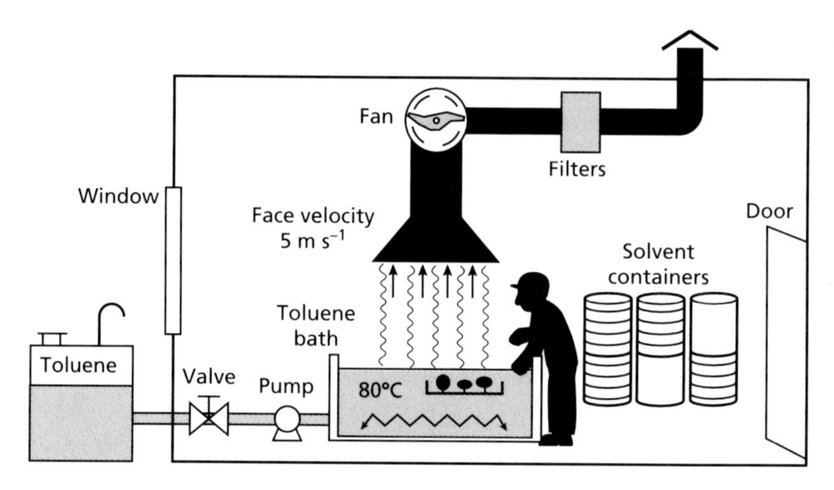

Figure 10.6 Metal cleaning shop with controls following COSHH assessment.

and it was assumed that the employee is certain to be killed, then this should correspond with the maximum tolerable level of risk (top of risk level B).

3 If the chance of the hazard being realized is 1 in 1 million per year, then this would represent the limit of 'broadly acceptable' risk (top of risk level D).

Example. Risk assessment using the risk calculator. The process of metal degreasing involves the use of toluene (Fig. 10.6). Special valves are placed in a basket and then dipped in a heated toluene bath (80°C) which is ventilated using a local exhaust ventilation (LEV) system. The metal cleaning shop is also used for the storage of chemical drums which contain toluene for topping up the bath. Toluene has a boiling point of 111°C, flash point of 4°C and explosive limits of 1.3–7.0%.

A structured and systematic risk assessment can be workplace based, activity based, or both. For example, the analysis of the ventilation system and the cleaning tank is workplace based, while tasks such as filling both tanks and dipping the valve basket into the cleaning tank are activity based. The hazard identification and analysis worksheets, shown in Tables 10.3 and 10.4, are examples of a more open-ended approach to risk assessment. Table 10.3 analyses the metal cleaning shop ventilation system, and evaluates the risks associated with potential hardware failures and human error. The risk levels identified in the table are obtained using the risk calculator.

For example, the risk associated with ventilation power failure is estimated as follows.

- The probability of power failure is judged as occasional (1 in 1000).
- The proportion of time the operator is inside the shop is about 8 h per day and 5 days per week. This would result in exposure to the hazard 25% of his/her time.
- The consequences of exposure to an increase in the toxic/flammable

Table 10.3 Example of hazard identification and analysis worksheet (equipment based).

Machine/process/activity: Metal cleaning shop — Hazard analysis study reference

Activity type	Hazardous events, error/failure	Possible causes	Consequences
Ventilation system: to extract toluene vapour emitted from metal cleaning tank (face velocity, 5 m s^{-1})	Loss of ventilation	Power failure	Increased toxic and flammable concentration
		Filter blocked	Same as above
		Flue blocked	Same as above
		Ducting blocked	Same as above
		Fan bearing seizes	Fire/explosion
	Reduced flow	Corrosion of blades	Increased concentration (toxic and flammable)
		Leakages from ducts	Same as above
		Door + window open	Operator exposed to high concentration
		Filter partly blocked	Increased concentration
	Flow reversed	Fan incorrectly fitted	Same as above
		Incorrect wiring of fan	Same as above

Table 10.4 Example of hazard identification and analysis worksheet (activity based).

Machine/process/activity: Metal cleaning shop — Hazard analysis study reference

Activity type	Hazardous events, error/failure	Possible causes	Consequences
Filling cleaning tank with toluene	Overfilling tank	Operator does not switch pump off	Increased toxic and flammable concentration
		Pump fails to stop (electrical fault)	Same as above
Switch tank heater on	Toluene overheated	Thermostat fails	Major fire
	Toluene not heated	Thermocouple fails	Valves not cleaned
Dipping metallic components inside cleaning tank	Operator falls in tank	Loss of stability	Fatality
	Too many valves put in basket	Cut down cleaning time	Valves fall into tank/upper limb disorder
	Toluene may be contaminated	Tank topped up with other chemical	Possible reaction
		Delivery of toluene already contaminated	Possible high level of benzene, water, etc.
	Tank may leak	Lack of maintenance	Exposure to high concentrations
		Impact by mobile equipment	Same as above

concentration of toluene are judged to be severe (an ignition source is also needed to cause a fire), and the operator may be able to escape.

The risk calculator is used to convert these estimates into risk level B (Fig. 10.5). This risk level falls within the 'ALARP' region, and should warrant some action based on cost–benefit analysis.

Table 10.4 shows an example of an activity-based risk assessment. This approach will follow the operator throughout his/her tasks, and attempt to identify various hazards associated with each step of the task. For example, when the operator fills the tank with toluene, he/she will depress a start push-button. If the operator forgets to switch off the pump, the tank could overflow. The tank could also overflow due to an electrical failure in the pump start/stop mechanism.

The hazard identification and analysis tables propose certain corrective and preventive measures, which can be prioritized according to the level of risk. Following this assessment, there is a need to prepare an action plan in which these corrective and preventive measures should be implemented, controlled and monitored through a 'living' risk management system. As discussed previously, there are more structured and systematic techniques available for carrying out a risk assessment, e.g. HAZOP studies, but the degree of detail and depth of the assessment should be proportional to the level of risk and degree of interaction between individuals and the process.

Conclusions

Risk characterization is the final step in the risk assessment process which can be used to provide and develop control strategies. If the risk criteria used suggest that the level of risk is intolerable, corrective or preventive measures will be required to reduce the probability of occurrence of the hazard (by improving the system reliability) and/or to mitigate the consequences should the hazard occur. It is important, however, to ensure that, as a result of corrective measures, not only are all existing hazards controlled, but no new hazards are introduced into the process. If it is decided that the risk is acceptable/tolerable, it is important to ensure that the existing situation does not change by following up and continuously monitoring the system.

Following the risk assessment, which is at the heart of risk management, a package of control measures should be identified in order to reduce significant risks. The next step is to implement the action plan, i.e. to carry out the design changes and/or procedural development. There is a need at this stage to train personnel on new modifications and procedures and to organize the plan. The action plan needs to be controlled, i.e. by identifying who is responsible for the implementation and at what level within the organization. There will be a need to monitor the action plan. This is to ensure that the plan is working as intended. A range of reactive and proactive mechanisms are needed to ensure that targets are met. Finally, there will be a need to audit/review the system in order to incorporate a feedback mechanism for possible changes/modifications as a result of experience gained. Practical examples of the implementation of action plans are included in BS 8800 (*Guide to Occupational Health and Safety Management Systems*) (BSI 1996).

References

BSI (1988) *Code of Practice: Safeguarding of Machinery*. BS 5304. BSI, London.

BSI (1996) *Guide to Occupational Health and Safety Management Systems*. BS 8800. BSI, London.

Covello, V.T. & Merkhofer, M.W. (1993) *Risk Assessment Methods—Approaches for Assessing Health and Environmental Risks*. Plenum, New York.

HSE (1992) *The Tolerability of Risk from Nuclear Power Stations*. HMSO, London.

HSE (1995) *Generic Terms and Concepts in the Assessment and Regulation of Industrial Risks*. HSE Books, Sudbury, Suffolk.

Raafat, H. (1995) *Machinery Safety—The Risk Based Approach*. Technical Communications (Publishing), London.

Section 3 Risk management

Chapter 11 Prevention and control of exposures

Frank Gill

Introduction

Having decided that the risk of exposure is unacceptable and that some form of control is necessary, the options are wide within a limited framework of: (i) *software* methods; and (ii) *hardware* methods (Gill & Alesbury 1998). Software methods refer to management solutions, without resorting to the purchase of hardware, and are also known as organizational methods. Hardware methods include engineering aspects of control (Boleij *et al.* 1995). Within British legislation (Control of Substances Hazardous to Health (COSHH) Regulations 1988 and 1994), the methods are listed in what has become commonly known in the UK as the 'COSHH hierarchy'. As a general rule, the software/organizational solutions come at the top of the list, and are always preferred to the hardware/engineering solutions, which are not only expensive to purchase and run, but can be prone to breakdown and misuse. This chapter describes examples of both software and hardware methods of control, as well as their management.

Control techniques and applications

The greatest risk of exposure occurs when a substance is handled or transferred from one place to another. For example, raw materials are delivered to a process and must be transferred from the supplier to the user; once in the process, raw materials may be transferred from one part of the process to another. Often, the final products have to be packaged in bags, sacks, drums, bottles and the like. Normally, when materials are enclosed in a container, whether a bulk container, a 25-l drum or a paper sack, they are under control; it is not until they are disturbed or moved that the risk is run.

The degree of risk, in this case, will depend upon the type of enclosure: the probability that a paper sack will split is greater than the probability that a drum will be punctured or tipped over when open, which, in turn, is greater than the probability that a bulk container will leak. Thus the choice of handling and packaging method has a large bearing upon the risk of exposure, a decision which is best made at the design stage of the process. Unfortunately, some production engineers have little concept of the hazardous nature of the substances to be used, and may choose a handling method that is best for production but less good for the health of the operators. When the process is in production and the health risk is discovered, they protest that had they known they would have designed the process differently. Thus, an occupational health input to any design process is essential, and access to a health professional with a good knowledge of production processes and engineering methods is invaluable in this regard.

Software/organizational solutions

Software solutions can be listed in order of preference as follows:
- complete elimination of the process that leads to the exposure;
- complete elimination of the substance(s) causing the risk;
- substitution by a less toxic substance;
- substitution by the same substance, but in a form that reduces the risk of exposure;
- designing or redesigning the process so that exposure is minimized;
- suppressing the substance;
- other software methods.

These will be discussed in turn.

The *complete elimination of a process* is normally out of the question. If the operation is not necessary, it will not be performed; however, if the risk is particularly high, it may be worth buying in this stage of the process by subcontracting to another operator. This could be seen as passing the buck but, if proper control measures are likely to become excessively costly, it may be a financially viable option.

The *complete elimination of the substance* may well be possible. An example can be cited in which a product has to be painted for aesthetic or anticorrosion reasons. Most paints contain a mixture of volatile solvents formulated to achieve the correct surface finish at an optimum drying rate, and it is the solvent that provides the greatest risk of exposure. Eliminating the solvent will remove the hazard. Surface coatings can be applied dry, adhesion to the coated surface being achieved by electrostatic means or by applying the coating as a plasma. An added advantage is that the supplier has also eliminated the solvent. Such an expedient will have to be balanced against the increased risk of exposure to the dry material, which will be more liable to become airborne.

The *substitution by a less toxic substance* is a feasible solution. In the case of paints, it may well be possible to use less toxic solvents or even water. Much research has been devoted to the development of water-based finishes in the motor industry, hitherto a large user of solvent-based paints. Many cars are now finished using paints that contain as much as 50% water (S. Shackleton, personal communication, 1996). Reductions in exhaust emissions from underground diesel engines have been shown to occur when the fuel used is substituted for one with a lower sulphur content (Rogers *et al.* 1993). This has resulted in a 44% reduction in diesel particulates passing into the mine ventilation system. Degreasing and cleaning solvents have been under consideration; various changes have taken place over several years to find less toxic and more environmentally satisfactory cleaning solvents. Even the use of a solvent with a lower vapour pressure (see Chapter 5) will reduce the rate of evaporation, and hence the risk of exposure, if it can be shown to fulfil its function equally well.

The *substitution by the same substance, but in a form that reduces the risk of exposure* can make a significant contribution to the control of airborne substances. Many raw materials are produced in powdered form which, when transferred from one place to another, can result in dusty conditions being created. Often it is unnecessary for the substance to be in powdered form when pellets or tablets are equally satisfactory, but far less dusty. It is always worth examining the reasons why a raw material is supplied in powdered form to establish whether it can be substituted for a less dusty form and whether the supplier is prepared to change the form. Most suppliers are prepared to co-operate for fear of losing the order to a competitor. Where the process involves dissolving the powder in a solvent, as in paint making, or into water, e.g. in food manufacture, a pelleted form would normally be just as satisfactory.

Designing or redesigning the process so that exposure is minimized. Often without making any changes to the substances used, improvements in exposure can be generated by making simple adjustments to the way in which the job is performed. Significant reductions in exposure were shown in vehicle windscreen manufacture by making small changes in the layout of the workstation and the operator's work procedure (Piney *et al.* 1988).

When liquids, such as solvents, are transferred from a bulk tank into containers at the final packaging end of a manufacturing process, vapours are released due to turbulence from the discharge hose and emission of the headspace above the surface. If these sources can be reduced or eliminated, the risks will be decreased. The end of the filling hose can be placed at the bottom of the container to be filled; thus, for most of the time, it will be below the liquid surface, thus reducing the turbulence. The vapour-laden air venting out of the container can be directed back into the bulk tank replacing equally the volume of liquid discharged. This will involve a double tube arrangement, where one tube handles the liquid to be filled and the other handles the discharged air. If the connections can be made reasonably airtight, no emissions will occur during the filling operation. These alternatives are illustrated in Fig. 11.1.

The delivery of powders is often made via paper sacks, each holding perhaps 25 kg of material. They arrive on a pallet occupying a volume of approximately 1 m^3. Each sack is individually emptied by slitting open the top and hand tipping into a hopper; the empty sack is then dropped onto the floor to form a pile as the loading process continues. Eventually, the pile becomes too high, and has to be compressed to accommodate more empty sacks; finally, the sacks have to be removed for disposal. At each stage of the operation, dust will be released into

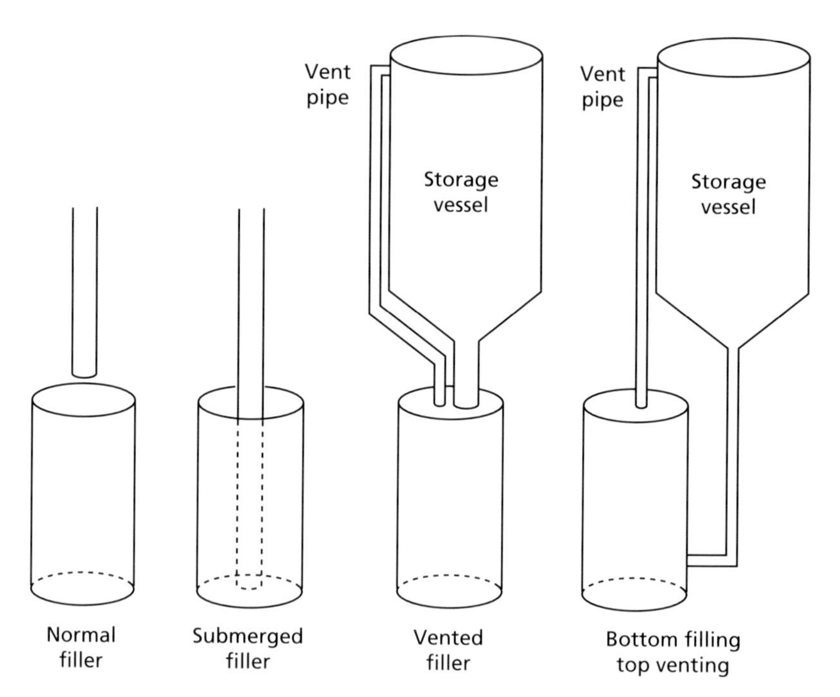

Figure 11.1 Alternative methods for drum filling.

the breathing zone of the operator. Sadly, such procedures are common, but unnecessary, as the operation can be better designed.

Several options are open to redesign the process. The material can be delivered in bulk bags with a small filler/discharge tube at the top through which the bag is filled by the supplier; this tube is tied closed. To empty the bag, it is inverted over the hopper, which is totally enclosed, but has a spigot at the top to which the tube can be positively attached. When connected the tie is undone and the powder is allowed to fall into the hopper with no release of dust. This technique is illustrated in Fig. 11.2. The bulk bag can be returned to the supplier for refilling, thus saving the need for paper sacks and the associated disposal problem. Negotiations will be needed to persuade the supplier to change to bulk bags, but, if successfully achieved, the supplier will also benefit by only having to fill one large bag rather than many small ones and by reducing his/her own dust problems. If negotiations fail, there is another alternative. Purpose built paper sack emptying machines are available which handle the splitting, emptying and disposal of the bags under total enclosure with negative pressure ventilation. In certain processes, it is possible to make the bags of an inert soluble material, which can be dropped into the process unopened, but which will dissolve releasing their contents without the emission of dust.

Suppressing the substance can be achieved in a variety of ways. Water is commonly used as a dust suppressant and can be applied in certain

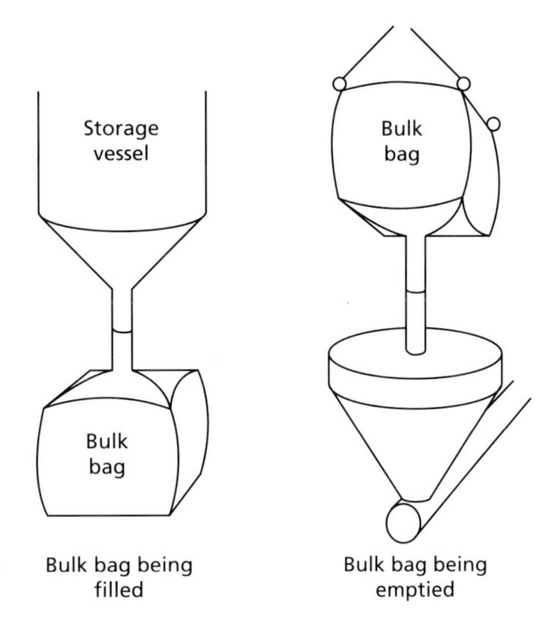

Figure 11.2 Use of bulk bag to minimize dust emissions.

situations. For example, in the stripping of asbestos lagging, presoaking of the material with water will entrap the fibres, thereby minimizing emission. In coal mining, water infusion is used to prewet the *in situ* coal before it is stripped from the coal face. This is done by drilling 50-mm diameter holes into the unworked coal, inserting a nozzle and pumping water at high pressure through the holes. Water disperses through the pores of the coal such that, when a coal cutting machine passes through, much of the dust has been suppressed. The disadvantages of both the asbestos and coal examples, apart from the cost of the machinery and labour, is that the wet material increases the humidity in what may already be a thermally unsatisfactory environment.

Surface works in mines and quarries in dry weather or in arid districts are often very dusty. To counter this, at regular intervals a water cart drives around the plant spraying water onto the ground thus laying the dust. This is only possible where a good supply of water is available, but is commonly used in mines in the outback in Australia where well water is available.

Water sprays on conveyor transfer points are used with limited success, as droplets of water are rarely successful in capturing airborne dust; however, they are more successful in damping down the dust that is lying on the conveyor.

Evaporation of vapour from volatile solvents in tanks can be suppressed by using a refrigerated strip just above the surface to create a cool layer of highly concentrated vapour, thus reducing further evaporation. In addition, surfaces of tanks can be covered with floating plastic spheres, known in some places as 'cruffles'. These allow the passage of products into and out of the tanks, but reduce the surface area available for evaporation. Low-density liquid surfactants can also be used by floating a layer on the surface of the tank.

Other software methods, such as good work procedures, training and worker awareness programmes, are important methods of control. The way in which a task is undertaken will have a bearing upon the risk of exposure and, within a group of workers undertaking the same tasks, the exposure will vary according to the method used to perform the task. Some will be careful in handling toxic materials; others will be more untidy and complacent about the hazards they are facing. Good work procedures backed up by good training and supervision will reduce the risks considerably. Regular reminders and retraining will reduce the risk of workers slipping back into bad habits.

Persuasion rather than discipline has been shown to be the best approach when encouraging workers to protect themselves (Ryckman 1990). A reduction in the duration of exposure can be used to reduce the accumulated 'dose' effect. Examination of the task will be required to establish how much time has to be spent in close proximity to the source of emission and how much can be spent in cleaner air. It may be possible to mix the tasks with other workers in less toxic surroundings, so that more workers are exposed for shorter periods of time. For example, if the worker need only spend half of his/her working shift in contact and the other half in unpolluted air, the chosen concentration for exposure can be doubled. This method is known as job rotation.

Hardware/engineering solutions

These involve total enclosures under negative pressure, partial enclosures with extract ventilation, extracted canopies, hoods or slots and general or dilution ventilation, the principles of which are described below. These devices require back-up equipment and machinery in the form of ducts and associated fittings, filters and air cleaners, fans or other prime movers and discharges to atmosphere with associated weather protection. Such solutions involving ventilation are inherently unsatisfactory in that they are difficult to design to provide good control and rely heavily on the operators using them properly (or at all) and the owners maintaining them in good working order.

It is sad to reflect that many industrial ventilation systems designed to reduce the risk of exposure to substances hazardous to health do not achieve their objective because of poor design or bad maintenance. The behaviour of air in front of suction inlets is not well understood by many designers of extract ventilation systems, despite being well understood by researchers in the field. There appears to be a gulf in communications between these two groups of people, which has only been bridged by a few designers. Most designers are ignorant of the research published in accredited scientific journals. Scientists should be encouraged to write readable accounts of their work in trade journals which are likely to be read by those in the sheet metal trade who profess to be industrial ventilation specialists.

Various types of enclosure, booth, hood, etc. are described below, with performance values quoted where applicable. Ventilation performance is defined as follows: air velocity v in metres per second ($m\,s^{-1}$), volume flow rate Q in cubic metres per second ($m^3\,s^{-1}$) and pressure p in pascals (Pa), where $1\,Pa = 1\,N\,m^{-2}$ (newton per square metre). The general equation for the volume flow rate is $Q = v \times A$, where A is the cross-sectional area of the point relating to v. If A is in square metres (m^2) and v is in $m\,s^{-1}$, Q will be in $m^3\,s^{-1}$.

Total enclosures under negative pressure

These are designed to reduce the risk of exposure from the most toxic of substances, such as cytotoxic and other drugs, radioactive materials, dangerous pathogens and very toxic substances, or for processes that produce large amounts of less toxic materials, but which need to be enclosed to minimize the nuisance. Examples of these include shot blasting and bead blasting enclosures. The pressure is maintained inside the enclosure below atmospheric pressure in order to ensure that, if the integrity of the enclosing fabric is broken, air will flow inwards so that nothing will escape to the outside. Examples of this type of device are given below.

Hot cells are used for radioactive materials; not only is a negative ventilation pressure provided, but the construction materials act as a barrier to radiation, including the observation windows. Manipulation of the work items inside is via levers operated from outside. Negative pressures are maintained by ventilation systems which discharge air via high-efficiency (HEPA) filters with radiation detectors on the discharge side. The pressure varies between 50 and 200 Pa below atmospheric, with indicators and alarms to show changes that might lead to failure.

The use of *glove boxes* allows operators to manipulate work items through flexible gloves which are sealed to apertures in the front. The negative pressures depend upon the construction materials, but are usually in the region of 25–100 Pa, the limit being the maximum the gloves or the fabric can withstand without bursting. Air flow rates are designed to ensure that, if a glove were to become detached, an inflow velocity of air exceeding $3\,m\,s^{-1}$ would be maintained. The volume flow rate required can be calculated from $Q = v \times A$, where A is the area of the glove port. Discharged air must be filtered to a high level of cleanliness depending upon the substance being handled.

Bead blasting cabinets are found in many workshops for the cleaning and polishing of items by jets of glass beads. They have replaced sand blasters which are prohibited in the UK. Access for the operator's arms is via two ports in the front, which have rubber seals through which glove-protected hands are inserted. Negative pressures are in the region of 100–200 Pa, with air flows achieving a velocity of $3\,m\,s^{-1}$ in the ports.

The volume flow rate required can be calculated from $Q = v \times A$, where A is the total area of the ports.

Shot blasting enclosures are found in foundries for fettling castings; they operate on either a batch process, where the enclosure is loaded and the doors closed, or continuously, where the castings pass through via some type of conveyor system. With the former, negative pressures of between 50 and 150 Pa can be maintained with minimal air flow. With continuous shot blasters, the integrity of the seals at the conveyor entry and exit points determines the maximum negative pressure that can be maintained, which is not normally much above 10 Pa. Air velocities through the openings should be above $2\ m\,s^{-1}$; therefore, the volume flow rate can be calculated from $Q = v \times A$, where A is the total area of the conveyor entry.

Partial enclosures with extract ventilation

These are devices in which the source of emission is enclosed on all sides, except that where access is needed; an air velocity is maintained at the opening, known as the face velocity, which must be sufficiently high to prevent the substances escaping through the opening. Typical devices of this type include spray booths and chemical fume cupboards. The face velocities chosen depend upon the energy of release of the pollutant inside the booth and can vary between 0.5 and $2.5\ m\,s^{-1}$. The lower value would be suitable for the gentle release of pollutants, typical of a laboratory fume cupboard; the higher value is more suitable for the high-energy release of paint particles in a spraying operation. The volume flow rates can be calculated from $Q = v \times A$, where A is the area of the face opening and v is the chosen face velocity.

Chemical fume cupboards used in laboratories normally have a sliding sash which pulls down over the face to reduce the area and to protect the face of the operator from possible splashes from reactions taking place within the cupboard. Changes in the position of the sash change the resistance and flow rate of the cupboard and may change the face velocity. Fume cupboard designs take this into account by fitting bypass arrangements to minimize the flow variations. When the sash is fully open all air passes through the front, but when the sash is lowered air flows through the bypass. Most fume cupboards also have a rear baffle to equalize the face velocity and to ensure good flow at the sill level.

Canopies, hoods and slots

When it is impracticable to enclose, a suction inlet has to be introduced as close as possible to the source of pollution to create sufficient air movement to draw the pollutant into the inlet.

Canopies are designed to draw air upwards, and are best suited to the capture of pollutants that naturally rise, such as hot gases. It is unwise to try to capture by means of a canopy pollutants that do not naturally tend to rise. The equation $Q = 1.4PVH$ can be used to calculate the required volume flow rate (American Conference of Governmental

Industrial Hygienists (ACGIH) 1995), where P is the perimeter of the area to be ventilated, H is the height of the canopy above the source and V is the chosen air velocity to flow around the perimeter. This can be between 0.25 and 2.5 $m\,s^{-1}$ depending upon the flow characteristics of the pollutant.

All other hoods are placed at the side or behind the source in relation to the worker, although side hoods appear to be more successful than rear hoods as they minimize the turbulence caused by the presence of the worker. The velocity required at the point of release is known as the *capture velocity*, which will vary with the momentum of the particle. Required capture velocities range from 0.25 to 10 $m\,s^{-1}$, the former being for a gently released source, such as a degreasing solvent or a painted item drying. The higher velocity is needed for a grinding wheel emitting heavy particles. Tables of capture velocities are published in various occupational hygiene texts (British Occupational Hygiene Society (BOHS) 1987; Gill 1995).

As the zone of influence of a suction inlet is essentially spherical, the face velocity will quickly decay with distance. For a circular or square hood, the velocity decays approximately inversely with the square of the distance; thus, with a circular hood, the velocity is only 10% of the face velocity one diameter away and, likewise, the velocity is 10% of the face velocity at a distance of the side dimension of a square hood. With rectangular hoods, this distance gets closer to the face the narrower the hood becomes. Various researchers (Fletcher 1977; Yousefi & Annegarn 1991; Garrison 1983) have related the dimensions of the suction inlet to the ratio of the actual velocity to the face velocity at a point distance X from the face for various dimensions of the hood. With an unflanged hood, air tends to be drawn from behind which serves no useful extract purpose; the addition of a flange increases the effectiveness of the hood (Fletcher 1978). These researchers have published equations relating the dimensions of the hood and the distance of capture to the ratio of the velocities. These equations can be inserted onto a spreadsheet computer program to give immediate face velocities and volume flows when the design parameters of the hood dimensions, capture distance and capture velocity are fed in. One worker (Fletcher 1977) provides a nomogram to assist in using his equations.

High-velocity, low-volume (HVLV) extraction is applicable to the emission of particles during the cutting, grinding and sanding of tools, where the particle is drawn directly from the point of release of the tool by a nozzle handling extremely high-velocity air. The chosen velocity must be higher than the tip speed of the tool (ACGIH 1995).

Dilution or general ventilation

This means of ventilation is applied to places where it is impracticable to use any of the above methods. It should be applied with care, and is not appropriate when the pollutant is highly toxic or is released intermittently in large amounts.

General ventilation in industrial premises is normally provided by means of roof extract fans designed to generate slow air movement through the workplace. Air enters at ground level, either by a purpose designed supply system linked with the heating or, more often, by percolating through the breaks in the building fabric unheated and unfiltered. This method of ventilation is not normally designed to dilute a particular emission, and is applicable to factory stores, general workshops and assembly areas where no significant amounts of toxic emissions occur; it may be provided in addition to some local extract ventilation.

With *dilution ventilation*, the purpose is to dilute known workplace emissions to safe concentrations where local exhaust ventilation cannot be applied. It has particular application to places in which large movable sources of emission are present. One example involves glass reinforced plastic (GRP) manufacturing shops where items are large, such as boat builders, large GRP components for the building trade (porticoes and pillars), nose cones for railway locomotives, etc. Dilution ventilation is also applicable to drying and curing rooms, where items are placed on trolley racks for drying, wheeled into one end of the room, gradually move across until dry and are removed at the other end. The method of introduction of the diluting air needs some consideration, as a high-velocity distribution through normal supply grilles may cause turbulence, which could blow concentrated pollutant into the face of the worker. A low-velocity method is preferred.

The aim should be to dilute the pollutant to a safe level before it reaches the breathing zone of any exposed person. In order to calculate the required volume flow rate to dilute the emitted substance, it is necessary to establish the rate of emission R and to select what is regarded as a safe concentration C. The selected concentration can be taken from government published standards (Health and Safety Executive (HSE) 1998) with a factor of safety applied; for example, in the UK, the HSE recommends designing to achieve about 25% of the published exposure limit (HSE 1989). The rate of emission is more difficult to obtain, and must be based on the usage of the substance being emitted. For example, in a drying room, if the items to be dried have been coated with a given amount of paint, and the volatile content of the paint is known, the amount of vapour produced during the production run can be calculated. The required volume flow rate Q is simply the ratio of R divided by C or $Q = R/C$. If C is expressed in milligrams per cubic metre ($mg\,m^{-3}$), it is useful to adjust the rate of emission R to milligrams per second ($mg\,s^{-1}$) to achieve a volume flow rate Q in $m^3\,s^{-1}$.

Example. Five kilograms of toluene-based ink, of which 80% is toluene and 20% is solids, is used in a printing process in 4 h; the printed items are dried on movable racks. How much air is required to dilute the toluene to a safe level?

Solution. The rate of emission of toluene is 80% of 5 kg in 4 h, i.e. 4 kg in 4 h, 1 kg h^{-1}, 1/3600 kg s^{-1} = 0.00028 kg s^{-1} or 280 mg s^{-1}. The chosen concentration for toluene from *EH40/98* is 191 mg m^{-3}; applying a 25% factor of safety, the chosen concentration is 48 mg m^{-3}. The required volume flow rate $Q = R/C = 280/48 = 5.83\ m^3\ s^{-1}$, say 6 $m^3\ s^{-1}$.

Displacement ventilation

Low-velocity displacement ventilation can be applied to the introduction of diluting air via very large supply grilles (1 m × 2 m) placed at floor level, introducing air at velocities not exceeding 0.2 m s^{-1}. The principle involves flooding the occupied area with clean air, which gently displaces the emissions upwards towards extract grilles or fans placed at ceiling level (Gill & Jones 1993).

Make-up air

If air is extracted and discharged to the outside, an equivalent amount of make-up air must be allowed to re-enter which, in most situations, will need to be heated and filtered. If not, air will percolate through breaks in the building fabric and enter unheated and unfiltered, and, in a tight building, will add an unnecessary restriction to flow. In a well-designed system, the make-up air can be part of the heating/air-conditioning system.

Management of control systems

Selection of controls

Earlier chapters (see Chapters 7–10) have shown how to establish whether a risk of overexposure to a toxic substance(s) exists in the workplace. A decision has to be made on whether the substance(s) requires control. An affirmative answer will pose the question: 'what methods of control are to be adopted?'. The checklist given below needs to be applied; it is based upon the 'hierarchy' covered in the first part of this chapter and poses a series of questions. If the answer is no to any question, pass to the one below.

- Do we need to undertake this task, or can we buy in or subcontract this operation?
- Do we need to use this substance?
- Can we substitute this substance for a less toxic one?
- Is the substance we are using in a form that exacerbates the exposure, or can we change the form to one that will reduce it?
- Can we suppress the substance?
- Can we redesign the process so that exposure is minimized?
- Are the operators following our written procedures?
- Are the operators supervised well enough?
- Is our training of the operators on this process satisfactory?
- Do we need to retrain the operators and their supervisors?

- Can the exposure time be reduced by moving workers to fresh air areas for part of the time?
- Can we rotate the tasks with operators in cleaner areas?

This checklist gives many options which can be tried and the exposure reassessed. If, after this exercise, exposure is still likely to be above the chosen concentration, hardware methods will have to be applied. These also have a hierarchy as follows.

- Total enclosure under negative pressure (glove boxes, closed chambers, etc.).
- Partial enclosure with local extract ventilation (booths or fume cupboards).
- Local exhaust ventilation (canopies, hoods, slots or HVLV).
- Dilution ventilation.
- General ventilation.

At this stage, it may be prudent to call in the company's ventilation expert, if one exists, or to engage a consultant. Application directly to a company of ventilation equipment suppliers may not be the wisest option, as they often have specific products to sell which they will try to adapt to the problem in question, often unsuccessfully. An experienced ventilation consultant will know the market, and can advise whether a proprietary product is suitable, or whether a more appropriate system needs to be designed. Money spent at this time may well save money later. The consultant can draw up a specification, with dimensioned sketches and the required technical performance criteria, from which tenders can be sought. Having chosen the best quotation, a contract can be drawn up holding the supplier to specific conditions with penalties for non-compliance. Sadly, many ventilation contracts are drawn up with very vague criteria from which no redress can be sought from the supplier in the event of an unsatisfactory installation.

Cost of control systems

As with most systems that improve the health and safety of workers, there are costs and benefits that may balance positively in favour of implementing the control system. The cost of controls in most cases can be divided into two components, i.e. capital costs and operational costs. The balance sheet of costs may have the headings given below:

- redesigning the work process;
- retraining the operators;
- capital costs of hardware and installation;
- reduction in productivity due to the interference of the control system during changeover;
- electrical power to drive a ventilation prime mover;
- heating energy for replacement air;
- routine maintenance and testing of control systems.

The benefits of successful control systems include:

- a saving in wastage and the use of less raw materials;
- improved health and well-being of staff due to a pollution-free environment, leading to:
  - reduced absenteeism;
  - reduction in the number of workers leaving to find more suitable work;
  - reduction in the number of workers taking early retirement;
- improved labour relations, leading to:
  - improved productivity;
  - fewer disputes;
- an increased demand to work in the improved area, leading to:
  - better quality staff;
  - better quality control;
- reduced compensation claims for work-related ill health;
- adherence to legal requirements where non-compliance may lead to disruption of production;
- reduced insurance premiums.

Few of the above headings can be accurately costed without case studies involving access to company files for individual production processes and people. Both capital and operational costs must be considered in order to compare different control options. For example, a personal protection programme not only requires a regular supply of new protective equipment, but also training, supervision, storage, maintenance and examination. When the costs of engineering controls are compared with those of personal protection, quite often the operational costs of a personal protective equipment programme are underestimated.

Costs of ventilation solutions

It is difficult to give guidance on the capital costs of ventilation systems as no two ventilation systems are alike. Compared with the costs of fans, filters and scrubbers, ductwork and hoods are relatively cheap. The operational costs of a ventilation system are made up of the electrical costs of operating the fan to overcome the resistance of the ventilation system and the heating costs to replace the heated air discarded to the atmosphere. The method of calculating costs has been shown elsewhere (Gill 1980). A reduction in ventilation hardware costs can best be achieved by reducing the total flow rate of air used, as this results in reductions in the sizes of fans, ducts and filters. Total and partial enclosure should be used instead of hoods wherever possible. Where hoods have to be used, the closer they are to the source, the lower the flow of air required. The sensible application of the principles of Fletcher (1977) and Garrison (1983) will reap benefits. Any reduction in the volume flow rate will have a knock-on effect regarding heating and power costs. Heat recovery systems are available, but are not normally a viable option in the UK as the grade of heat to be recovered is so low.

Reasons for poor ventilation performance

If an existing system is found not to provide satisfactory control, there may be many reasons, including faulty design, faulty installation and faulty maintenance and care. Some of the factors to be checked are given below.

Faulty design

Insufficient enclosure. The more enclosure that is provided, the better the control, i.e. a booth which provides enclosure around a source of emission is always an improvement on a hood which tries to draw the pollutants into itself. Total enclosure is ideal, but the necessary negative pressure must be provided. Localized draughts may disturb the flow of extracted air and prevent it from entering a hood; better enclosure will minimize this effect.

Low capture velocity or too great a distance between source and hood. The air velocity at the point of release of a pollutant may be insufficient to move it into the capture device. Alternatively, the distance of the hood from the point of release may be too great, such that the air velocity in front of the hood will have decayed to too low a value to move the pollutant.

Extracted air volume lower than the volume of pollutant released. Particularly when filling containers or opening oven doors, a finite volume of pollutant is released. If the extracted air volume is lower than the volume of pollutant released, some will not be captured and may escape around the sides of the hood or canopy.

Uneven velocity profile across the face of the capture device. Air will always take the path of least resistance; thus, hoods with extract ducts placed asymmetrically may have uneven face velocity profiles, the resulting pollutants not being drawn in on one side and being overextracted on the other.

Ducting too resistant. Ducts can be too narrow or too long, requiring high pressures to draw air through. The fan may not be capable of providing such pressures. The fan must be chosen to provide sufficient pressure (or suction) to overcome the resistance of the duct. However, there is an upper limit. Duct air velocities can become impracticably high when trying to force too much air through them.

Fan of the wrong type or size. The fan should be chosen after having designed the rest of the system. Its duty to provide the necessary flows must be calculated knowing the dimensions and associated pressure losses of all the components. Fans have characteristics that must be correctly matched to the requirements of the system.

Fan entry conditions unsatisfactory. The performance of some fans is affected by a poor velocity profile as the air enters. For example, a bend or a damper close to the fan inlet may reduce its performance. A straight, unrestricted duct is preferred at the inlet to the fan.

Air discharge to atmosphere affected by outside winds. It is best to discharge air vertically, so that it is normally at right angles to the direction of the wind. Under certain wind and weather conditions, horizontal discharges will have outside air blowing into them unless suitably protected. Weather shields must not restrict the flow of air away from the discharge point such that polluted air is re-entrained into the building.

No provision to allow make-up air to replace that extracted. If no properly designed make-up air system is provided, air entry may be restricted by the fabric of the building. Air entering uncontrolled and unheated in winter may cause unacceptable draughts, leading to complaints or systems not being used.

Faulty installation

A well-designed system may be spoiled by poor installation as described below

Ductwork damaged, obstructed or badly connected and supported. Careless installation may result in ducts being dented or joints damaged or not properly made, resulting in restriction and/or leakage. Poor and insufficient duct support may cause the ducts to sway or sag, resulting in breaks and distorted joints. Sometimes a careless installer may leave rubbish and waste inside the duct, causing a restriction. Wrapping material and clothing have been found inside ductwork systems, sometimes having been carried on the air stream to lodge against a damper or on the fan blades.

Multibranched systems not balanced. Multibranched systems, unless inherently balanced at the design stage, will need to be balanced by means of flow controlling dampers to ensure the correct amounts of air flow in each branch. Balancing is normally carried out at the commissioning stage after the plant items have been completely installed. If this is performed carelessly or the balancing dampers are not properly locked into place, incorrect flows will occur and unsatisfactory extraction will ensue.

Fans badly installed and electrically connected. Fans may be installed the wrong way round or rotating in the wrong direction, or two stages may oppose one another. Some of these faults may not be noticed, resulting in poor extract performance. Fans running in reverse do not necessarily result in reversed air flow, but will always give poor performance.

Faulty maintenance and care
Some of the occurrences mentioned in the section 'Faulty installation' can also occur due to faulty maintenance. Continued use over a period of time can cause problems simply due to wear and tear of the plant items.

Restricted, blocked or damaged ducting. Materials carried on the air stream may deposit on the walls and horizontal sections of the ducting. This is particularly true if the velocity inside the duct is below the *transport velocity* of the materials being conveyed, e.g. dust. With dust extraction systems, it is vital to ensure that the correct velocity is provided so that the dust remains airborne until it reaches the filter. The range of transport velocities lies between 15 and $25\,m\,s^{-1}$, depending upon the size and density of the dust being conveyed.

Ducting may be damaged by the movement of vehicles or by items being conveyed by overhead cranes, resulting in dents and broken joints. Control dampers may become dislodged, damaged or corroded, resulting in unbalanced flows.

Fan blades dirty, corroded or motors seized. Dust is inclined to deposit on the blades of fans gradually changing their shape and hence their performance. In extreme cases, fan blades can wear away or corrode. Some fans have their electric motors in the air stream and, if incorrectly selected for dust extraction or if handling corrosive air, may seize up and no longer rotate. The use of bifurcated axial flow fans or centrifugal fans will prevent this.

Filters and air cleaners blocked. Fabric filters need to be cleaned at regular intervals depending upon the dust loadings. Automatic cleaning systems, such as shakers, reverse jets and pulses, are designed to do this. If they fail, the filter fabric will quickly fill and block. Even with good cleaning arrangements, a time comes when fabrics no longer release the deposited dust and a replacement filter medium is required. Blocked filters result in greatly reduced air flows. This may occur quite soon after installation if the wrong medium is chosen for the collection of the dust, e.g. a sticky dust or if the air has a high water vapour content.

All filters including non-fabric filters, such as cyclones and electrostatics, need to have their collecting bins emptied regularly or they will gradually fill up and block.

New workstations added at a later date. It is tempting to install further extract points on an existing system without adjusting the fan performance to suit. This results in all other extract points being denuded of air to the detriment of capture. If it is known that extra points are likely to be added later, the system can be suitably designed and the fan chosen to be uprated when required.

Organizational problems. Some ventilation systems are used on demand by shop floor personnel, either by having the facility to turn them on and off at will, or to bring a branch into use by means of a control damper. There is always the danger of the system not being turned on at all or, if on, not closed down when the workstation is out of use. Good training and supervision will limit these problems. However, some systems are so badly designed that they create excessive noise or uncomfortable draughts, and may be turned off by disgruntled operators.

No ventilation system should be under the control of a shop floor worker. Ideally, the system should automatically run whenever the process is running, i.e. it should be electrically coupled to the machinery of the process, or, if run throughout the shift, should be on a time switch to turn on and off to coincide with shift times. Furthermore, unless specially designed for the purpose, no multibranched system should have branches that can be turned on and off at will.

Checking performance

When managing the performance of a ventilation system that controls substances hazardous to health, it is necessary to identify the most important function for which the system was designed. Some examples are given below.

- An enclosure must be structurally sound with no cracks or breaks in its construction, and must be under negative pressure; if gloves are used, they must be positively attached to the casing and must be free from leaks.
- A booth or fume cupboard must have the correct face velocity, which should be measured in a series of equidistant positions across the face to obtain the true mean; no single reading should be more than 20% above or below the mean.
- A hood or slot must provide the correct capture velocity at the point of release of the pollutant.
- A dust extraction system must not only provide the correct capture velocity, but must maintain the correct transport velocity in the ducting from the hood to the filter; in addition, the pressure across the filter must be monitored to indicate the condition of the filter medium.
- A dilution ventilation system must maintain the designed volume flow rate of air.
- All systems should ensure that the concentrations of the pollutants to be controlled are well below the occupational exposure limits in the breathing zone of the worker in the workplace being controlled.

Ideally, the system should be fitted with a continuous monitor showing the value of the parameters, with an audible or visual alarm to warn of malfunction. In the most critical situations, where malfunction could result in serious exposure, this is essential. In less important situations, a notice should be placed alongside the indicator denoting the correct value and stating the action to be taken in the event of deviation from the norm However, it is often sufficient to test the performance of the system at regular intervals. In some countries, this is required by law. In the UK, for example, systems that control substances hazardous to health and, in particular, local exhaust ventilation systems must undergo a thorough examination and check at intervals not exceeding 14 months, and more frequently for some systems (Health and Safety Commission (HSC) 1994); coal mine ventilation must be checked monthly (Mines and Quarries Act 1956).

The methods used to make a judgement on the performance of ventilation systems include visual observations, pressure measurements, air flow measurements, dust lamp studies, air sampling and filter integrity tests (HSC 1994). Records should be kept of the results of these examinations and tests. The methods involved are listed and described below.

- Visual methods involve an inspection of the physical condition of all the items comprising the ventilation system to identify damage, corrosion, leaks, breaks, etc.
- Static pressure measurements should be taken behind each hood or extraction point, at the inlet, outlet and across a filter and at the inlet to a fan. The static pressure is the difference in pressure between the inside and outside of a duct or filter chamber measured at right angles to the direction of flow.
- Air flow measurements should be taken at the face of a hood or booth, in a duct to determine the volume flow and transport velocity and at a filter and fan to determine the volume flow. Air flow measurements involve the use of an anemometer or air velocity indicator at the point recommended. Volume flow measurements involve the selection of a measuring station free from turbulence and obstructions, the determination of the average velocity across it and the multiplication of this value by the cross-sectional area of the station, i.e. using the equation $Q = v \times A$ mentioned above.
- A dust lamp should be used on a dust extraction system to highlight the emitted particles of dust and to ensure that they are being satisfactorily drawn into the capture device.
- Air sampling of the airborne concentration of a substance can be used to determine whether good control is being achieved. This should be done in the breathing zone of a worker by personal sampling equipment (see Chapter 8). The results should be compared with the government published standards relevant to the country in question. The results should be well below these values.

Where possible, the results of any measurements should be compared with what is required by acceptable good practice, which has been outlined above in the section: 'Hardware and engineering solutions'.

Gathering and recording information

It is advisable to follow published Codes of Practice (HSC 1994) regard-

(a)

RECORD OF VENTILATION PLANT (in accordance with COSHH Regulations)
Name and address of company
Department or site
Location of plant
Identification of plant
Hazardous substances controlled by plant
Type of plant (for sketch see page 2)

Fan details: maker: serial no.:	Fan speed rev min^{-1} *Anti clockwise (from drive side)
Fan type (e.g. guide vane, bifurc, forward bladed, etc.) Axial: dia mm Centrif: dia mm	Max design speed rev min^{-1}
Drive type (e.g. direct, V-belt)	Motor: maker speed rev min^{-1}
If V-belt drive, number of belts: pulley dia: drive mm, fan mm	Motor power kW
Duty: Volume flow rate $m^3 s^{-1}$ Static or total press Pa Air power kW	Voltage phase
Inlet dia: mm Outlet dimens: mm	Full load current amp

Primary air cleaner details: type:		Static press.	
Maker		inlet	Pa
Serial no.:		outlet	Pa
Filter area:	m^2	across	Pa
Design volume flow	$m^3 s^{-1}$	change at	Pa

Second air cleaner details: type:		Static press.	
Maker		inlet	Pa
Serial no.:		outlet	Pa
Filter area:	m^2	across	Pa
Design volume flow	$m^3 s^{-1}$	change at	Pa

* Delete 'anti' where applicable.

(b)

Sketch of plant layout, label ventilation plant items and indicate measurement positions ○

Extract points, showing as far as possible the design values of performance (see sketch)

Point no.	Type (e.g. hood, booth, etc.)	Face dimensions (mm)	Duct dia. (mm)	Area (m^2)	Face vel. ($m s^{-1}$)	Duct vel. ($m s^{-1}$)	Flow rate ($m^3 s^{-1}$)	Comments

Figure 11.3 Ventilation system: basic information record form.

(a)

Extract plant (hood, slot, enclosure, etc., see sketch and initial details in Fig. 11.3(b))

Identification of plant:

Point	Date	Static pressure (Pa)	Air velocity ($m\ s^{-1}$)	Volume flow ($m^3 s^{-1}$)	Instrument used	Comments

Results of visual inspection
Describe below any defects found in any parts of the ventilation system and state what remedial action is required

Measurements/inspection made by Name:	Employer's name and address:

(b)

Air monitoring results (state units e.g. mg m^{-3} or ppm)

Is exhaust air returned to workplace? yes/no

If yes give below returned air concentrations (state substance and units, e.g. Xylene 450mg m^{-3})

Date	Concentration	Date	Concentration	Date	Concentration

Are these concentrations satisfactory? yes/no
If no state remedial action required

Concentration of substances (in workers' breathing zone at extract points, give duration of sampling)

Test point	Date	Duration	Subs.	Conc.	Subs.	Conc.	Subs.	Conc.	Subs.	Conc.
1										
2										
3										
4										
5										
6										
7										
8										
9										
10										
11										
12										
13										
14										
15										

Name of Occupational Hygienist or organization

Do any of the results above show concentrations exceeding the OES or MEL? yes/no
If yes give details

Figure 11.4 Ventilation system: routine measurement record form.

ing what information needs to be collected and recorded with respect to the main components of the ventilation system. The essential headings are listed below.

- *Enclosures/hoods*: maximum number to be in use at any one time; location or position; static pressure behind each hood or extraction point; face velocity.
- *Ducting*: dimensions; transport velocity; volume flow rate.
- *Filter/collector*: specification; volume flow rate; static pressure at inlet, outlet and across the filter.
- *Fan or air mover*: specification; volume flow rate; static pressure at inlet; direction of rotation.
- *Systems which return exhaust air to the workplace*: filter efficiency; concentration of contaminant in the returned air.

Record forms detailing this basic information should be drawn up. A typical form is shown in Fig. 11.3.

Difficulties can be experienced in obtaining this basic information for existing systems, as often no written specification exists, either because it was not asked for originally or it has been lost. It is advisable when ordering a new system to give a blank form to the supplier and ask him/her to complete all the information on it as far as it applies to the system being installed.

With existing systems, much of the information can be gathered by a detailed inspection by reading details from cover plates on fans, drive motors and filters, although designed flow rates may not be available. The advice here is to take measurements of all the performance parameters, record them and regard them as the specification as found. At the same time, the typical time-weighted average concentration in the breathing zone of the affected worker can be measured, and a judgement can be made as to whether the system provides adequate control. If it does, the record can be used as the specification. If it does not, the system will need to be upgraded and the new performance will become the specification.

Records of routine measurements can be kept on forms, such as that shown in Fig. 11.4. The results should be compared with the specification to detect any deterioration in performance.

References

ACGIH (1995) *Industrial Ventilation*, 22nd edn. American Conference of Governmental Industrial Hygienists, Cincinnati, OH.

BOHS (1987) *Technical Guide 7, Controlling Airborne Contaminants in the Workplace*. Science Reviews, Leeds.

Boleij, J., Buringh, E., Heederik, D. & Kromhout, H. (1995) *Occupational Hygiene of Chemical and Biological Agents*. Elsevier Science, Amsterdam.

Fletcher, B. (1977) Centreline velocity characteristics of rectangular unflanged hoods and slots under suction. *Annals of Occupational Hygiene* 20, 141–146.

Fletcher, B. (1978) The effect of flanges on the velocity in front of exhaust

ventilation hoods. *Annals of Occupational Hygiene* **21**, 265–269.
Garrison, R.P. (1983) Velocity calculation for local exhaust inlets—empirical design equations. *American Industrial Hygiene Association Journal* **44**, 937–940.
Gill, F.S. (1980) The energy implications of ventilation systems—an introductory outline. *Annals of Occupational Hygiene* **23**, 423–434.
Gill, F.S. (1995) Ventilation. In: *Occupational Hygiene* (eds. J.M. Harrington & K. Gardiner), pp. 378–403. Blackwell Science, Oxford.
Gill, F.S. & Alesbury, R.J. (1998) Industrial hygiene engineering. In: *Encyclopedia of Environmental Science and Engineering* (eds. J.R. Pfafflin & E.N. Ziegler), 4th edn., pp. 554–567. Gordon and Breach Science Publishers, New York.
Gill, F.S. & Jones, M.D. (1993) Control of solvent vapours in the workplace. *Safety and Health Practitioner* **11** (8), 13–17.
HSC (1994) *Control of Substances Hazardous to Health Regulations 1988 and 1994 and Associated Codes of Practice*. HMSO, London.
HSE (1989) *Guidance Note EH42 (Rev). Monitoring Strategies for Toxic Substances*. HMSO, London.
HSE (1998) *Guidance Note EH40/Year. Occupational Exposure Limits*. Updated annually. HMSO, London.
Piney, M., Gill, F.S., Gray, C.N., Jones, D. & Worwood, J. (1988) *Air Contaminant Control: The Case History Approach. Ventilation 88*. Pergamon, Oxford.
Rogers, A., Davies, B. & Conaty, G. (1993) Diesel particulates—health effects, measurement and standard setting. *Proceedings of the Twelfth Annual Conference of the Australian Institute of Occupational Hygienists, Terrigal, NSW*. AIOH, Melbourne.
Ryckman, R. (1990) The power of persuasion: how to motivate workers to wear PPE. *Occupational Health and Safety Canada* **6** (1), 64–68.
Yousefi, V. & Annegarn, H.J. (1991) *Aerodynamic Aspects of Exhaust Ventilation. Ventilation 91*. ACGIH, Cincinnati, OH.

Chapter 12 Economics of risk management

Ian Wrightson

Introduction

Risk management can be defined as the eradication or minimization of the adverse effects of the pure risks to which an organization is exposed (Bamber 1990a). Risk management is a wide-ranging subject, and relates to all the risks and potential losses which an organization can incur and which can arise from personal injury accidents, property damage or loss (buildings, plant, equipment, finished goods, money), lost production and sales, lost profit and near-misses. A risk management programme therefore involves the safeguarding of all the assets of an organization. Loss control, on the other hand, can be defined as a management system which is designed to reduce or eliminate all aspects of accidental loss that lead to the wastage of an organization's assets.

Risk management

Risk management in industry and commerce (Carter & Doherty 1974) is seen to:

- consider the impact of certain risky events on the performance of the organization;
- devise alternative strategies for controlling these risks and/or their impact on the organization; and
- relate these strategies to the general decision framework used by the organization.

Risk management involves the identification of hazards and risks, the evaluation of these risks and the introduction of systems and procedures to eliminate, reduce or control these risks. These principles form the basis of a number of recent regulations made under the Health and Safety at Work, etc. Act 1974. The Control of Lead at Work Regulations 1980 introduced the concept of risk assessment. The concept was developed thoroughly in the Control of Asbestos at Work Regulations 1987, the Control of Substances Hazardous to Health (COSHH) Regulations 1989 (now replaced by the 1994 COSHH Regulations) and the Noise at Work Regulations 1989. The principles of risk management are now firmly enshrined in the Management of Health and Safety at Work Regulations 1992 and other regulations applying to manual handling operations, display screen equipment and personal protective equipment.

Risks can be identified by health and safety inspections or audits, job safety analysis, accident analysis, management/employee discussions or other techniques, such as 'what if?' or hazard and operability (HAZOP) studies. The evaluation of the risks can be based on legal, social and humanitarian or economic considerations. Legal considerations should include the constraints from compliance with all relevant legislation, codes of practice and current standards. Social and humanitarian considerations should include the well-being of employees, members of the public who may be affected by the organization's activities and consumers of the organization's products. Economic considerations should include the cost of insurance, the uninsured costs of accidents, the cost of non-compliance with legal requirements and the overall effect on the profitability of the organization. The probability of the frequency of each occurrence and the severity of the outcome, including the maximum potential loss, will need to be included in the evaluation. Having identified and evaluated the risk, control strategies can be considered.

Risk control strategies can be grouped into four main categories: risk avoidance, risk retention, risk transfer and risk reduction.

Risk avoidance involves a deliberate decision being made by an organization to avoid a specific risk completely by no longer undertaking the operation that gives rise to the risk. Examples include the removal of asbestos from the manufacture of insulation material and from the friction linings used in the braking and clutch systems of motor vehicles. There are many examples of hazardous chemicals, such as benzene and other carcinogens, which have been taken out of use or have been replaced by other chemicals that either have a reduced risk potential or have no known risks associated with them. The replacement of solvent-based paints and inks in the engineering and printing industries by water-based materials has not only removed health risks, but has eliminated fire risks and has led to environmental benefits. In order to avoid risks from their most hazardous operations, some large organizations now contract out these operations to smaller and more specialized companies.

Risk retention is when an organization retains a risk and finances any consequential loss itself. This can either be done with knowledge or without knowledge. Risk retention with knowledge involves a deliberate decision being made by an organization to retain the risk within its own financial operations. This involves either self-insurance or the use of deductibles. Risk retention without knowledge arises from a lack of knowledge of the existence of a risk or the failure to take out appropriate insurance.

Risk transfer involves the legal transfer or assignment of the cost of particular potential losses from one organization to another. The most common way of achieving such a transfer is by insurance. In such circumstances, the insurer (an insurance company) undertakes, within the terms of the policy, to compensate the insured (an organization) for losses resulting from an event or incident specified in the policy (e.g. a fire, accident, etc.). Some insurance policies, such as employers' liability and public liability, cover third party liabilities, and provide compensation to the individual or organization that has incurred a loss resulting from an event or incident.

Risk reduction involves the reduction of risk within an organization by means of a loss control programme, the aims of which are to protect the organization's assets by preventing accidental loss and wastage. A loss control programme needs as much information as possible on the losses arising from accidents in order to establish a programme of improvements. The first stage involves the reporting and investigation of accidents which lead to injury or ill health, damage to property and products and near-misses, where there has been no injury or damage. This stage is known as loss prevention. The second stage of development towards risk reduction or loss control is the gathering of information from other areas of potential or actual loss arising from fires, theft, pollution, products or business interruption together in a co-ordinated manner. The aim is to reduce all accidental losses arising out of or in connection with an organization's activities.

The combination of risk reduction (loss control) and risk transfer (insurance) is risk management.

Loss control

Loss control, as defined above, is the management system which is designed to reduce or eliminate all aspects of accidental loss that lead to the wastage of an organization's assets. Loss control is about the application of sound management techniques to the identification, evaluation and economic control of losses in an organization.

Bird and Loftus (1976) suggested that loss control management involves the following:

- the identification of risk exposures;
- the measurement and analysis of exposures;
- the deterioration of exposures that will respond to treatment by existing or available loss control techniques or activities;
- the selection of appropriate loss control action based on effectiveness and economic feasibility; and
- the management of the implementation of the loss control programme in the most effective manner, subject to economic constraints.

This approach uses the economic argument to persuade management to make improvements and to enhance the overall viability of the organization.

The theories on which loss control are based were first developed in 1931 by Heinrich (1959). He suggested that an accident prevention programme should seek to prevent all accidents, not just the more serious ones which resulted in major injury. Heinrich's emphasis was on accidents rather than injuries, because major injuries were a small proportion of all accidents. He demonstrated this by developing ratios between different types of accident. His study was based on the examination of 5000 accident cases from organizations which were insured by a particular insurance company. He demonstrated that, for every major or lost-time injury, there were 29 minor injuries and 300 no-injury accidents (or near-misses). These ratios are represented in the accident triangle in Fig. 12.1. He concluded that accident prevention should be based on the analysis of the causes of all accidents, rather than just on those involving major injuries. Heinrich also developed a method of costing accidents (see section on 'The cost of accidents'), and suggested that the economic argument should be used as a tool to promote accident prevention.

Bird (1974) carried out a second accident ratio study in 1969 involving 1 753 498 accidents reported by 297 co-operating organizations which represented 21 types of industrial activity. The study included accidents which led to property damage. Bird concluded that, for every serious injury, there were 10 minor injuries, 30 property damage incidents and 600 other accidents with no injury or damage. This ratio is depicted as an accident triangle in Fig. 12.2.

Fletcher and Douglas (1971) adopted and extended Bird's approach to loss control, and applied it in one organization operating 50 plants in 12 countries. Their analysis indicated that for each major injury, there were 19 minor injuries and 175 damage only and no-injury near-misses. This ratio is shown as an accident triangle in Fig. 12.3. Further

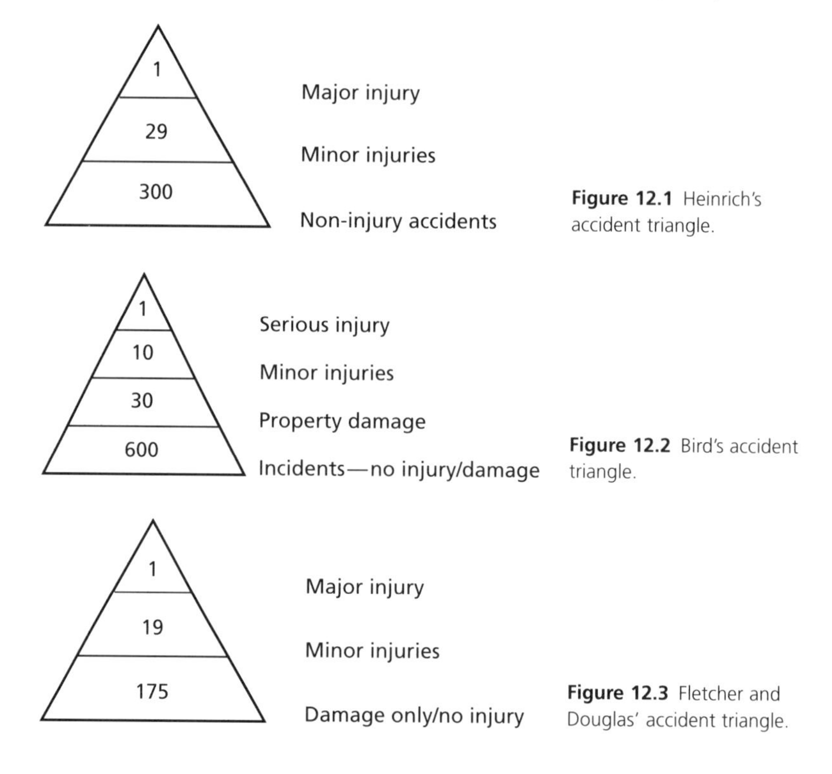

Figure 12.1 Heinrich's accident triangle.

Figure 12.2 Bird's accident triangle.

Figure 12.3 Fletcher and Douglas' accident triangle.

studies of accidents have been performed by Tye (1976) and the Health and Safety Executive (HSE 1993), and their findings in terms of accident ratios are depicted as accident triangles in Figs 12.4 and 12.5.

All of these triangles involve the measurement of different parameters derived in widely different circumstances. Nevertheless, they all illustrate a preventive opportunity. If the underlying failures which lead to each type of accident are the same, by investigating and dealing with the causes of the incidents at the base of the triangle, the total losses, including personal injuries, will be reduced. This approach assumes that most accidents can result in both property damage and personal injury. This is not always the case, as some accidents are unlikely to lead to property damage and others lead to property damage but have no potential to cause personal injury. It is, however, the underlying principle of a preventive approach which is important.

For an injury prevention programme (which includes the prevention of occupational ill health), it is necessary to have in place a management system which ensures compliance with health and safety legislation through the provision of a health and safety policy, procedures for hazard identification and risk assessment, safety training, safe systems of work, control measures, safety inspections, safety audits and accident reporting and investigation. The HSE (1991) advocates the establishment of a management system based on loss control and total quality management. Its approach establishes five key elements for successful health and safety management: policy; organization; planning and implementation; measurement of performance; and review of performance (including auditing).

Damage control involves the protection of assets in terms of raw materials, plant and machinery and finished goods. It is essentially a direct extension of an injury prevention programme, and the same principles as outlined above can be applied. The principles of damage

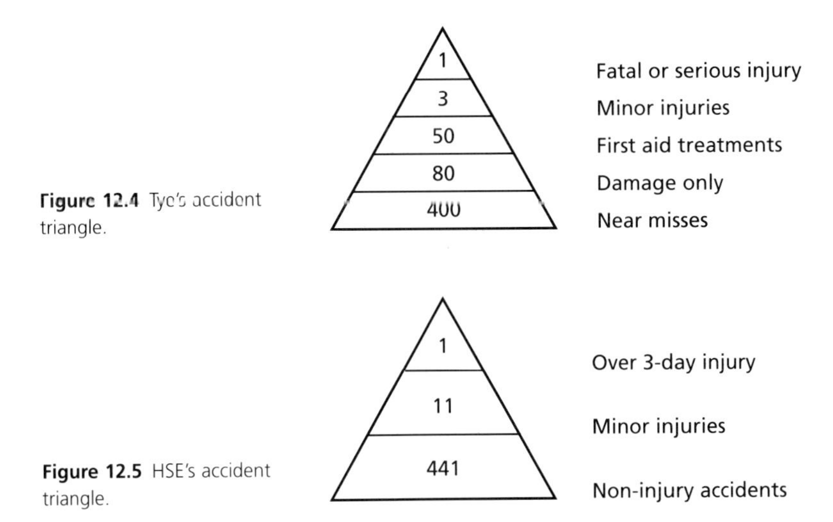

Figure 12.4 Tye's accident triangle.

Figure 12.5 HSE's accident triangle.

control have been set out in detail by Bird and Germain (1966) and Bird and Loftus (1976). To complete the establishment of a loss control programme, similar general principles can then be applied through the management organization to prevent losses arising from fires (fire prevention), theft (security control), pollution (pollution prevention), products and business interruption.

Fire prevention is a special form of damage control, as it involves the protection of raw materials, plant and equipment and finished goods. It also involves the protection of the manpower asset, as fire can cause injury to employees as well as property damage. Fire damage can be a costly item. In 1990, the total cost of fire insurance claims in the UK was £1005 million. Fire prevention involves the elimination or control of sources of ignition and the provision of fire-resisting structures to prevent the spread of fire, fire detection and alarm systems, fire-fighting equipment (including sprinklers), fire safety training, fire escape routes and fire assembly points. Special consideration should be given to the storage and use of explosives, highly flammable liquids, flammable gases, explosive dusts and other readily combustible materials, such as cellular plastic. Sources of ignition, such as naked flames used in hot work (cutting, burning and welding), and the use of smoking materials need to be strictly controlled.

Security control protects raw materials, methods and procedures, finished goods and money from theft. Security is included in loss control because of the financial implications. Losses due to theft are not usually considered to be accidental. A security control programme should involve the security of the premises, procedures for the collection, handling and distribution of cash, the prevention of theft by intruders or by pilfering, the special storage of valuable and attractive goods, the protection of confidential and commercially sensitive information and procedures and the use of accounting procedures to prevent fraud. Security control can also have an impact on damage control in terms of the prevention of vandalism and sabotage.

Pollution prevention or control involves the protection of the environment both inside and outside the workplace. The control of pollution from airborne emissions and liquid and solid wastes can prevent damage to the environment and injury to both employees and members of the public. It can also indirectly protect the financial assets of the organization by preventing enforcement action under environmental legislation, claims for damages and associated adverse publicity.

Product control provides protection to all consumers of the organization's products or services. It is primarily concerned with the protection of the financial asset. This asset may suffer losses due to increased insurance premiums arising from compensation payments. Indirect losses may also occur from any adverse publicity arising from problems associated with the products or services. Product control involves ensuring the integrity and safety of the product or service from its initial design, through its development or manufacture, to its final presentation to the consumer. Product control can be achieved through formal quality assurance procedures.

Business interruption takes into account the fact that lost production or service costs money, and that this impacts on the overall profitability of the organization. Business interruption is therefore concerned with the protection of the financial assets. A business interruption control strategy should include the securing of a continuous supply of raw materials, planned preventive maintenance of plant and equipment, the securing of an uninterrupted supply of essential services (gas, steam, electricity, etc.), the availability of key personnel and a reliable distribution system for the product.

An effective loss control programme requires the commitment of senior management and the co-ordination of management activities in order to ensure a constant and consistent approach. Such an approach leads to a reduction in accidents and occupational ill health, compliance with health and safety legislation, the minimization of other losses and, ultimately, increased profitability. Many managers consider the reduction of operating costs as the prime motivator. The economic argument is therefore likely to be more persuasive than either the legal or the moral (humanitarian) arguments for the provision of good standards of health and safety.

Loss control (risk reduction), when combined with insurance (risk transfer), leads to risk management. In recent years, there have been a number of developments that have led to both loss control and risk management becoming more important issues (Wrightson 1995). The factors involved include:

- the increasing cost of liability insurance;
- the evaluation of the real cost of accidents;
- the changing approach to the enforcement of legislation; and
- the increased level of criminal penalties.

These factors all have actual or potential economic effects upon organizations, and need to be considered within risk management programmes. It is also important to consider the costs associated with risk improvements, and the benefits which will accrue as a result of their implementation.

Employers' liability insurance and its cost

Employers have a duty of care towards their employees and, if they breach their duty and this results in employees suffering injury or ill health, the employees are entitled to sue their employers for damages to compensate them for the injury or ill health which they have suffered. To ensure that sufficient funds are always available to pay such compensation, the Employers' Liability (Compulsory Insurance) Act 1969 requires all employers to take out an insurance policy with an authorized insurer to cover their legal liability to their employees. There are exemptions to this requirement which are covered in the Employers'

Liability (Compulsory Insurance) Exemption Regulations 1971. The main exemptions include nationalized industries, local authorities, policy authorities, nuclear power installation operators, various other bodies financed by public funds and employees who are close relatives of the employer.

Employers who fail to obtain such insurance can face a fine of up to £2500 per day for each day for which they did not have insurance cover. Where the offence is committed with the consent, connivance or by the neglect of a director, manager, secretary or other officer, that individual can also be punished along with the body corporate. Employers are required to display a copy of the insurance certificate, send a copy of it on request to an inspector and show a copy of the certificate and their insurance policy to an inspector on request. Failure to comply with these requirements can lead to a £1000 fine.

The annual premium of employers' liability (EL) cover is based on a rate percentage applied to the wages paid to employees, and takes into account the type of industry, the risks associated with the industry and the claims experience. The insurer expects the insured to disclose all relevant facts about their business, and to take appropriate steps to prevent accidents and occupational ill health so that claims of negligence by employees can be prevented (or minimized). If a claim arises, the insurer looks to the insured to provide evidence to refute the claim. The existence of a health and safety or risk management system would provide a framework for such evidence to be available.

The value of the UK market for EL insurance in 1993 was worth £650 million (Association of British Insurers 1995). Insurance companies account for nearly 80% of the market in terms of gross premium income. The Lloyd's market supplies approximately 15%. Some 50 insurance companies write EL insurance, but the top five insurance companies account for approximately 64% of the company gross written income for EL. It is estimated that 10% of gross premium is involved in reinsurance.

The cost of EL claims has risen dramatically in recent years and this, together with several other factors, has led to increases in the cost of insurance. There have been sharp increases in the number of claims arising from both accidents and occupational ill health.

During the period 1981–1990, the number of claims rose by 48% from 103 000 to 152 000. However, since 1990, the claims have fallen back by 20% to 123 000. The nature of claims has changed. Although there have been more claims for accidents, the number of claims for occupational diseases has become more important, and accounted for 55% of all claims in 1993. Most of these claims involve noise-induced hearing loss. There have also been significant increases in the number of claims for asbestosis, occupational asthma and occupational cancers.

The recent reduction in the number of claims may be due to a number of factors. Places of work have generally become safer as a result of greater safety awareness on the behalf of employees. Over the last 20 years, the total number of fatalities each year has been reduced from approximately 650 in 1974 to 240 in 1993. There has also been a shift away from the more traditional and more hazardous industrial sectors to the service industries where employment has increased by 80%.

The overall increase in the number of claims since 1981 has resulted from a greater awareness of the right of individuals to claim for compensation. This is due to a number of reasons, including the availability of free legal advice given by Trade Unions to their members, the advertising of services by solicitors, higher awards being ordered by courts and increased publicity and media attention. In some areas, in addition to advertising in the press, some solicitors hold public meetings to acquaint individuals with their rights and to offer services. The advent of the 'no win, no fee' service offered by solicitors may give rise to further increases in claims in the future.

Inflation has a major effect on claim settlement costs. For reasons outside the control of insurers, it can take many years to settle some EL claims. This is especially significant in the case of severe injury, which is not only extremely costly, but medical prognosis may not be known for a number of years. Today's premiums must provide for settlement of these claims, and take into account the fact that the eventual settlement, perhaps 5 or 6 years later, will be based on the levels which are applicable at the date of settlement.

In the case of many occupational diseases, there is often a time delay between the exposure to harmful chemicals or fibres and the manifestation of the disease; this can be up to 50 years. This time delay is called the latency period, and hence the description of EL insurance as a 'long tail' class of business. Examples of such diseases include asthma, asbestosis, mesothelioma, pneumoconiosis, bladder cancer, byssinosis, noise-induced hearing loss, vibration white finger and bronchial carcinoma. This so-called long tailed nature of the business creates a major problem for EL insurers. The reason for this is that EL insurance is written on a causation basis, and this leads to claims being made in relation to the time of the exposure, i.e. when the disease was contracted. Such a claim may not necessarily be lodged with the current insurer, but with the insurer who provided cover at the time of the occurrence or when the exposure took place. Insurers find themselves in a dilemma, having to predict levels of claims for occupational ill health which may not yet have manifested themselves (and have not been reported), and allowing for adequate reserving for these future claims. Whilst it may not be possible to forecast precisely any future liabilities, this situation highlights the need for premiums to reflect future claims potential and not simply to be based on past and current claims.

Legal costs and expert's fees continue to rise. Legal costs vary from case to case and can represent a significant proportion of the final settlement cost. Even a successful defence may mean that an insurer does not cover his/her own legal costs, particularly when the claimant has no money and is legally aided.

Between 1981 and 1990, the value of claims paid and those outstanding almost tripled from £221 million to £613 million (Association of British Insurers 1995). The value of these claims fell back to £567 million in 1993. In direct response to the rising cost of claims, EL insurers increased their premiums from £203 million in 1981 to £646 million in 1993. During much of this period the claims paid and outstanding exceeded premium income and many insurers made an underwriting loss. Overall, insurance companies made an underwriting loss of £588 million between 1987 and 1992 on EL insurance. As a consequence, some EL insurers either withdrew from the market (e.g. Builders' Accident Insurance) or now only write EL insurance as part of a much wider commercial package of insurance. In 1993, the gross written premium exceeded the value of claims paid and outstanding for the first time since 1981. Whilst this is an improvement, it does not necessarily indicate an underwriting profit, as the figures do not include the costs and expenses incurred as part of the business.

The Employers' Liability (Compulsory Insurance) Act 1969 requires a minimum of £2 million insurance cover per occurrence. In practice, up until 1995, insurers provided unlimited cover to employers. However, insurers have experienced a number of substantial problems relating to increased injury awards, long-term disease claims, the number of claims made because people are more litigious and improved medical techniques which can identify work-related injuries and diseases. These problems led to the underwriting loss suffered by EL insurers. In addition, reinsurers have become reluctant to provide protection on an unlimited basis in the light of a number of large claims, such as those arising from the Piper Alpha disaster. Some reinsurers have withdrawn from the market, and there are fewer reinsurers on which EL insurers can spread the risk.

Piper Alpha opened the eyes of the reinsurers to the so-called 'accumulation' risk that they had faced in the past, but which had never received the consideration it deserved by underwriters. Accumulation is where a large number of employees, often employed by different organizations, are exposed to risks from one serious or disastrous incident. Accumulation can occur on oil rigs offshore, oil refineries, chemical works, large construction sites and large multioccupancy office complexes.

Direct EL insurers have therefore been forced to protect their balance sheets by limiting liability. From 1st January 1995, standard EL policies have been capped and limited to £10 million per occurrence, costs inclusive. If the insured requires additional cover beyond a £10 million liability, a further premium is required. Such excess cover is not subject to the requirements of the 1969 Act and does not have the same terms as the primary policy. Consequently, excess policies can exclude cover for certain types of claim, e.g. disease claims, which is not permitted under the primary policy.

In order to minimize the cost of EL insurance, it is essential to prevent the occurrence of accidents and occupational ill health and the consequential claims of negligence. Insurers can offer financial rewards for those employers whose risk management systems have enabled them to keep claims to a minimum. For example, Eagle Star policy holders can be rewarded through an optional renewal bonus scheme, which provides a bonus on a sliding scale of up to 25% of premium for a claim-free history (Wrightson 1994). Companies with good claims records are benefiting from their savings on premiums.

EL insurers can also help their insured by providing advice on risk management in order to reduce claims, so that both parties can remain commercially viable. Some specialist EL insurers have their own staff who carry out EL risk management surveys to assist the insured. The service can be free, but is usually provided within the premium. On some occasions, an additional fee is charged. Other insurers simply undertake surveys to provide underwriters with an up-to-date assessment rather than to provide advice to the insured. Insurers often make enquiries about health and safety at the inception or renewal of EL policies to help them quantify the risk. Major insurance brokers also employ their own specialist staff to provide risk management advice to their clients in order to improve their performance and prevent claims.

There has been a move in recent years for companies, particularly those with effective risk management systems, to seek alternatives to the normal EL insurance with a view to reducing their costs. This involves companies retaining more of their own insurance risks, but still having a degree of EL insurance provided by an insurance company in order to meet legal requirements under the 1969 Act. Many insurers offer alternative approaches in the form of deductible schemes, aggregate schemes and retrospective rating schemes.

A deductible scheme allows an employer to pay the first part of a claim up to a predetermined level (i.e. the deductible) and the EL insurer pays the balance. Consequently, the premium is reduced and the employer has an incentive to reduce his/her own contribution to low-level claims through good risk management.

An aggregate scheme is a type of deductible which operates at a high level. The employer pays claims up to an agreed figure arising from a single claim or an aggregate of smaller claims. The insurer pays the balance.

A retrospective rating scheme allows the employer to share the total cost with the insurer. A minimum premium is charged at the outset and a maximum premium is agreed and set aside until the end of the insurance period. The actual premium is the charge at the end of the period after all the claims are known. As with deductible and aggregate schemes, the employer is charged a reduced premium. The amount of saving depends on the minimization of claims through good risk management.

The financing of the employer's share in these risk retention schemes can be from the employer's normal operating budget, or from a fund managed by a captive insurance company set up specifically for the purpose by the employer or a group of employers.

The operation of effective risk management systems does not necessarily mean that the use of such risk retention schemes is the most cost-effective form of insurance. As shown earlier, companies with effective risk management systems can achieve substantial savings on their EL premiums for standard policies. To determine which is the most cost-effective method, each case must be judged on its own merits.

Damages arising from injuries and ill health

Claims for compensation or damages under the EL insurance policies, which arise from personal injury or ill health suffered as a result of an employee's work, are heard at civil courts. The employee, or claimant, has to prove that the employer has either committed a breach of statutory duty or has been negligent in the duty of care to the employee, and that this led directly to the injury or ill health suffered. In many cases, a settlement is reached before the case comes before the court. In these circumstances, the full costs of legal action are avoided. Damages are usually paid by the insurer. If, however, the employer's EL policy involves either a deductible or aggregate scheme, the employer will pay part or all of the damages, depending on the terms of the policy.

Damages awarded for injury or ill health are made up of general damages and special damages.

General damages relate to the pain, suffering and any continuing effects. The level of general damages for various injuries is based on information given in the book, *Guide Lines for the Assessment of General Damages in Personal Injury Cases*, prepared for the Judicial Studies Board (1994). Some examples of the general damages given in these guidelines are shown below:

- paraplegia: £80 000–£90 000;
- severe brain damage: £105 000–£125 000;
- total blindness: £90 000;
- loss of sexual function: £55 000;
- loss of thumb: £15 000–£22 000;
- amputation of large toe: £12 500.

These guidelines are based on settlements which have been paid in previous cases for similar injuries. The precise amount of general damages paid in any settlement depends on the circumstances of the individual case.

Special damages relate mainly to the injured person's loss of earnings, both at the time of the claim and in the future. The major components of claims are often for loss of earnings and other special damages. For example, a young man in his thirties with a wife and family to support who suffers an injury which restricts him to light duties or makes him unable to work again is likely to have a substantial proportion of his damages paid as special damages. In such circumstances, his damages will be for a much higher amount than the specific figures quoted above.

Some examples of actual claims settled recently are given below.

- £1.2 million was awarded to 14 policemen for post-traumatic stress in an out of court settlement following the Hillsborough football disaster in 1989 in which 96 persons were killed. During the chaos, the policemen had tried to rescue Liverpool supporters.
- £175 000 was awarded for work-related stress to a Northumberland social worker after he suffered two nervous breakdowns.
- £211 000 was awarded to four laboratory technicians for occupational asthma after they had had to give up their jobs caring for laboratory animals.
- £167 000 was awarded to a former naval fitter after he contracted leukaemia arising from his work on nuclear submarines.
- £88 000 was awarded to a 64-year-old man who had been exposed to asbestos for 16 months during the Second World War.
- £72 000 was awarded for a work-related upper limb disorder to an operator who made parts for Trident submarines.

Up until October 1997, if an award of damages was made in excess of £2500, the Compensation Recovery Unit of the Department of Social Security recovered from the claimant any state benefit which had been paid from the excess above £2500. When damages were below £2500, the claimant did not have to repay any state benefit. The £2500 bar for the repayment of state benefit has now been removed, and it is likely that this will lead to an increase in the cost of EL insurance, mainly due to the additional administration imposed on insurers. If, in the future, the state industrial injury benefit system were to be abolished, there would be an increase in the number of claims and this, in turn, would lead to an increase in the cost of EL insurance.

Other insurances

An employer owes a duty of care to persons who are not his/her employees, but who may be affected by the activities of his/her undertaking. If such a person suffers injury, ill health or property damage as a direct result of that undertaking, he/she is entitled to sue for compensation for the harm or damage done. In order to protect themselves against such claims, employers can take out a public liability insurance policy to ensure that cover is available to provide compensation. Public liability insurance, unlike EL insurance, is a voluntary insurance.

Public liability policies specify a limit of liability, often £1 million, but cover up to £5 million is readily available. For large, complex organizations, policies with liabilities up to £100 million can be purchased.

The premiums of public liability policies are based on the risks associated with the premises (including the processes and activities), the risks arising from any work activity undertaken away from the site and the risks associated with the products of the undertaking. Product liability insurance may also be purchased as a stand-alone policy. Where appropriate, relevant claims experience is taken into account when setting the premium.

Public liability insurance policies exclude the liability arising from the ownership, possession or use by or on behalf of the insured of a mechanically propelled vehicle, vessel or craft. With regard to motor vehicles, the employer is required by the Road Traffic Act 1972 to have compulsory motor insurance to cover his/her third party liability to persons who may be killed or injured as a result of the use of the vehicle on the road.

Public liability insurance excludes pollution other than that which is caused by a sudden, identifiable, unintended and unexpected incident which takes place in its entirety at a specified time and place during the period of insurance. Gradual or ongoing, known releases, emissions or discharges which lead to insidious pollution are not covered by public liability insurance. Damage to the policy holder's own property is not covered by public liability insurance. Such pollution can be covered by environmental impairment liability insurance, but there is a very limited market for this type of insurance and, in any event, it is not a general insurance; it is site specific and is subject to a detailed environmental survey.

The cost of public liability insurance over recent years has increased. This increase has been very modest compared with the increases in the costs of EL insurance mentioned earlier. Because of the voluntary nature of public liability insurance and the paucity of statutory reporting procedures, there are no detailed statistics readily available to give general information about claims and the costs of incidents.

The cost of accidents

Losses arising from major fires, explosions and other incidents involving the loss of life are all too apparent. Some of the most well-known events have been costed on an individual basis. The explosion on the Piper Alpha oil platform in the North Sea in 1988 involved the loss of 167 lives, and has been estimated to have cost £2 billion, including £746 million paid out in insurance claims. British Petroleum (BP) have estimated that the fire at their Grangemouth refinery in 1987, in which one person died, cost £50 million in property damage and £50 million in business interruption. The fire at a chemical warehouse at Allied Colloids Ltd., Bradford in 1992 did not involve the loss of life, but is estimated to have cost £6 million.

There are many other accidents, which either injure or kill people, and cases of occupational ill health which do not make the headlines. The precise costs of these events are not always clear or well understood. Very few organizations examine costs in a systematic or detailed way. In most cases, the direct costs of accidents are known in terms of wages paid during an absence, plant and equipment damage caused and any loss of product. On the other hand, managers do not know the extent of the indirect or hidden costs. A number of attempts have been made to quantify these costs.

Heinrich (1959) undertook the first detailed study of the costs of accidents in 1931. This study was based on the examination of 5000 accident cases from organizations which were insured by a particular insurance company. Heinrich classified the costs of accidents in terms of visible direct and invisible indirect costs. These costs were represented as an iceberg, with the direct costs (20%) being visible and above the water and the indirect costs (80%) being invisible and below the water (see Fig. 12.6).

Andreoni (1986) showed that the estimated hidden costs of accidents varied between 0.5 and 20 times the wage costs incurred during the absence due to the accident. In an Australian study (Oxenburg & Guldberg 1988), it was estimated that the hidden costs of accidents were between zero and 3.5 (medium, 1.75) times the employees' compensation. These hidden costs were based on overtime payments, extra staffing, training, employee turnover and lost production time. A number of known hidden costs, such as additional management time, plant and product damage, downtime and personal losses suffered by those injured, were not included.

Oxenburg (1991) proposed two models for the costing of injury absence based on insurance considerations and productivity. The productivity model takes into account the various extra hidden costs which were not considered in the previous study (Oxenburg & Guldberg 1988). Oxenburg used the productivity model in a wide range of case studies to demonstrate the cost effectiveness of health and safety improvements.

A number of other authors have explored the links between the cost of accidents and the management of health and safety (Brody *et al.* 1990; Soderqvist *et al.* 1990; Veltri 1990; Wright 1990; Sachs 1991). Others have argued that the key principles in quality management, including quality costing, have direct relevance to health and safety management (Salazar 1989; Whiston & Eddershaw 1989; Fisher 1991; Pardy 1991). Fisher (1991) classified the costs of quality and safety

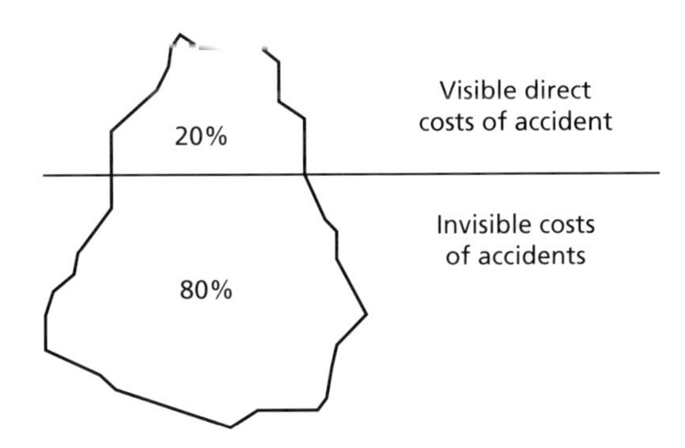

Figure 12.6 Heinrich's iceberg.

functions into prevention, appraisal and failure costs. He also explored the links between the management of quality and health and safety. He concluded that failure costs can be greater than the combined costs of prevention and appraisal.

The costs of accidents can be divided into those which are covered by insurance and those which are not insurable. In the case of injuries at work and occupational ill health, the insurance costs are covered primarily by the EL policy which is compulsory. Other insured costs can be covered, to a large extent, by public liability, fire, engineering, motor and business interruption policies, all of which are voluntary.

When an accident occurs which causes injury to an employee, there are a number of costs which cannot be offset by EL insurance. Uninsured costs were listed by Bamber (1979) and his list was extended by Wrightson (1994). Examples of such costs are:

- cost of injured person's lost work time;
- cost of wages paid to persons who go to the assistance of the injured person;
- cost of wages paid to persons who stop work out of curiosity or sympathy;
- cost of wages paid to persons who are unable to continue work because they rely on the injured person's aid or output;
- cost of damage to material;
- cost of damage to plant;
- cost of supervisor's time spent in assisting, investigating, reporting, reassessing work and making necessary adjustments;
- cost of instructing a replacement worker;
- cost of first aid or medical facilities;
- cost of time spent by administration staff in processing investigations and reports;
- cost of any action taken by the enforcing authority, including legal costs; and
- cost of any adverse publicity.

In the UK, the costs of accidents were studied by the HSE (1993) during 1990 and 1991 in five different areas of employment. The activities chosen involved a construction site, a creamery, a transport company, a North Sea oil production platform and a National Health Service hospital. Each site chosen employed between 80 and 700 persons. Each participating organization displayed an average or better than average health and safety performance in their sector of industry. The study period at each site varied between 13 and 18 weeks.

The HSE study costed all accidents which fell within their definition. An accident was regarded as any unplanned event that resulted in injury or ill health of people, or damage or loss to property, plant, materials or the environment or a loss of a business opportunity. It was found that only a small proportion of these costs were covered by insurance costs. This ratio was represented by an iceberg, which showed the actual insured costs above the water line and the uninsured costs below the water line. The insured costs covered all insurance premiums during the study period, including EL. The uninsured costs were found in four of the case studies to be between 8 and 36 times greater than the cost of the insurance premiums (see Fig. 12.7). The ratio of the insured/uninsured costs could not be calculated for the hospital, because the National Health Service is self-insured.

The study showed that accidents cost:

- one organization as much as 37% of its annualized profits;
- another the equivalent of 8.5% of the tender price; and
- a third organization 5% of its running costs.

During the study, there were no accidents at any of the five organizations which involved a death, major injury or large-scale loss due to fire or explosion. There were no prosecutions or significant civil claims to swell the basic figures. The HSE study also concluded that the average cost to the employer of injuries of all types was £75. The average cost of non-injury events was almost three times higher at £224.

These figures alone do not have a significant impact. In order that an organization can recognize the full cost implications of accidents, the total number of accidents and non-injury events must be considered. In a hypothetical case of a factory employing 500 persons, that has 160 recorded accidents and 200 non-injury events, the costs can be calculated using HSE's figures.

- Uninsured cost of all accidents: 160 × £75 = £12 000.
- Uninsured cost of all non-injury events: 200 × £224 = £44 800.
- Total accident cost: £12 000 + £44 800 = £56 800.

If a hypothetical EL insurance premium of £112 500 (based on 1.5% of wages) is added, the total cost increases to £169 300 or £339 per person per year. This total does not include any capital expenditure on health and safety projects, safety department costs or the cost of safety equipment and personal protective equipment. When the total cost of accidents is compared with other business costs, such as production, sales and distribution, the true drain on the organization's resources can be appreciated. These accident costs can have a significant impact on the overall profitability of an organization.

The HSE (1993) publication, *The Costs of Accidents at Work*, provides a methodology for estimating the costs of accidents, together with costing proformas which can be freely reproduced by organizations wishing to do their own costings.

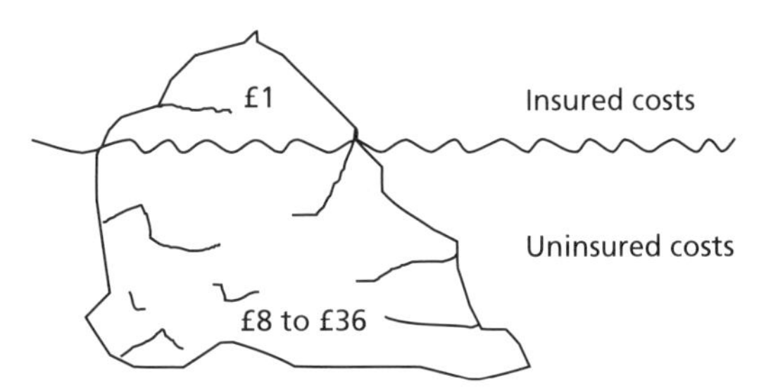

Figure 12.7 HSE's accident cost iceberg.

A second study was commissioned by the HSE in 1993 to trial a simplified costings methodology, particularly for small and medium sized establishments, which included the reworking of data from three of the original case studies (New 1996). Six organizations were chosen:

- a prison with 220 employees;
- an engineering company with 60 employees;
- a college with 150 employees;
- a paint distributor with 25 employees;
- a plastics company with 150 employees;
- a manufacturer of soft drinks with 100 employees.

The study lasted for 1 month and confirmed the lessons learnt from the first study in terms of the relationship between insured and uninsured costs. As a result of this second study, the HSE published its leaflet for small firms: *Be Safe, Save Money!—The Costs of Accidents—A Guide to Small Firms* (HSE 1995). The aim of the leaflet was to raise awareness and spread the message about the cost of accidents by giving some examples of actual costs, rather than to precipitate further detailed costing exercises.

The health and safety supplement to the 1990 Labour Force Survey (Stevens 1992) indicated that, in England and Wales, there had been 1.6 million injury accidents at work in the previous 12 months and 2.2 million persons suffered ill health caused by or made worse by working conditions. The outcome of these injuries and ill health was that 30 million working days were lost and some 20 000 persons had to give up work permanently.

In a further study by the HSE in 1994, the costs of work-related accidents and ill health were estimated for individuals, employers and society (Davies & Teasdale 1994). The basic statistics used were from the 1990 Labour Force Survey, and the costings suggested, therefore, relate to 1990 prices.

Individual workers who suffer injury due to accidents and work-related ill health are estimated to lose about £1 billion because of reduced incomes and additional expenses. Workers and their families also have a loss of welfare in terms of pain, grief and suffering. The HSE used various methodologies to estimate this loss, and concluded that it was of the order of £4.3 billion, but this needed to be offset in part by the civil compensation received of about £650 million. The net cost to the individual was estimated to be about £5 million.

The cost to employers of injuries from work activities and work-related ill health was estimated to be around £1.5 billion. This was made up of £900 million for accidents and £600 million for ill health. Losses arising from non-injury incidents were estimated to be between £2.9 billion and £7.7 billion. The total cost of all accidents to employers was therefore estimated to be between £4 billion and over £9 billion (including insurance). This equates to around 5–10% of all UK industrial companies' gross trading profits, and averages between £170 and £360 for every person employed.

The total cost to the British economy of all work activity injuries and work-related ill health was estimated to be between £6 billion and £12 billion each year. This includes property damage, reduced output, medical costs, administrative costs and Department of Social Security costs. The total cost to society as a whole is estimated to be between £11 billion and £16 billion, and includes the loss of welfare resulting from pain, grief and suffering for victims and their families. The total cost to society is equivalent to between 1 and 2% of the total gross domestic product.

Accidents and occupational ill health are a significant drain on the resources of any organization. There are more days lost through accidents and ill health than through industrial disputes. Accidents are expensive events which should be avoided. However, the costs of accidents are often regarded as part of the organization's normal operating costs and are, in effect, written off. Accident costs are not usually included in departmental budgets and, consequently, there is a lack of financial accountability at departmental level. The inclusion of accident costs in a departmental budget is an effective way of achieving accountability. Budgets can be used to set targets for the reduction of accidents and occupational ill health. These targets can be considered as part of the manager's annual job appraisal review. There are major savings to be made by preventing accidents and occupational ill health. The savings on the hidden costs of accidents can far exceed those which are recoverable from insurance policies. The implementation of good risk management procedures to prevent the occurrence of accidents and occupational ill health is an economic necessity.

The enforcement of health and safety legislation

The enforcement of health and safety legislation by inspectors of the HSE has changed gradually over recent years, from detailed workplace inspections to a more wide-reaching examination of the approaches of organizations to the management of health and safety.

This new approach was confirmed in the Health and Safety Commission's (HSC's) *Plan of Work for 1993/94 and Beyond* (HSC 1993), where it is stated that one of the main priorities will be the securing of more competent and effective management of health and safety by employers. This approach was reiterated in the HSC's *Plan of Work for 1994/95* (HSC 1994). Priority is given to ensuring that employers accept the importance of assessing risks as an essential part of sound safety management. The HSE is pursuing a variety of new approaches to improve its effectiveness. These include inspection initiatives, campaigns and more extensive auditing of health and safety management systems. The HSE is placing great emphasis on the costs of accidents and occupational ill health as a key factor in raising employers' awareness of health and safety issues and achieving compliance with legal requirements.

In May 1995, the HSE launched its largest ever campaign, 'Good Health is Good Business', with the aim of reducing ill health in the workplace. This campaign will last for 3 years, and hopes to raise awareness amongst managers and to persuade them to take positive action to prevent ill health. The principal objective is to improve employer's competence in the management of occupational health. The first phase of the campaign focused on noise, musculoskeletal disorders and respiratory sensitizers. The campaign is supported by a pack of free literature and a range of on-sale publications.

The underlying messages of this campaign are to achieve compliance with legal requirements, to reduce the costs of sickness absence and sick pay, to lower labour turnover and to reduce the costs of recruitment and initial training. These benefits will then lead to increased productivity, improved product quality and, therefore, to improved commercial viability.

The HSE points out in its publicity material for the campaign that 2.2 million people suffer ill health which is caused by or is aggravated by their work activities. The quality of life of these people and their families is affected, and their treatment places a heavy burden on the National Health Service. The HSE emphasizes the cost to the economy in terms of the loss of 13 million working days annually at a total cost of £4.5 billion.

In June 1996, the HSE launched a further campaign for 2 years to reduce accidents involving slips and trips. The HSE again emphasized the cost of such accidents to the individual, to the employer and to society as a whole.

In addition to the programmes of special visits associated with these campaigns, inspectors from the HSE and local authorities will continue to make their routine inspections of workplaces and to undertake audits of organizations' management systems. It is important, therefore, for any organization to demonstrate that it is complying with its legal obligations.

The avoidance of criminal penalties

In order to avoid formal enforcement action by the HSE or local authorities, it is important to have an effective management system in place in order to comply with health and safety legislation. If a prosecution is taken against an organization, as well as any financial penalties which might be imposed by the courts for the failure to comply with legal requirements, there will be other legal costs. Such costs could include the fees for legal representatives, arising from briefings, discussions, the preparation of mitigation or defence arguments and court appearances, and the prosecution's costs. There will also be the costs of any remedial actions or improvements to ensure compliance with legal requirements, whether or not improvement or prohibition notices are served. The cost of management time associated with enforcement actions must also be taken into account.

The maximum fine which can be imposed in a magistrates' court for each offence under Sections 2–6 of the Health and Safety at Work, etc. Act 1974 is £20 000. This maximum also applies to the failure to comply with an improvement or prohibition notice of a court remedy order. The maximum fine for other offences is £5000. Magistrates also have the power to imprison individuals for up to 6 months for breach of an improvement notice, prohibition notice or court remedy order.

At the Crown Court, individuals can be imprisoned for up to 2 years for breach of an improvement notice or court remedy order, as well as for offences concerning explosives, licensing regimes or breach of a prohibition notice. For breaches of the Health and Safety at Work, etc. Act 1974, or of relevant statutory provisions under the Act, the Crown Court can impose unlimited fines.

At magistrates' courts, the maximum penalty is not always served, but there is an increasing willingness by the courts to impose stiffer penalties. Companies, directors and employees (including managers) are routinely prosecuted both by the HSE and local authorities. Some recent examples of penalties imposed at magistrates' courts are given below.

- £20 000 for a company who failed to display a warning notice for an asbestos cement roof. A production foreman who had worked for the company for 30 years fell through the roof and was killed.
- £15 000 for a power station whose poor working procedures led to employees being exposed to ozone levels eight times higher than the occupational exposure standard.
- £12 500 for a local council who failed to ensure the protection of two workers who were exposed to asbestos during work on a council building.
- £6000 for a company who exposed an employee to hydrogen sulphide.

At the Crown Court, large fines have been imposed for health and safety offences. The highest fine imposed to date was £500 000 against BP following a fire at their Grangemouth refinery in 1987. In February 1991, J. Murphy & Sons, a firm of civil engineers, were fined a total of £160 000 plus £28 000 costs following the death of a worker from electric shock when drilling through a cable. Allied Colloids Ltd. were fined £100 000 following a fire at their chemical warehouse in Bradford in 1992. In February 1995, Associated Octel were fined £150 000 plus £142 655 costs following a fire at their chemical works at Ellesmere Port in February 1994.

In January 1996, a freelance demolition contractor was sentenced to 3 months in prison by Bristol Crown Court for failing to prevent the spread of asbestos. The contractor also had to pay £4000 costs. The prosecution case was brought under the Asbestos (Licensing) Regulations 1983 and the Control of Asbestos at Work Regulations 1987. This was the first custodial sentence to be given by a court, previous sentences having either been suspended or having involved community service. Some company directors have been disbarred from being directors as a result of convictions for health and safety offences.

In April 1996, two former company directors were both jailed for 4 months at Bradford Crown Court after pleading guilty to contravening prohibition notices served by HSE inspectors. The notices had been served after an employee had lost his arm as he had been cleaning machinery.

It must be pointed out that insurance cannot be obtained against penalties which may be imposed by courts. Some insurance policies are, however, available to provide cover for possible legal costs which may be incurred by companies, directors or officers in the event that a prosecution or other legal action is taken against them. Such policies would add to the known costs incurred by an organization.

These new penalties now provide a powerful incentive to ensure compliance, and send a clear message to senior management that high standards must be achieved and maintained. Higher penalties are now being imposed by the courts, and these often result in damaging publicity and the consequential stigma of a criminal record. Adverse publicity will clearly have an impact on an organization in terms of its prestige and image with the public, clients and customers. Lost contracts arising from prosecutions can easily be costed, but the loss of potential future contracts is less easy to quantify. Individuals who have been convicted for health and safety offences could have their long-term prospects and earning potential severely impaired, and may experience great difficulties in securing future employment. It clearly pays to avoid prosecution and the penalties which can be imposed.

Cost–benefit analysis

Cost–benefit analysis is a technique which is used to assist in decision making on risk management by comparing the costs of a project to reduce or eliminate risk with the benefits which can accrue. Cost–benefit analysis is used in relation to proposed legislation and in the formulation of strategies for risk management within organizations.

Modern health and safety legislation is based on the cost vs. benefit equation through the phrase: 'so far as reasonably practicable'. Since 1982, the HSC, as part of government policy, has required that cost–benefit analyses are carried out on all major proposals for revised or new health and safety legislation. Such analyses are included in all Consultation Documents on proposed legislation. The costs of the proposed legislation are usually quantified, but it is not always possible to quantify the benefits. However, the benefits are always listed. In order for the proposed legislation to proceed, the benefits must be seen to outweigh the costs. Cost–benefit analysis has been extended to the consultation procedure for maximum exposure limits (HSC 1996).

Within any organization, the undertaking of a cost–benefit analysis requires that the following questions (Bamber 1990b) are answered.

- What costs are involved to reduce or eliminate the risk?
- What degree of capital expenditure is required?

- What ongoing costs will be involved, e.g. regular maintenance, training?
- What will the benefits be?
- What is the pay back period?
- Is there any other more cost-effective method of reducing the risk?

The various cost factors associated with poor risk management have been discussed in previous sections. The cost of insurance premiums and, where appropriate, the contributions towards the cost of damages have been discussed in the sections on: 'Employers' liability insurance and its cost', 'Damages arising from injuries and ill health' and 'Other insurances'. The costs of accidents, both the insured and uninsured costs, have been discussed in the section on: 'The cost of accidents'. Fines and associated legal costs have been discussed in the section on: 'The avoidance of criminal penalties'. Where possible the actual and potential costs should be quantified, and then the cost of the necessary risk improvements can be assessed using the above questions. The cost of risk improvement projects can usually be assessed relatively accurately as there is little difference between the investment requirements of risk management projects and those of any other project.

The benefits arising from risk management projects may be more difficult to quantify than the investment. Where possible, monetary values should be given to all the benefits which can accrue. Benefits of effective risk management (Bamber 1990b) include:

- fewer claims resulting in lower insurance premiums;
- less absenteeism;
- fewer injury and damage accidents;
- better levels of health amongst employees;
- higher productivity and efficiency;
- better utilization of plant and equipment;
- higher morale and motivation of employees; and
- reduction in cost factors.

Other benefits arising from effective risk management have been listed by Bibbings (1995), and include contributions to good business practice by:

- enhancement of quality and reliability programmes;
- enhancement of the public image;
- enhancement of the recruitment image and training programmes;
- enhancement of industrial relations;
- reduction of waste;
- promotion of effectiveness; and
- promotion of a culture of excellence.

The costs of the project can then be balanced against the benefits, and a decision can be made as to whether or not to proceed with the project. Consideration will probably be given to the potential return on investment in terms of the pay back period. It is worth noting that the pay back period for most risk management projects is of the order of 2–5 years (i.e. the medium term).

In any cost–benefit analysis, there are a number of costs which cannot be precisely quantified. The most significant problems relate to the value of a human life and good health. Over the years, economists have sought to set values for the cost of a fatal injury or other injuries to individuals based on the amount that people are prepared to pay to reduce the risk of being killed or injured or, conversely, how much they are prepared to accept for a small increase in risk. In 1987, the Department of Transport commissioned a review of the previous studies on the willingness of people to pay to reduce the risk of death (Dalvi 1988). The value of a life based on this review, and which is now used by the Department of Transport for avoiding a road fatality, is £750 000.

This value of a life was used by Davies and Teasdale (1994) in their study of the cost to the British economy of work accidents and work-related ill health. They used £750 000 as a measure of the cost to injured workers and their families of fatal injuries and premature death from occupational ill health. They calculated the cost of other injuries and occupational ill health using a 'relative utility loss index', which describes the relative disutility of different states of injury or disability in comparison with normal health (Jones-Lee *et al.* 1993). Monetary values can then be ascribed to different states of injury or disability by applying the indices to the value of a life. The HSC (1996) has used the 'relative utility loss index' in the cost–benefit analysis as part of its consultation procedure on maximum exposure limits.

Problems also arise in ascribing realistic monetary values to other benefits. Some benefits may arise immediately and others may occur at unspecified future dates. Other benefits, such as the effect of a project on the morale of individuals or on the reputation of an organization, are less tangible and difficult to quantify. This is a very subjective area, and can lead to disagreements about individual values which have been allocated. However, those who disagree can put forward arguments to the decision makers who can make judgements about the various arguments (Lammin 1995).

Cost–benefit analysis is a useful tool in decision making, but it is important that the limitations outlined above are fully understood and taken into account within the decision-making process.

The needs of the employer

In order to demonstrate compliance with his/her legal obligations (both in criminal law and common law), to reduce the costs relating to accidents and insurance and to avoid criminal penalties, an employer needs to establish a systematic approach to the management of risk. The employer needs to have four key systems (Wrightson 1994) in place:

- a regime of gathering information to enable risks to be identified;
- a method of assessing risks and formulating acceptable risk controls;
- a programmed evaluation of risk controls; and
- a procedure for the investigation and correction of deficiencies.

These key systems must form a management framework which must be capable of generating commitment by the whole workforce. To ensure that the framework is successful, the employer must provide the following:

- a positive policy on the assessment and control of risks, involving the participation of both management (at all levels) and employees in all systems;
- a progressive risk reduction programme;
- safe systems of work and operating procedures;
- agreed disciplinary procedures;
- periodic safety inspection/audits;
- investigation of all accidents, dangerous occurrences, near-misses and cases of occupational ill health;
- annual evaluation of health and safety performance and the setting of future objectives by senior management;
- clear records to demonstrate achievements on all the above matters, including decision-making processes, with permanent retention; and
- periodic liaison with the insurer to update the state of knowledge.

The employer needs to be able to demonstrate that he/she has discharged his/her duties and obligations to both insurers and the enforcing authority and, more importantly and ultimately, to the courts. This can be done to a large extent by following the guidance in either the HSE (1991) publication, *Successful Health and Safety Management*, or the British Standard BS 8800, *Guide to Occupational Health and Safety Management Systems* (British Standards Institution (BSI) 1996).

Conclusions

Risk management has become increasingly important in recent years and provides forceful economic arguments which can be used to persuade managers that the prevention of accidents and occupational ill health and the protection of an organization's assets are essential. Effective risk management can lead to substantial potential cost savings in terms of insurance premiums and accidents and the avoidance of criminal penalties. The adoption of effective risk management procedures can also lead to other benefits and improvements in business practice which, in turn, will contribute to the commercial success of any organization.

The views expressed in this chapter are those of the author and do not necessarily reflect those of his employer.

References

Andreoni, D. (1986) *The Cost of Occupational Accidents and Diseases.* Occupational Health and Safety Series No. 54. International Labour Office, Geneva.

Association of British Insurers (1995) *The UK Employers' Liability Insurance Market—Information Sheet.* Association of British Insurers, London.

Bamber, L. (1979) Accident prevention—the economic argument. *Occupational Safety and Health* 9 (6), 18–21.

Bamber, L. (1990a) Principles of the management of risk. In: *Safety at Work* (ed. J.R. Ridley), 3rd edn., pp. 143–158. Butterworth–Heinemann Ltd., Oxford.

Bamber, L. (1990b) Risk management: techniques and practices. In: *Safety at Work* (ed. J.R. Ridley), 3rd edn., pp. 159–172. Butterworth–Heinemann Ltd., Oxford.

Bibbings, R. (1995) Selling safety. *Occupational Safety and Health* **25** (11), 45–49.

Bird, F.E. (1974) *Management Guide to Loss Control.* Institute Press, Longville, GA.

Bird, F.E. & Germain, G.L. (1966) *Damage Control.* American Management Association, New York.

Bird, F.E. & Loftus, R.G. (1976) *Loss Control Management.* Institute Press, Longville, GA.

Brody, B., Letourneau, Y. & Poirer, A. (1990) An indirect cost theory of work accident prevention. *Journal of Occupational Accidents* 13, 255–270.

BSI (1996) *Guide to Occupational Health and Safety Management Systems.* BS 8800. British Standards Institution, London.

Carter, R.L. & Doherty, N. (1974) *Handbook of Risk Management.* Kluwer-Harrap, London.

Dalvi, M.Q. (1988) *Value of Life and Safety; a Search for a Consensus Estimate.* Department of Transport, London.

Davies, N.V. & Teasdale, P. (1994) *The Cost to the British Economy of Work Accidents and Work-related Ill Health.* HSE Books, Sudbury.

Fisher, T.A. (1991) A 'quality' approach to occupational health, safety and rehabilitation. *Journal of Occupational Health and Safety—Australia and New Zealand* 7 (1), 23–28.

Fletcher, J.A. & Douglas, H.M. (1971) *Total Loss Control Within the Industrial Environment.* Associated Business Programmes, London.

HSC (1993) *Plan of Work for 1993/94 and Beyond.* HMSO, London.

HSC (1994) *Plan of Work for 1994/95.* HSE Books, Sudbury.

HSC (1996) *Proposals for Amendments to the Control of Substances Hazardous to Health Regulations 1994 and the Approved Code of Practice: Control of Substances Hazardous to Health (General ACOP).* Consultative Document CD103. HSE Books, Sudbury.

HSE (1991) *Successful Health and Safety Management.* Health and Safety Series Booklet HS(G)65. HMSO, London.

HSE (1993) *The Cost of Accidents at Work.* Health and Safety Series Booklet HS(G)96. HMSO, London.

HSE (1995) *Be Safe, Save Money!—The Costs of Accidents—A Guide to Small Firms.* IND (G)208L. HSE, London.

Heinrich, H.W. (1959) *Industrial Accident Prevention: A Safety Management Approach*, 4th edn, pp. 13–16. McGraw-Hill, New York (5th edn., 1980, revised by D. Peterson *et al.*).

Jones-Lee, M., O'Reilly, D. & Phillips, S. (1993) *The Value of Preventing*

Non-Fatal Road Injuries: Findings of a Willingness to Pay National Sample Survey. Transport Research Laboratory Contractor Report 330. Department of Transport, London.
Judicial Studies Board (1994) *Guide Lines for the Assessment of General Damages in Personal Injury Cases*. Blackstone Press Limited, London.
Lammin, S. (1995) The role of cost–benefit analysis in formulating strategies for improving safety and health at work. *The Safety and Health Practitioner* **13** (1), 18–20.
New, N.H. (1996) Measuring accident losses. Paper presented at the *IIR Ltd. Conference on Human Factors of Health and Safety Management, June 27, 1996, London*. IIR Ltd., London.
Oxenburg, M. (1991) *Increasing Productivity and Profit Through Health and Safety*. CCH Australia Limited for CCH International, North Ryde, NSW.
Oxenburg, M. & Guldberg, H. (1988) *Economic Impact of Draft Safe Manual Handling Code of Practice*. The National Occupational Health and Safety Commission (Worksafe Australia), Sydney.
Pardy, W.G. (1991) Do the right thing. The safety/quality relationship. *Canadian Occupational Safety* **29** (5), 10–12, 14.
Sachs, B. (1991) Accidents—an avoidable waste. *Safety Management* **17** (2), 23.
Salazar, N. (1989) Applying the Dening philosophy to the safety systems. *Professional Safety* **34** (12), 22–27.
Sonderqvist, A., Rundrno, T. & Aaltonen, M. (1990) The cost of occupational accidents in the Nordic furniture industry (Sweden, Norway, Finland). *Journal of Occupational Accidents* **12** (1–3), 79–88.
Stevens, G. (1992) Workplace injury: a view from HSE's trailers to the 1990 Labour Force Survey. *Employment Gazette* 100, December.
Tye, J. (1976) *Accident Ratio Study 1974/75*. British Safety Council, London.
Veltri, A. (1990) An accident cost impact model: the direct cost component. *Journal of Safety Research* **21**, 67–73.
Whiston, J. & Eddershaw, B. (1989) Quality and safety—distant cousins or close relatives? *The Chemical Engineer* **461**, 97–102.
Wright, E.L.G. (1990) True costs of accidents are not assessed. *Australian Safety News* **61**, 11.
Wrightson, I. (1994) An insurer's approach to health, safety and environmental issues. In: *The Laboratory Environment* (ed. R. Purchase), pp. 27–45. The Royal Society of Chemistry, Cambridge.
Wrightson, I. (1995) The growing importance of risk management—an insurer's view. *Loss Prevention Bulletin* **123**, 15–18.

Chapter 13 Emergency response

Chris Whitmore

Introduction

This chapter deals with emergencies—events which occur after all the precautions and control measures have failed. The effects of emergencies can be mitigated by careful consideration, planning and implementation of response arrangements. However, if these actions are not taken, an emergency can quickly escalate into a 'crisis', with consequences which can cause potential long-term or even permanent damage to the organization, affecting its corporate image and its ability to continue operating. In this chapter, we look at examples of how effective emergency response arrangements can be developed and put in place so that, hopefully, a crisis will never occur.

Emergencies

An emergency is any unplanned event which requires urgent action to be taken in order to prevent injury or loss of life, damage to plant and equipment or damage to the environment. In many cases, a threat to the corporate image or the future business of an organization may also be considered as an emergency (e.g. in the case of product liability).

Emergencies vary significantly in their nature and extent: an injured person on the shop floor may be the most serious emergency experienced by one company; a massive fire and explosion with fatalities and serious environmental pollution may affect another. The scale of response therefore needs to be matched to what the organization may be expected to deal with.

Emergencies tend to fall into the following categories:

- *operational*: fire, explosion, gas leak, etc.;
- *environmental*: oil spill, chemical leak, etc.;
- *health*: outbreak of disease, fatality, injury, etc.;
- *transport*: air crash, rail crash, vessel sinking, road accident, etc.;
- *security*: bomb threat, kidnapping, extortion, criminal damage, civil disturbance, etc.;
- *product*: product tampering, failure to meet specification, etc.;
- *natural disaster*: earthquake, flood, hurricane, etc.

Effective emergency response depends on a careful assessment of the risks to the organization and its operations, the consideration of all likely scenarios and the development of arrangements to mitigate the effects of the emergency. These arrangements include the organization's own response, together with that of external emergency services, when these are required. The interfaces between the organization and the external agencies, and between the external agencies themselves, must be carefully defined.

Hence, as in other areas, the process starts with a risk assessment to determine what might happen; nevertheless, the prime objective must be to take all reasonable preventive measures to try to ensure that an emergency does not occur in the first place. Having to activate the emergency response arrangements should be regarded as a failure of other primary Health and Safety Executive (HSE) management arrangements.

Statutory requirements

Statutory requirements governing emergency response vary from country to country—many have no specific legislation. However, because of a number of major industrial incidents in recent years—Bhopal, Seveso, Piper Alpha, Chernobyl, Flixborough—the UK, Europe and other countries have put in place legislation which addresses the response to industrial emergencies. In the UK, the main items of legislation which are relevant are given below.

- The Control of Industrial Major Accident and Hazard (CIMAH) Regulations 1984 for onshore hazardous facilities.
- The Offshore Installations (Prevention of Fire and Explosion, and Emergency Response, PFEER) Regulations 1995 for offshore facilities.

The CIMAH Regulations deal with planning considerations, safety assessments and contingency plans. They apply to chemical and petrochemical plants which have, on site, dangerous substances in quantities specified in the CIMAH Regulations. The plant operator is required to produce on-site emergency plans, in conjunction with local authorities and emergency services. The local authorities have responsibility for off-site emergency planning, but the operator must provide them with information to enable them to make the necessary off-site arrangements.

The PFEER Regulations affect offshore oil and gas installations, where the need for good emergency response arrangements is made particularly critical by the adverse conditions, high personnel density in a potentially hazardous environment and the remoteness from emergency support should things go wrong. The PFEER Regulations take account of the experience gained from the Piper Alpha disaster, and replace the legislation which existed prior to that event.

In addition to the above specific regulations, the issue of emergency response is effectively covered by the employer's general duty of care as defined in the Health and Safety at Work, etc. Act 1974, in particular Section 2.1, namely:

It shall be the duty of every employer to ensure, so far as is reasonably practicable, the health, safety and welfare of all his employees.

As well as a duty to employees, employers have responsibility for visitors, contractors and the general public.

In simple terms, the ability to administer first aid to a heart attack victim, or to evacuate people from a blazing office, are examples of emergency response arrangements which need to be in place to meet the above requirement of the Health and Safety at Work, etc. Act 1974.

There are other non-legislative, but nevertheless powerful, documents which influence emergency response planning. A good example is contained in:

- *Guidelines for the Development and Application of Health, Safety and Environmental Management Systems*, Report No. 6.36/210, published by the Oil Industry International Exploration and Production Forum (E & P Forum 1994).

The E & P Forum is the international association of oil companies and petroleum industry organizations, formed in 1974 to represent its members' interests at the International Maritime Organization and other specialist agencies of the United Nations, European Union, governmental and other international bodies. The E & P Forum is made up of 38 oil companies and 14 national oil industry associations operating in 60 different countries. The guidelines referred to above are in the nature of a code of practice for use in a hazardous industry, and the sections relating to emergency response are as follows:

Contingency and Emergency Planning

The company should maintain procedures to identify foreseeable emergencies by systematic review and analysis. A record of such identified potential emergencies should be made, and updated at appropriate intervals in order to ensure effective response to them.

The company should develop, document and maintain plans for responding to such potential emergencies, and communicate such plans to:

- command and control personnel;
- emergency services;
- employees and contractors who may be affected;
- others likely to be impacted.

Emergency plans should cover:

- organization, responsibilities, authorities and procedures for emergency response and disaster control, including the maintenance of internal and external communications;
- systems and procedures for providing personnel refuge, evacuation, rescue and medical treatment;
- systems and procedures for preventing, mitigating and monitoring environmental effects of emergency actions;
- procedures for communicating with authorities, relatives and other relevant parties;

- systems and procedures for mobilizing company equipment, facilities and personnel;
- arrangements and procedures for mobilizing third party resources for emergency support;
- arrangements for training response teams and for testing the emergency systems and procedures.

To assess the effectiveness of response plans, the company should maintain procedures to test emergency plans by scenario drills and other suitable means, at appropriate intervals, and to revise them as necessary in the light of experience gained.

Procedures should also be in place for the periodic assessment of emergency equipment needs and the maintenance of such equipment in a ready state.

Thus, there is plenty of guidance material available to assist those responsible for developing and implementing emergency plans.

Risk assessment

The precursor to the development of appropriate responses to emergencies is to carry out risk assessments covering all the activities of the organization. Most organizations are reluctant to consider the negative things that might happen to them, yet this is essential to the risk assessment process. Those events which could conceivably happen should be examined, the consequences determined and the actions necessary to respond to them established. Events which are considered too unlikely to occur can be rejected, but those involved should try to imagine what their response should be were they to occur.

For example, an organization operating in a country with limited medical facilities should consider the actions to be taken in the event of serious injury or illness to an employee. What immediate help is there? Where does the person need to be taken for further treatment? How quickly can they be transported there? What prior arrangements need to be in place to get them there? Answering these questions may lead to the inevitable conclusion that, if satisfactory emergency medical evacuation arrangements cannot be made, the organization may have to provide comprehensive medical facilities at the location.

The best results from the risk assessment process are achieved by getting together all the key people with a knowledge of the organization's business and operational activities, and 'brainstorming' all the 'what if?' situations which could occur. An outsider, experienced in emergency planning, but with little knowledge of the organization and its activities, can help immensely in this process by challenging and testing the organization's assumptions. By adopting this approach, plans and arrangements will be produced which will be appropriate to the organization's needs.

Additional information will be available from other sources, such as a CIMAH case or safety case, and this should be taken into account.

Levels of response

The organization needs to have different levels of emergency response which can be mobilized according to the type and severity of the incident. For example, one extreme would involve first aid given to an injured person at the workplace, with initial attempts to fight fire, clean up spillage, etc.; the other extreme would involve the mobilization and co-ordination of the entire emergency response organization, together with the external emergency services.

The procedures must enable the level of severity of an emergency incident to be clearly identified and communicated, such that the appropriate level of response is mobilized. However, whenever there is any doubt, the response should be greater rather than less; it is easier to stand resources down than to try to mobilize additional resources later, and hence lose valuable time in responding.

For example, major oil companies with oil spill response arrangements in place use a 'tiered' response, normally three tiers, with the number of tiers mobilized dependent on the size and nature of the spill.

Some form of predetermined classification of emergency severity can be helpful as shown below.

Level 1. An incident which can be handled by the persons at the site without additional help. There is unlikely to be danger to life, the environment or to company assets.

Level 2. An incident which can be handled by persons at the site, but which requires assistance from external emergency services. There may be danger to life, the environment or to company assets.

Level 3. A serious incident which requires the involvement of extensive resources and of government and external agencies. There will be one of the following:

- death and/or serious injury;
- significant environmental damage;
- significant damage to assets;
- significant media interest.

Emergency organization

The emergency organization is usually arranged in a hierarchy—from front-line response at the scene of the incident to corporate response covering topics such as media response, government liaison, overall strategy, etc.

It is common for the emergency response to be organized in up to four levels, depending on the nature and size of the organization, namely:

- on-site response;
- local emergency management;
- national emergency management;
- corporate emergency management support and crisis management.

The key to an effective response to emergencies is to have a preestablished organization, on call and capable of mobilizing and responding to the extent required by different levels of emergency. It should be staffed with competent individuals and organized into teams, with allocated and defined roles, and practised in those roles. As far as possible, responsibilities within the emergency teams should be as close as possible to those which the team members hold in their normal day-to-day activities, i.e. a team member with responsibility for logistics would normally be involved in the logistics function. Examples of typical members for each level of emergency response team are outlined below.

For each of the emergency management teams, a logkeeper needs to be provided. This is an important role. The logkeeper must have an understanding of the technicalities of the business, and works under the direction of the team leader to record the status of events as they unfold. Keeping accurate information on the status boards is critical as major decisions may be made on the basis of the information displayed. New arrivals in the team can gain a quick update of the status of events by reviewing the status boards in the emergency room. In addition to the status boards, it is often the practice to keep a running log of all events. This log simply records everything that is happening, with no attempt

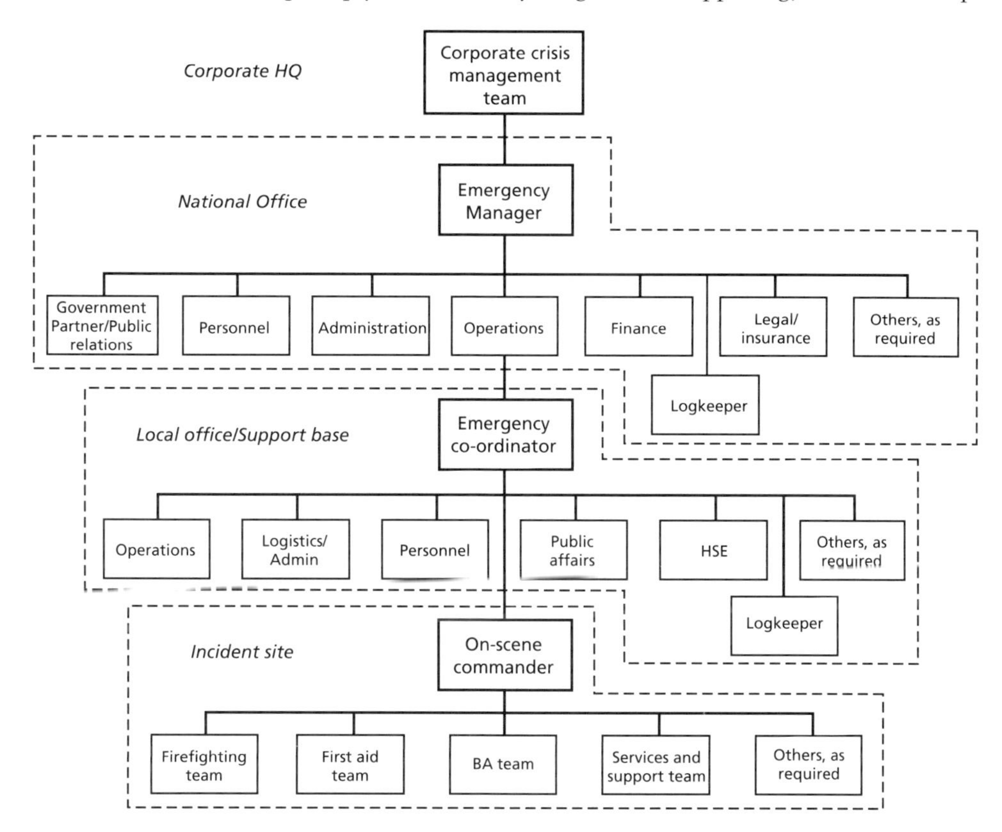

Figure 13.1 Typical emergency organization.

made to separate out the significant information. It is used as a historical record, rather than as an up-to-date status display. There may therefore be a requirement for two logkeepers, each with an entirely different function to perform.

An additional important factor in the selection and training of emergency personnel was highlighted in the Cullen Report into the Piper Alpha disaster in the North Sea in 1988 (Cullen 1990). This is the ability of the person in charge of the emergency scene to take command and make decisions under pressure. Lives may depend on decisions made at the scene, and therefore exceptional qualities of leadership may be required. Such qualities are also required of leaders of the supporting emergency teams.

Figure 13.1 shows a typical hierarchical emergency organization for a multinational company with major operations within a country remote from its corporate headquarters.

Figure 13.2 shows the communication lines and external interfaces which the organization has to handle.

Typically, the higher level teams work on a much longer timescale of events than those nearer to the incident. For the latter, the incident may be over in a couple of hours or less. For the corporate team, the consequences may need to be dealt with over days, weeks, months or even years.

On-site response team

The on-site response team (or teams) is that which takes the immediate actions to respond to an incident. In a large complex environment, there may be several on-site teams covering fire-fighting, breathing apparatus (BA) and rescue and first aid. Their function is to take all the immediate actions required pending the arrival of the supporting emergency services. The risk assessment should have considered the extent of an incident which might be experienced at the site, the level of support available from the local emergency services and the time required for them to respond. In a remote rural location (where hazardous plants are often deliberately built), this time can be significant, and the organization's on-site teams may have to deal with a major incident involving multiple casualties, rescue and fire-fighting without any immediate support.

The risk assessment should also have taken into account whether or not the organization adopts a 'burn-down' philosophy, i.e. no major attempts are made to protect assets once all personnel have been safely rescued. This can be an option for cost reasons, or simply so that personnel are not put at further risk. The result of the risk assessment determines the level of competence required of the on-site team, and therefore the extent of training required. The on-site team is usually under the command of an on-scene commander, who directs its activities and liaises with external emergency services and the emergency management team.

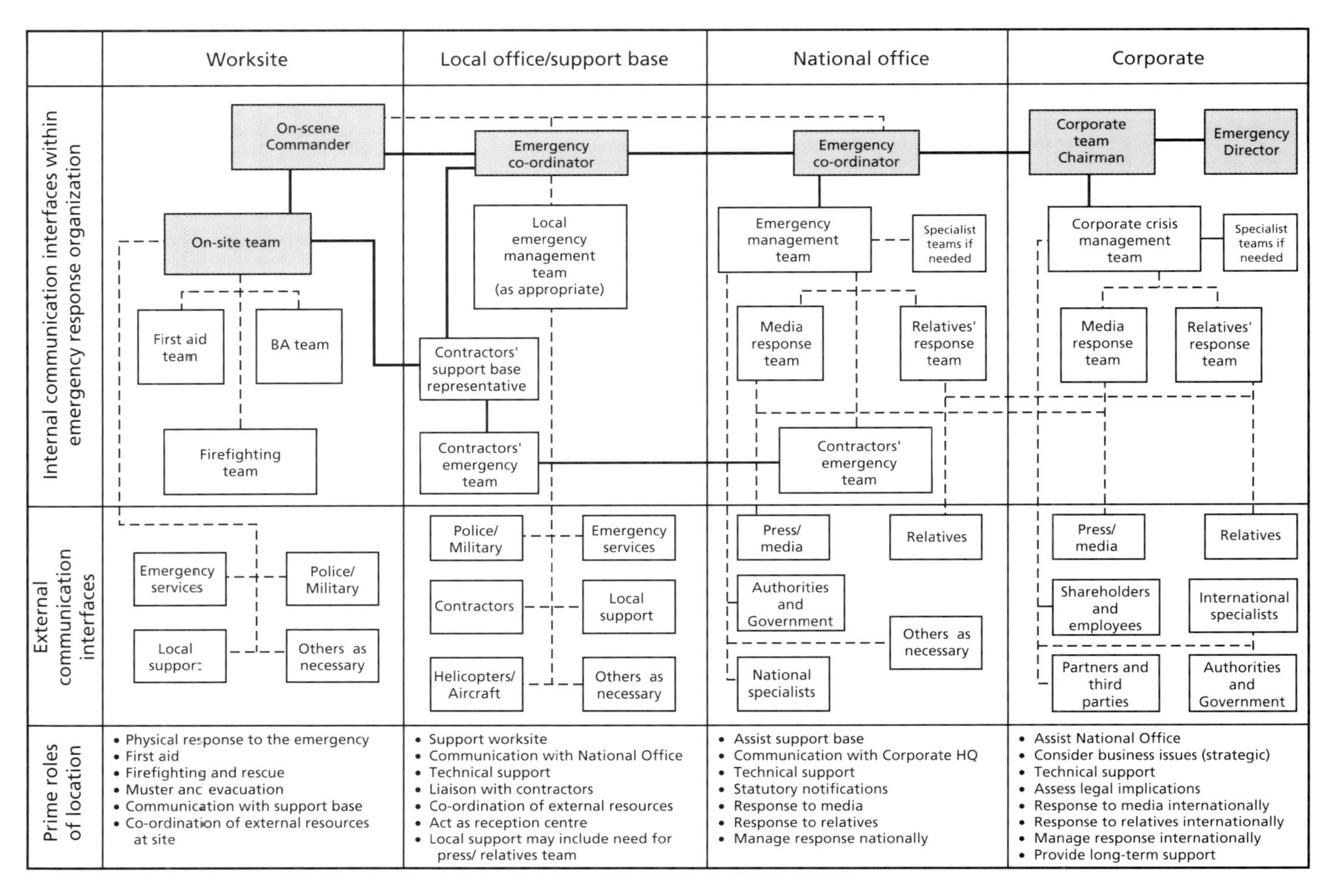

Figure 13.2 Emergency response overview. ——, denotes primary lateral lines of communication; - - - - -, denotes other lines of communication.

An important duty of the on-site team is to ensure that emergency personnel coming onto the site are informed about, and protected from, hazards which may exist on the site. The on-scene commander must ensure that information on hazards, such as chemicals, is transmitted to the external emergency services. One way of doing this is to assign a knowledgeable and informed person to meet the emergency services at the entrance to the site. The on-site commander must also ensure that the plant is made as safe as possible to enable rescue and fire-fighting activities to take place. This means ensuring that plant is shut down and isolated. In certain situations, electrical isolation of entire areas will be necessary to allow the use of firewater.

Local emergency management team

At the location of the incident, or at the base from which the operation is run, an emergency management team is usually established. Its function is to liaise with the on-site team, the rest of the organization, representatives of the emergency services and other external organizations. Not being directly involved in the actions taking place at the scene, it is able to take an overview of how well the response is working, and can take actions, such as mobilizing additional support, providing technical advice, etc., if these are required. Most importantly, the team is the focal point for the collection and assimilation of information coming directly from the on-site team and from other sources, such as the media. A major site, such as a chemical plant, will have such an on-site management team. The team leader is often called the emergency co-ordinator.

The emergency management team is usually provided with its own dedicated facilities or, at worst, with a room, such as a conference room, which can be quickly set up to be used as an emergency control centre. Team members have their own dedicated roles within the team, such as dealing with the media, logistics, technical back-up, operational support, etc. Each team member must ensure that he can access the information required and additional back-up and support to help him fulfil his role, particularly outside of normal working hours. This means that each function represented in an emergency response team will have its own departmental procedures detailing how it will support the team in the event of an incident.

Typically, an emergency management team might include the following:

- team leader;
- operations;
- logistics/administration;
- health, safety and environment;
- personnel;
- public affairs;
- technical;
- logkeeper.

It is vitally important that the emergency management team does not interfere with the ability of the on-site team to handle the events at the scene. It must not try to run the on-site response, and it must not make excessive demands for information. It should try to ensure that it provides support, and should try to remove unnecessary pressure from the on-site team members, e.g. by dealing with enquiries from outside agencies.

The emergency co-ordinator needs to be a person with the ability to direct the activities of a multidisciplined team—setting priorities, summarizing key information, delegating tasks, anticipating events, ensuring that no important issues are overlooked, etc. It is good practice for the emergency co-ordinator to call for 'time-outs' at regular intervals (e.g. every 15 min) so that the team can take stock of what is happening. During these time-outs, all phone conversations are halted, the co-ordinator summarizes what is happening and where they are going, asks each team member to contribute anything he/she wants to add, and makes sure everyone is clear about what is being done. In this way, nothing gets overlooked under the pressure of events.

National office emergency management team

The organization's national office in a country (other than where its corporate headquarters are located) needs to have its own emergency management team to deal with issues resulting from the emergency which have implications for its operations in the country. Typically, this would involve dealing with governmental bodies and similar groups, dealing with corporate headquarters if in another country and, most importantly, providing the necessary back-up and support to the local emergency management team. The national office will be concerned with protecting the organization's business interests in the country and its ongoing operations there by, for example, controlling the issue of press releases. The team would normally take responsibility for the official notifications to governmental authorities.

As for the local team, the national team should ensure that it does not interfere with the proper operation of the local team by, for example, making excessive demands for information. Rather, it should take a supporting role and, wherever possible, try to take the pressure off the local team.

In addition to some of the functions represented in the local team, the national team is likely to include representatives of legal, finance and insurance functions.

Corporate emergency management team (or crisis management team)

Most major international organizations have in place arrangements to mobilize a team of their senior people to form a corporate emergency management team, more commonly named a crisis management team.

Its primary responsibility is to look at the unfolding emergency events and consider what needs to be done to protect the organization's corporate image and to minimize any 'corporate damage' which may be caused by the emergency. Examples of corporate damage are the eventual withdrawal from UK operations of Occidental Petroleum following the Piper Alpha disaster, the effect on sales when benzene traces were found in Perrier mineral water and the long-term damage to the reputation of Exxon caused by the oil spill disaster at Valdez.

The types of issue that the team would consider include:

- the effectiveness of the organization's response to the emergency, particularly whether there have been any management failures;
- any additional back-up and support required;
- strategic issues affecting the organization's future operation;
- how the organization is being portrayed by the media and how it is seen by the outside world;
- whether or not a senior person should travel to the site of the incident (an important decision—after Bhopal, Union Carbide's president, Warren Anderson, flew to India and was promptly arrested, thus removing him completely from the emergency response effort just when he was needed).

Back-up teams

Depending on the type of emergency and the nature of the organization affected, different back-up teams may be called out and mobilized to assist the main emergency teams. These could include:

- engineering/technical support teams;
- public affairs' teams to answer media calls;
- personnel response teams to answer relatives' calls;
- medical, environmental or other teams to provide support as required.

Common to almost all emergencies is the need for good support from the organization's switchboard staff. They need to be fully trained, briefed and updated, and need to be able to mobilize additional help and support for themselves as necessary.

Callout and mobilization

The names and contact details of all emergency team members must be published and kept up-to-date by nominated persons responsible for the emergency response arrangements at all locations. A duty rota is essential, with adequate availability of deputies.

All personnel on duty are responsible for ensuring that they are contactable, available and able to respond to an emergency callout for the duration of their duty period. This will mean individuals carrying the necessary equipment (e.g. pager) and documentation. All pagers and other communications devices should be tested at the start of the duty period. Individual team members are responsible for ensuring that their equipment is working at all times, and particularly that batteries are charged. If an emergency team member is personally unavailable for any part of his duty period, he must ensure that he hands over properly to his deputy, and that *all* relevant persons are notified of the change.

An all-too-frequent occurrence is the partial or complete failure of an organization's carefully planned emergency response, simply because a key individual (or individuals) is unable to be contacted when an incident has occurred.

Arrangements should be made to relieve duty personnel after an appropriate time when the emergency is long running. This means having preplanned alternative personnel available who can be called upon.

Ideally, the callout will be initiated using the following, in order of preference:

- pager;
- office/home telephone number;
- mobile telephone number.

Communications

An effective response to an emergency is heavily dependent on the ability to communicate details of the incident quickly to the emergency organization, for the organization itself to be able to mobilize quickly and for the emergency plans to be quickly activated as required. Therefore, it is essential that good reliable communications are provided and that duty personnel are able to be contacted quickly and able to mobilize quickly. Where communications are less than ideal, e.g. in many countries, consideration must be given to the provision of dedicated communications for emergency use. These will probably need to include the use of fixed or portable satellite links. Even in a country with good communications, a major disaster can cause such an increase in communications traffic that a normally effective system cannot cope. This is what happened in the case of the San Francisco earthquake.

Consideration should also be given to the security of emergency communications, as much information passing may be of a confidential nature, and possibly damaging if allowed to fall into the hands of the media or similar groups. For example, in the Three-Mile Island nuclear incident, a journalist using a scanner was able to tune into the radio-frequencies being used by emergency personnel.

Emergency facilities

Emergency personnel need to have access to adequate facilities from which to control the response. In a major plant, the front-line response is often run from a control room, with management support and back-up either from a dedicated emergency response room or from a room, such as a conference room, which can be quickly converted into a suitable location for running the response. This is often achieved by having

Table 13.1 Typical emergency response facilities.

Emergency response rooms	A suitable location from where events can be controlled, such as: • mobile command and control vehicle • plant control room • dedicated emergency response centre • conference room, easily adapted into emergency room Reception centre for evacuees/casualties Separate rooms for dealing with relatives and media Press/relatives' holding area (e.g. local hotel)
Callout equipment (to call off-duty personnel)	Pagers and/or mobile phones Spare batteries and chargers, as required
Emergency equipment	The emergency equipment will depend on the operation and may include some or all of the following: • fire-fighting • breathing apparatus • first aid/medical • oil spill containment and cleanup
Communications	Telephones with direct lines/VHF radios/mobile phones for team members Mobile phones (with charged batteries) as back-ups Satellite links independent of local phone system Speaker phone (with duplex transmission) Tape recorder for recording phone calls, if required Fax machine on dedicated number (must not be able to receive routine traffic) E-mail, if in normal use
Clocks	Digital clocks, one on local time; others on location times, if different
Status board	Plain white board with usable pens for recording key information White board premarked up for recording key facts and events, particularly notifications Flipcharts, and means of displaying sheets around rooms

Continued

an 'emergency cupboard' in the room, or nearby, which contains telephones, documentation, status boards and all the other equipment needed to convert a normal room into an emergency control centre.

Adequate and well-maintained facilities and communications are essential for effective emergency response. Because of the potential speed of events during an emergency, preplanning is essential to ensure that adequate facilities and equipment are available and in place. This also applies to what may be regarded as of minor importance prior to an event (e.g. stationery, maps, etc.), but which could cause unnecessary problems if absent during a real emergency.

Table 13.1 gives examples of typical facilities and equipment. It should not be considered to be comprehensive, as other items unique to the location may be required.

Table 13.1 *Continued.*

Documentation	Emergency procedures (including those of other locations, as appropriate) Up-to-date lists of personnel and their locations Next of kin details for all personnel Contractors' emergency procedures Contingency plans Technical and operating procedures (particularly emergency shutdown) for all facilities Up-to-date list of all duty personnel (including contractor, etc.)* Technical data regarding status of operations* Operational and logistical data (e.g. up-to-date weather forecasts)* All necessary contact numbers, e.g. hospitals, doctors, contractors, etc.* (NB. It will be necessary for the information marked * above to be updated in the emergency control room at regular intervals, e.g. daily) Material safety data sheets Detailed maps covering all areas of operation, marked with travelling times between locations. Other relevant information could include access routes to beaches, riverbanks, etc., for personnel, heavy equipment, etc. Aerial photographs for environmentally sensitive areas Checklists for each team member (consider placing these on wall charts) Press packs and holding statements for distribution to media
Administrative	PC for wordprocessing event log and e-mail, if used Overhead projector Stationery: logsheets, pens, etc. TV/video and radio (for monitoring media broadcasts)

Plans and procedures

When the risks facing the organization have been assessed and the various scenarios evaluated, much work is required to develop effective plans for dealing with the events which may occur and affect the organization. Typical activities which need to be considered include:

- the emergency organization;
- the duty rota;
- the first-line response, and the availability and readiness of personnel and equipment;
- the support available from the local and national emergency services, and from specialist contractors;
- the technical issues which need to be dealt with, and the availability of information (such as chemical data sheets) and specialist expertise (such as oil spill cleanup experts).

It is essential that the plans and procedures are properly documented and controlled, both for communication purposes and to ensure that the correct actions are taken. Emergency procedures should be handled as controlled documents under the organization's quality assurance system. In addition to the detailed definitive procedures, easy-to-use checklists and contact lists (possibly with simple flow charts) should be made available for all key emergency staff and, if possible, on the organization's computer network system, e.g. intranet.

Typical contents in an emergency procedure manual would include:

- classifications of emergencies;
- emergency organization and duty personnel;
- alarm, callout and mobilization;
- emergency facilities;
- communications;
- checklists for specific emergencies;
- notifications to authorities;
- contact lists.

Training and exercises

When the emergency arrangements have been put in place and clearly documented in procedures, comprehensive training of all personnel must be carried out. Personnel must obviously be given detailed training in how to perform their own particular duties, but, in addition, they will be able to perform far more effectively if they can see how they fit into the overall emergency response organization and can see what others will be doing. Therefore, a clear description of the overall response should be given to all those involved.

Training needs will depend upon the nature of the organization and the types of incident which will have to be dealt with. Typical examples of the types of training required are given below.

Initial familiarization

When the emergency response arrangements have been initially set up, a familiarization session should be run for all staff involved at the location. This should stress the importance of being ready and able to respond to an emergency, and should inform all personnel of the arrangements in place.

All employees and visitors should be made aware of the existence of the emergency response arrangements, particularly the alarm system, the escape routes and the muster points.

Initial training is vital to ensure that emergency response arrangements work effectively, and that personnel know how to use the facilities and equipment. Follow-up training must also ensure that the competence in emergency response is maintained to a suitable level at all times, especially for key personnel.

Specific training for team members

For those directly involved in the emergency response organization, specific training should be given in their individual roles and responsibilities, and how these relate to others in the organization. In particular, special training may be given to team leaders and those managing emergencies in how to handle conflicting priorities and stress in crisis situations. Courses are available which put participants under extreme pressure. These include being presented with scenarios where there is inadequate information and conflicting or irreconcilable issues, but at the same time calling for positive decisions and judgements to be made.

Depending on the likelihood and possible extent of fire, fire teams will need specific training in fire-fighting techniques. The competence required of the teams will also depend upon the speed with which the local fire brigade can respond to an incident at the site. On offshore oil installations, for example, the fire teams need to be totally self-sufficient, as it is unlikely that any back-up fire-fighting capability is going to be available. Specialized training therefore needs to be carried out at a training institution, or specialist training can be provided at the site. Usually, however, special facilities are required, such as smoke chambers and firegrounds, which may not be appropriate to have on site.

First aid training is essential for all members of the first aid teams, and will involve, as a minimum, training similar to St. John's Ambulance or Red Cross first aid courses, including techniques of cardiopulmonary resuscitation (CPR).

Where fire, hazardous gases or a lack of a breathable atmosphere is likely to be encountered, rescue teams need to be trained in the use of breathing apparatus and in associated rescue techniques.

Plant operators need to know how to make the plant safe in emergency situations and what will be expected of them in response to the scenarios identified. The operating procedures for the plant must include how it can be shut down safely in abnormal conditions. In industries involved in hazardous transport, drivers need to be trained in the first-line response, i.e. the actions that need to be taken prior to the arrival of the emergency services to prevent further escalation of the incident and to protect the public and the environment.

Where the emergency could result in damage to the environment, specific training should be given in techniques to prevent or mitigate the effects of such damage, e.g. in oil spill containment and cleanup.

Exercises

The testing and validation of training are generally performed by simulating emergency situations. There are several types of exercise commonly used. Each type of exercise requires a different level of involvement by the participants and the use of different internal and external resources.

Desk top exercise

This is a simple run through, by either the emergency co-ordinator or an external specialist, of a simulated emergency. This would normally be held in the emergency response room, allowing personnel to familiarize themselves with the facilities, plans and communication arrangements. It is primarily a means of assisting personnel to identify the tasks expected of them against the backdrop of an emergency. The usual duration may be of the order of 1–2 h.

Simulated exercise

This is an exercise in which emergency events are simulated externally. Role players simulate the actions, responses and activities of individuals, external agencies, organizations, officials, relatives and the media. In many cases, professionals are used, e.g. journalists, which adds realism to the events. The normal duration is of the order of 2–4 h, but this may vary.

It is normal to hold a post-exercise debriefing session with those personnel involved in the exercise, both participants and role players. The aim of the debriefing session is to identify the strengths and weaknesses of the response and where improvements can be made. A formal report, detailing the findings, is usually prepared and submitted to the person sponsoring the exercise. No external resources need to be mobilized in this form of exercise.

Live exercise

This is similar to the above, but would normally only be used where major operations exist. External personnel and organizations are used to perform the roles that they would execute during a real emergency. This may, for example, involve the mobilization and flying of helicopters to the incident site, the mobilization of and liaison with emergency services, dealing with the police, the organization and attending of press conferences, etc. Realistic injuries may be simulated by role players (such as those provided by Casualty Union) to test the first aid and medical response. The duration of such an exercise may be substantially longer than that of a simulated exercise—typically 2–3 days. Exercises of this type are organized at regular intervals by local authorities in the UK, often in conjunction with a major company, such as the operator of a hazardous plant in the authority's area. They can involve many other organizations, such as voluntary agencies.

Media response

Whenever an emergency situation occurs nowadays, the media are quick to respond. They will often have better information about what is happening than the organization itself. In the past few years, the improvements in communications, both local and worldwide, have resulted in major changes in how organizations handle events when dealing with emergency situations. It is easy for a media representative, local to a developing scenario, to have access to better information about the event than the organization's management, who may be at another location. In addition, with the ease of communication nationally and internationally with mobile phones and satellite links, the information can be transmitted to a wide audience, even while events are actually happening at the scene. It is therefore not credible for the organization to deny that anything is happening, or to try to hide behind a statement such as 'no comment'. The media and their audience can see for themselves what is happening and, for the organization to suggest that there is nothing going on, will quickly give the impression, rightly or wrongly, that it does not know what is happening and is therefore not in control.

If the media know that there has been an incident, a response of 'no comment' will quickly make them hostile to the organization—their objective is to get the facts about what has happened and what is being done and to produce a story. If the organization is not prepared to help in this regard, they will go elsewhere for their material, and may obtain inaccurate or damaging information from sources which may not have the organization's best interests at heart. Therefore, the organization must be prepared to help as best as it can.

It is easy for the organization to quickly discredit itself in the eyes of the outside world, giving an image of being uncaring, incompetent, reckless, with a total disregard for safety, etc. The damage which can be inflicted on the organization's ongoing business or its corporate image can have serious long-term implications. Therefore, the organization's ability to respond effectively to the media and the outside world is a critical part of its overall response.

General information about the organization is a good starting point—it gives the journalists something to work with. A 'holding statement' should be issued quickly when the existence of an incident is confirmed. Such a statement should be worded in the following manner:

> I am sorry that we have no information that we can give you at the moment. Please call back in 30 min when we may be able to help.

Such a message demonstrates a willingness to co-operate. At the same time, general information about the organization and its activities contained in 'press packs' can be made available.

A facility needs to be set up quickly to deal with enquiries. This would be the typical 'press office'. There needs to be sufficient trained staff to deal with the volume of enquiries, and these staff must be clearly instructed in what information they are allowed to release. This will normally be restricted to the information contained in the 'press packs' and in authorized press releases. The importance of being able to compile and authorize press releases quickly cannot be overemphasized—this is a critical part of the organization's response. The public, i.e. the media, want to know what is going on. In order to be able to tell them, the organization must know, firstly, what is happening at the scene in as much detail as possible, and, secondly, what its position is on the incident and how it is to be presented to the outside world.

Therefore, there is a need to have as much accurate factual information available as possible on which to make decisions relating to the incident and the response, and on which to base the information to release. The validation of the information received is essential as, if factually incorrect information is given out, serious damage to the organization's credibility and reputation can be done, which can be difficult to rectify. A soundly based emergency response organization and good plans and procedures go a long way to ensuring that reliable information is collected, validated and correctly assessed.

The organization's switchboard and security staff need to be given clear guidance and training about what to do in response to media enquiries, particularly in the early stages of an incident when information may be sketchy and confused.

It is also important that senior managers in the organization, particularly those at remote locations, are trained in how to handle media interviews and are given the authority to talk to the press. It should also be widely known that only authorized persons are allowed to speak to the media. At the national or corporate headquarters, a skilled person should be nominated to act as the media spokesperson. This may not necessarily be the most senior person; rather, the person who will portray the organization and its actions in the best possible light. Training for all those who may have to face the media needs to be intensive, and must include appearing in front of film/TV cameras, with feedback and coaching as required.

Relatives' response

In an incident in which the organization's own employees have been involved, possibly as casualties, or where members of the general public have been involved, there will inevitably be enquiries from concerned relatives and other interested parties (some genuine, others frivolous or even malicious). Therefore, the organization needs to have in place a system for answering calls from relatives. In the case of a major emergency involving members of the general public, the police (certainly in the UK, but not necessarily in other countries) will usually provide a response service for relatives, and issue the numbers to call through the media. A major organization experiencing an emergency involving its own personnel needs to have effective procedures in place and staff trained to operate them.

Contingency planning

A contingency plan is a plan to cope with the effects of an emergency, while, as far as possible, enabling normal operations to continue, e.g. rerouting pipelines to maintain production, arranging other means for product distribution, etc.

A classic example of how contingency plans can be brought into play was the Apollo 13 mission to the Moon, where the spacecraft experienced a potentially catastrophic explosion which damaged many of its essential functions and threatened the safe return of the three astronauts to Earth. The National Aeronautics and Space Administration's (NASA's) emergency response arrangements rose to the occasion—teams of back-up engineers were mobilized and set to work on different aspects of the problems threatening the spacecraft, all under extremely tight time pressures. The ingenious contingency plans which were developed, such as the use of the Lunar Excursion Module as a virtual lifeboat, saved the lives of the astronauts.

Recovery planning

A recovery plan is a plan to restore as many of the normal operations as possible following an emergency. Although not the subject of this chapter, business recovery plans also form an essential part of the overall emergency response plans. An example of how well these can operate was given by the speed with which institutions in the City of London were able to resume business following the terrorist bomb which destroyed many of the buildings. Alternative accommodation was quickly made available, and important computer systems were able to function because of the sensible back-up strategies which were in place.

Investigation and follow-up

When the incident is over and the emergency response organization has been stood down, it is essential that a thorough investigation is carried out to determine the cause of the initial incident, the way in which the emergency developed and possibly escalated and how well the organization's response to the emergency worked. This needs to be performed with a view to preventing a similar event from occurring in the future, and to making any necessary improvements to the emergency response arrangements. It is important to ensure that the incident site is not disturbed until a proper investigation has been carried out (in some situations, there are statutory requirements regarding disturbances to an incident site). In addition, where there has been loss of life, a police investigation will normally be carried out (certainly in the UK). The incident should be carefully analysed to determine its potential for more serious consequences and what changes to the emergency arrangements need to be made to mitigate such consequences. In this way, the loop is closed.

References

Cullen, W.D. (1990) The Public Enquiry into the Piper Alpha Disaster, 2 vols. Department of Energy. HMSO, London.

E & P Forum (1994) *Guidelines for the Development and Application of Health, Safety and Environmental Management Systems*. Report No. 6.36/210. Oil Industry International Exploration and Production Forum (E & P Forum), Oxford.

Chapter 14 Risk perception

Anne Spurgeon

Introduction

An essential part of the risk management process is the communication of necessary information to the workforce. There is, however, increasing recognition that the process of communicating risk is a complex matter, requiring an understanding of a range of psychological and social factors which may influence the effectiveness of the communication. Of central importance is an understanding of the process of risk perception, which is concerned with the ways in which people interpret and evaluate the information they receive in order to arrive at their own assessment of any risk.

It is clear that different people perceive similar risks differently, and that the perception of the public or, in this case, the workforce may often be at variance with the perception of experts employing, for example, mathematical modelling techniques. The study of risk perception grew out of the realization that there was very little correspondence between the judgements of lay people and statistical estimates of the frequency of deaths from different causes (Fischhoff *et al.* 1981). This does not necessarily imply that a firm distinction can be made between 'subjective' decisions and the so-called 'objective' assessment arrived at by reference to statistical data. All hazard identification and subsequent risk assessment depend, to a certain extent, on human values; for example, judgements are made about the importance of what may be threatened by a particular hazard (health, environment, economy) or about what constitutes an acceptable number of individuals who might be affected within a certain timescale. However, 'objective' assessment and the workforce's perception of risk may differ in terms of the nature and perhaps the extent of the subjectivity involved.

In the workplace, a risk assessment will be carried out by individuals with a certain level of knowledge and expertise. In attempting to communicate the results of this assessment to the workforce, it is important to understand the factors likely to influence the worker's perception of the risks involved, and how these factors may differ from those that influenced the persons who carried out the assessment. Without an appreciation of these factors, the effective communication of risk to the workforce may be considerably reduced.

The study of risk perception

Information about the factors involved in risk perception has largely been gathered using an approach referred to as 'expressed preference' (Slovic 1987). Essentially, this involves asking different groups of people, typically via questionnaires and rating scales, what activities they consider to be risky, how risky they consider them to be, which hazards they feel cause them a threat and how acceptable they find these various different risks. This is in contrast with an earlier approach which employed a method known as 'revealed preference' (Starr 1969). Here, the analysis of currently 'accepted' accident levels was used to infer the existing trade-offs which a society implicitly made between the risks and benefits of any particular hazard. This approach assumed that the way in which individuals or societies actually behaved towards a risk reflected their perception of that risk or, expressed in another way, 'accepted' risk was the same as 'acceptable' risk. Furthermore, the assumption was made that people arrived at decisions about risk by rationally trading off costs against benefits. The 'expressed preference' approach, on the other hand, revealed that people's perceptions were derived from a whole range of qualitative factors, rather than from a quantitative estimate of ill health or fatalities occurring within a unit of time. Research using the 'expressed preference' approach began in the late 1970s (Fischhoff *et al.* 1978) and, since then, has identified a range of factors which have the potential to influence the individual's perception of risk. It has also become clear that a distinction must be made between the perceptions of an individual and those of larger groups or society in general. Most recently, interest has focused on the means by which the perception of risk may be amplified within certain groups or societies. One important outcome of these findings is the recognition among policy makers and legislators that public attitudes towards the 'tolerability' of risks should be an integral part of the risk assessment process itself, placing social scientific considerations alongside technical considerations in arriving at any decision (Health and Safety Executive (HSE) 1988). The emphasis here, however, is on the importance of these factors for subsequent risk communication. Once a risk assessment has been made in a workplace, the process becomes one of attempting to bring the worker's perceptions of risk more into line with those of the health and safety professionals. This process, which is largely dealt with in Chapter 15, will be considerably aided by a prior understanding of the perceptual process.

How do individuals perceive information?

It has long been recognized that perception is different from simply receiving information via the sense organs. The individual is not simply a passive converter of such information, but actively interprets it in order to construct its meaning. This interpretation is carried out by reference to an enormous amount of information stored in the memory about past experiences and perceptions, as well as information derived second hand from other individuals. These various types of information are integrated into what are usually termed 'schemas', or knowledge structures which individuals use to interpret the world around them. These structures also help to develop attitudes and belief systems which, in turn, feed into future interpretations.

Perception is also a selective process. Before individuals have begun to interpret the information they receive, they will have already unconsciously selected, on the basis of attitudes and beliefs, which information they will attend to and which they will ignore. For example, the assimilation of new information from a second-hand source, as opposed to direct experience, will depend on the perceived credibility of that source. Research in Europe (Jungermann *et al.* 1996) has demonstrated that groups, such as medical practitioners, scientists and government officials, differ markedly in terms of both their perceived competence and their perceived truthfulness in the eyes of the general public, with government officials scoring lowest on both counts.

Although much initial research on perception focused on the individual, it is now recognized that particular social and cultural groups are likely to share certain belief systems. Furthermore, attitudes within societies change over time, and these are both reflected in and influenced by the media and the growth of pressure groups. Therefore the following section will consider, firstly, those facts known to influence individual perceptions, namely the characteristics of the individuals themselves and the context in which the potential hazard occurs. Secondly, it will consider the social and cultural influences which appear to amplify risk in the collective consciousness of groups.

Factors influencing the perception of risks

The characteristics of the situations and individuals involved

Voluntary vs. involuntary activities or exposures

One of the first observations made in relation to risk perception was that individuals were more likely to regard risks as acceptable if they involved activities in which they participated voluntarily (Starr 1969). Perhaps the most obvious example of a voluntary risk is that of smoking, although this also involves another factor, that of immediate vs. delayed consequences (see below). Examples of involuntary risks in the wider society include exposure to pesticides, electromagnetic fields and emissions from motor vehicles. The notion that individuals regard as highly unacceptable those risks from exposure to factors over which they feel they have no control is of particular relevance for the workplace. Exposure via the inhalation of toxic chemicals provides the clearest example. The importance of the perceived lack of control also relates to health outcomes. For example, exposure to a known carcinogen may involve a health outcome which cannot be removed by the subsequent cessation of exposure.

Responsibility for the hazard and its control
Associated with the issue of voluntariness is that of attribution (Royal Society 1983). One part of the process of interpreting information involves attributing causes to events or situations. In the workplace, this may be translated into responsibility or, more negatively, blame. Workers are likely to perceive that the responsibility for producing and therefore controlling exposure to hazards lies with the management. This is particularly the case where, as in many modern industries, technology has become extremely complex and the workers feel remote from the responsibility for the process. Risks which are seen as the responsibility of someone else to control tend to be regarded as less acceptable. Attitudes towards responsibility or blame tend to be enhanced by a range of additional factors, such as the perceived motivation of the persons deemed to be responsible and whether they are regarded as sufficiently competent to assume that responsibility. The attribution of responsibility therefore represents a further aspect of limited control, and often results in a high rating of unacceptability for the risks involved.

Uncertainty about the consequences of exposure
People frequently lack personal experience with a particular risk and lack information about a hazard or its potential consequences. Inadequate provision of this information often leads them to draw on other indirect sources, which may be misleading or inaccurate. The acceptance of such sources will depend on their credibility as perceived by the worker. However, it should be noted that people seek out information from sources which they have already preselected as being credible. In general, therefore, fear of the unknown can have the effect of elevating the perception of risk and hence reducing its acceptability.

Familiarity with the hazard
While a lack of personal experience and fear of the unknown may lead workers to overestimate risk, familiarity with a hazard frequently has the opposite effect. Research has confirmed what seems intuitively plausible: workers perceive less risk from those hazards to which they are continually exposed (Slovic *et al.* 1980). However, the relationship is not always straightforward. Three factors appear to be important in determining the perceived risk from repeated exposure. First is the well-established principle of adaptation. Repeated exposure to the same information leads the individual to assume that all future exposures will follow the same pattern, thus reducing anxiety and producing a reinterpretation of information and a reassessment of risk. Secondly, repeated exposure without apparent cost tends to emphasize for the individual the benefits of the process relative to the costs. A third factor associated with familiarity, however, may have the effect of increasing or decreas-

ing risk acceptability depending on the circumstances. There is evidence that, in some situations, a hazard's general availability to the perceptual process, because of the frequency of occurrence, makes it more memorable and more vivid, and may therefore result in an overestimation of the associated risks. The particular circumstances in which this becomes important and overrides the principle of adaptation are not currently well understood, but may, for example, occur in the presence of intermittently, but frequently occurring, hazards, such as exposure to high noise levels or vibration.

Immediate vs. delayed consequences
Risks with delayed consequences are often perceived as being less important than those with immediate outcomes (Royal Society 1983). This is likely to be related to the frequency and visibility of the consequences, but may also result from equivocal information regarding long-term effects. Many workplace hazards are associated with both acute (short-term, reversible) and chronic (long-term, irreversible) effects. Often, however, the acute effects are much better documented, less controversial and more firmly tied to exposure levels than are the potential chronic effects. Typical examples include a variety of organic solvents where the short-term effects of overexposure, such as drowsiness, dizziness and nausea, are well known and well accepted by managers and workers alike. Added to this, they are likely to affect the majority of workers. Chronic effects, such as irreversible damage to the nervous system, on the other hand, are not universally accepted and, like other long-term risks, e.g. cancers, are likely to affect only a proportion of the workforce. Clearly, the 'it can't happen to me' principle may come into play here. This is particularly the case amongst younger workers for whom the risk may be especially remote, and can be rationalized by reference to the contradictory information available and the expectation of only a short period of employment in the industry concerned.

Two further factors should be considered, however, before an assumption is made that delayed consequences are almost always perceived as being less of a risk than immediate outcomes. Firstly, the nature of the hazard is important. Specifically, it would appear that the genetic effects of exposure, which are likely to affect future children or, in the wider sense, generations, are usually perceived as being highly unacceptable and important to eliminate (Otway & Winterfeldt 1982). Similarly, fears of immediate effects on pregnancy outcomes, such as those which, at one stage, were suspected of being associated with exposure to visual display units, are difficult to allay, despite evidence to the contrary (Pearce 1984). Research into environmental risk perceptions has demonstrated that risks to vulnerable groups, particularly children, are perceived as being highly unacceptable. This was clearly demonstrated in the debate which followed the controversial evidence regarding the effects on children of environmental lead exposure (Spurgeon 1992).

This heightened concern to protect young children may partly explain the difference between the perception of genetic and reproductive risks and that of other long-term outcomes.

A second factor which should be mentioned briefly in relation to the perception of delayed and immediate consequences is that of individual personality and consequent behaviour patterns. Although difficult to take account of in the workplace, it should be noted that individuals are known to vary by age, social class and personality in terms of their future time perspectives (Royal Society 1983). Furthermore, the distinction between risk-seeking and risk-avoiding individuals is well established in the psychological literature (Eysenck & Eysenck 1978).

Numbers exposed

In addition to the characteristics of the hazard itself and the potential consequences, the perception of risk appears to be strongly related to the number of individuals exposed. It has been noted, for example, that the exposure of a few people which results in most of them being affected is less likely to increase the perception of risk than the exposure of many people where few or none are affected (Reissland & Harries 1979). This seems contrary to the findings related to major incidents (see below). However, this may be explained in terms of the vividness and media coverage associated with catastrophes, which may not occur in the case of smaller events.

Infrequent but catastrophic consequences

Despite the above, the occurrence of major dramatic incidents appears to increase risk perceptions significantly. Some of the earliest research (Slovic *et al.* 1979) has demonstrated that individuals tend to perceive a greater risk from specific events which happen infrequently, but which result in a large number of deaths, than from frequent events with fewer deaths. This is partly due to the dramatic nature of catastrophes and the tendency for detailed news reporting as noted above. This increases the memorableness of the event, as mentioned above, and hence the availability to the perceptual process. As individuals cannot attend to all the information which they encounter, they tend to select for future storage on the basis of vividness and interest. An additional factor is that which is usually referred to as 'named lives' (Reissland & Harries 1979). As a result of media coverage, specific individuals involved are often identified and, in these circumstances, the risk becomes less remote to those not involved. It has been noted, for example, that a large amount of public expenditure has often been diverted to guard against the repetition of dramatic disasters where relatively few lives were lost and where a reoccurrence was highly unlikely. Rational considerations would dictate that spending on alternatives, for example in the National Health Service, would save many more lives. This demonstrates, however, the principle that dramatic events considerably heighten the perception of risk, regardless of their likely future occurrence. This is an important consideration in industries where fatalities have occurred in the past.

Who benefits?
Risks which appear to be imposed for the benefit of others, and therefore not for the benefit of those taking the risk, not surprisingly, tend to be viewed as being less acceptable (Royal Society 1983). This is particularly the case when those enjoying the benefits are not themselves exposed to the potential hazard. In the workplace, therefore, it is important that workers are convinced of the necessity of employing a particular process, or using a particular substance, and also feel a sense of participation in the risk–benefit process.

Characteristics of assessors

Reference has been made above to the question of responsibility in relation to the management of risk. The perception of risk by the workforce and their acceptance of a risk assessment process are likely to be considerably influenced by their perception of the people carrying out that process. In this context, individuals tend to rate others in two dimensions: (i) competence; and (ii) truthfulness or partiality. Research carried out in Europe (Jungermann *et al.* 1996) has examined people's attitudes to different officials and professionals in relation to these two attributes. The results fairly consistently indicate that medical personnel and scientists are more likely to receive high ratings in both dimensions than government officials or company managers. Clearly, the situation is likely to vary from company to company, but the underlying point is that the perceived trustworthiness of the health and safety professionals is likely to influence significantly the way and extent to which hazards are perceived. Associated with this, it should be noted that, in the wider public arena, risks which are seen to arise from 'secret' activities, such as in the field of defence, are regarded as being much greater and less acceptable than risks for which there is a perception of more information being available. By applying this principle to the workplace, it is clear that any impression of secrecy is likely to elevate the workers' perception of risk.

Individual vs. societal risk perception

It has been demonstrated that there are considerable differences in the way in which individuals evaluate risks to themselves personally and risks to society as a whole (Royal Society 1983). The latter appears to be based on wider moral values, while the former is based on personal interest. For the majority of individuals, the issues appear to be separate and do not overlap. In the workplace, therefore, there are likely to be differences in the way in which workers may perceive the risk to the environment arising from the activities of the company and the risk to themselves in their everyday working lives. Although, in both cases, many of the factors discussed above will come into play, in relation to personal risk, the question of moral values is unlikely to be a significant factor.

Gender differences in risk perception

There is a considerable amount of evidence that women are more concerned about risk and are more likely to rate risks as unacceptable than men (Schmidt & Gifford 1989). However, this evidence comes mainly from environmental research and, as such, tends to be more concerned with risks to the wider environment, and hence to society as a whole, rather than with personal risks. As noted above, societal risk assessment tends to be based on different perceptual processes than is individual risk assessment. The relevance of the research findings to the workplace is therefore questionable. However, in some cases, the hazard being investigated has posed a potential risk to individuals as well as to wider society, e.g. the movement of radiological waste (McBeth & Oakes 1996). Here, the findings again indicated a perception of a higher level of risk among women than among men. Furthermore, a more recent study carried out at the Sellafield Nuclear Reprocessing Plant also observed that women were more cautious in their attitudes towards potential hazards than men (Lee *et al.* 1993). Given the fact that women, in general, are known to be more concerned with health issues than are men, it is worth considering that females in the workforce may have a different perception of risk than their male counterparts.

Age differences in risk perception

As in the case of gender, much of the research which has been carried out in relation to age is related to environmental issues and may not therefore be directly applicable to the workplace. However, it is interesting to note that some findings indicate that younger people are more concerned about environmental issues, while older people are more concerned about the health and safety of individuals (Fischer *et al.* 1991). This may reflect the changes in attitude towards the environment which have taken place during the last 20 years, but may also reflect some of the factors noted in the section on 'Immediate vs. delayed consequences'. Regardless of the source of this difference, the indications are that the attitudes of younger workers towards risks may differ from those of their older workmates. It is also possible that older workers may underestimate the risk because of the familiarity factor, although evidence for this is anecdotal only.

Social group differences in risk perception

At group level, a number of social factors may affect risk perception.

Lower risk acceptance has been shown in those belonging to professional groups, such as medicine, social work, science and arts-related occupations. In contrast, higher risk acceptance is associated with industrial and agricultural workers (Vlek & Stallen 1981). There is also evidence that a higher income and education are associated with a lower acceptance of risk (Jones & Dunlop 1992). Again, however, the focus of concern has been mainly on the wider environment rather than on the workplace, and it seems likely that the factors noted in the section on 'The characteristics of the situations and individuals involved' are of much more relevance in understanding the risk perception process in the working environment. Recently, it has been shown that workers from different cultures perceive risk levels differently, even within Western societies (Jungermann *et al.* 1996). For example, individuals from different European countries differ in terms of their perceptions of the credibility of information sources. In the UK, for example, companies were ranked higher as a credible source of information than in other countries such as Belgium and Germany, although most countries gave low ratings to politicians and government officials. As noted earlier, the perception of the credibility of those responsible for risk management is crucial to the risk communication process, and cultural factors have a role to play in this perception.

The social amplification of risk

In recent years, attention has been paid to a range of social, cultural and institutional factors which may operate to increase or reduce the perception of risk. These factors, although once again studied largely in the context of the general public's perception of wider environmental issues, have relevance to the workplace. The process, which has become known as social amplification, was initially described in the late 1980s (Kasperson *et al.* 1988) using ideas borrowed from communication theory. In electronic communication, amplification refers to the process of intensification or attenuation of signals during the transmission of information. An information source sends out a number of signals forming a message to a transmitter. This transmitter alters the original message by intensifying or attenuating the incoming signals, adding to them or subtracting from them, to form new signals. These are then sent to the next transmitter, where further decoding occurs. In the social amplification process, the heightening or attenuation of risk perception in the individual occurs as a result of the operation of various amplification stations. These include the scientist or health and safety professional who communicates the risk assessment, government agencies, the news media, cultural groups, pressure groups and other interpersonal networks.

The process of the social amplification of risk may begin with an event or the discovery of a hazard in the working environment. Individuals select certain characteristics of the event or hazard to attend to, and interpret these characteristics according to their own knowledge structures, beliefs and attitudes. Many of the factors described in the section on 'The characteristics of the situations and individuals involved' will be included in this process. The interpretations which are made at this stage are communicated to other individuals and groups (amplification stations), who then respond to the information, acting to heighten or reduce the perception of risk. Therefore, the individual evaluation of risk, which depends on beliefs and attitudes, also operates within a framework of the social group to which an individual belongs, e.g. as an employee, manager, professional scientist or physician, pressure group member, journalist, civil servant or politician. All of these groups have norms and expectations that determine the way in which they operate and how they respond to information. Appropriate behaviour within the group tends to be reinforced by training and by material and social rewards.

The social amplification approach also incorporates the notion that secondary effects are likely to occur as a result of the responses of individuals and groups, which may, in turn, affect future risk perceptions. These include the development of enduring attitudes, such as distrust of technology and of the risk management process, economic consequences for the industry, political pressure for change and an impact on the acceptance of other technologies which may be unrelated to the hazard in question.

Research within the framework of social amplification theory is currently at an early stage. However, the approach has already begun to enhance the understanding of the risk perception process in demonstrating the importance of social influences, as well as personal factors, in determining how individuals arrive at their own assessment of risk.

Risk perception and risk communication

As noted at the beginning of this chapter, the processes involved in risk perception have important implications for effective risk communication. Perhaps the most important of these is that the communication of information must take into account, first, how the receiver of the information already perceives the risk and, second, what factors have been important in forming that perception, i.e. the frame of reference of the individuals concerned. It is likely that this will be different from that of the health and safety professionals who may have carried out the formal risk assessment. In addition, there may be many different groups within a workforce, each with its own reference frame. The perceptions of different individuals will be derived both from personal belief systems and also from the interpretations placed on the information by the particular social groups to which the individual belongs. In addition to the perceived characteristics of the hazard, a central issue is the question of trust in those responsible for risk assessment and management in situations in which such management is outside the personal control of the individual. Effective risk communication will therefore depend, to a large extent, on the perception of competence and truthfulness of those responsible for managing risks in the workplace.

Given an understanding of the various factors involved in risk perception, is it possible to predict perception on the basis of the characteristics of the hazard and the individuals involved? Work carried out in the USA suggests that it is. Wandersman and Hallman (1993) found that the presence of various characteristics of certain hazards of the type discussed above ('The characteristics of the situations and individuals involved') did in fact predict the subsequent risk ratings of the individuals exposed to these hazards. Therefore, a knowledge of the perceptual processes is increasingly becoming an integral part of the development of risk communication programmes.

References

Eysenck, S.B.G. & Eysenck, H.J. (1978) Impulsiveness and venturesomeness: their position in a dimensional system of personality description. *Psychological Reports* **43**, 1247–1255.

Fischer, G.W., Morgan, M.G., Fischhoff, B., Nair, I. & Lave, L.B. (1991) What risks are people concerned about? *Risk Analysis* **11**, 303–314.

Fischhoff, B., Lichtenstein, S., Slovic, P., Derby, S.L. & Keeney, R.L. (1981) *Acceptable Risk*. Cambridge University Press, Cambridge.

Fischhoff, B., Slovic, P., Lichtenstein, S., Read, S. & Combs, B. (1978) How safe is safe enough? A psychometric study of attitudes towards technological risks and benefits. *Policy Sciences* **9**, 127–152.

HSE (1988) *The Tolerability of Risk from Nuclear Power Stations*. HMSO, London.

Jones, R.E. & Dunlop, R.E. (1992) The social bases of environment concern. Have they changed over time? *Rural Sociology* **57** (1), 28–47.

Jungermann, H., Pfister, H.-R. & Fisscher, K. (1996) Credibility, information preferences and information interests. *Risk Analysis* **16** (2), 251–261.

Kasperson, R.E., Renn, O., Slovic, P., *et al.* (1988) The social amplification of risk: a conceptual framework. *Risk Analysis* **8**, 177–187.

Lee, T.R., Macdonald, S.M. & Coote, J.A. (1993) Perceptions of risks and attitudes to safety at a nuclear reprocessing plant. Paper presented at *Society for Risk Assessment. Fourth Conference (Rome)*. Quoted in Means, K. & Flin, R. (1993) Risk perception in hazardous industries. *The Psychologist* **9** (9), 401–404.

McBeth, M.K. & Oakes, A.S. (1996) Citizen perceptions of risk associated with moving radiological waste. *Risk Analysis* **16** (3), 421–428.

Otway, H.J. & Winterfeldt, D. (1982) Beyond acceptable risk: on the social acceptability of technologies. *Policy Sciences* **14**, 247–256.

Pearce, B.G. (1984) *Health Hazards and VDTs*. Wiley, Chichester.

Reissland, J. & Harries, V. (1979) A scale for measuring risks. *New Scientist* **13 September**, 80–81.

Royal Society (1983) *Risk Assessment. A Study Group Report*. Royal Society, London.

Schmidt, F.N. & Gifford, R. (1989) A dispositional approach to hazard

perception: preliminary development of the environmental appraisal inventory. *Journal of Environmental Psychology* **9**, 57–67.
Slovic, P. (1987) Perception of risk. *Science* **236**, 280–285.
Slovic, P., Fischhoff, B. & Lichtenstein, S. (1980) Facts and fears: understanding perceived risk. In: *Societal Risk Assessment: How Safe is Safe Enough?* (eds. R.C. Schwing & W.A. Albers), pp. 181–216. Plenum Press, New York.
Slovic, P., Lichtenstein, S. & Fischhoff, B. (1979) Images of disaster, perception and acceptance of risks from nuclear power. In: *Energy Risk Management* (eds. G.T. Goodman & W.D. Rowe), pp. 222–245. Academic Press, London.
Spurgeon, A. (1992) Is there an adverse effect on the intellectual development of children exposed to low levels of lead. *Indoor Environment* **1**, 300–307.
Starr, C. (1969) Social benefit vs. technological risk. *Science* **165**, 1232–1238.
Vlek, C.J.H. & Stallen, P.J.M. (1981) Judging risks and benefits in the small and in the large. *Organisational Behaviour and Human Performance* **28**, 235–271.
Wandersman, A.H. & Hallman, W.K. (1993) Are people acting irrationally? Understanding public concerns about environmental threats. *American Psychologist* **48** (6), 681–686.

Chapter 15 Risk communication

Frank Rose

Introduction

Most, if not all, societal judgemental processes are based on some form of risk management. This may involve a complex mathematically modelled risk assessment, or may be a relatively simple expert decision point. In either case, the process and outcome will need to be communicated to the stakeholders involved, i.e. those who will be bearing the risk.

The process of risk communication has attracted increasing attention in recent years, with regulatory bodies and industrial corporations emphasizing the need for the improved communication of risk. A number of factors underlie this increased interest, notably the greater awareness of industrial hazards by the general population, the speed with which information is disseminated globally, raised levels of concern about adverse effects, particularly from newer technology, and a loss of trust in those traditionally seen as credible sources of information. In particular, governments and industry have lost trust and credibility and yet, at the same time, are perceived as the most knowledgeable sources of information.

Key to the process of risk communication is an understanding of risk perception, which has been covered in Chapter 14. The findings from risk perception research hold several potential implications for risk communication, and a number of publications offer advice in this regard (Covello & Allen 1988; Covello *et al.* 1988). There is a significant difference in the perception of risks by 'experts' who carry out the risk assessments and those who are subject to the risk and need to understand it. Failure to take these underlying perception differences into account when planning risk communication will make the outcome much less satisfactory. Overviews of many of the key contributions to risk communication are provided by Krimsky and Plough (1988), the US National Research Council (NRC 1989), Handmer and Penning-Rowsell (1990) and Kasperson and Stallen (1991). The aim of this chapter is not to provide a comprehensive review of this literature, but to raise practical issues relevant to the development, implementation and evaluation of the risk communication programme.

The risk communication process

What is risk communication? A number of partially overlapping conceptual approaches to risk communication can be identified in the literature. The simplest definition is an exchange of information about risk. Covello (1992) takes this further. Risk communication is not only about the exchange of information, but also the different aspects of risk: the nature, the magnitude and, in particular, the acceptability of the risk. The concept of the exchange of information is important because it represents the two-way process of listening to the needs of those to be communicated to as well as the response to those needs. Making the distinction between nature, magnitude and acceptability is necessary, because different forms of communication are required for these different elements.

As soon as we start to discuss acceptability, it is no longer adequate to talk only about the magnitude of risk. Many other factors influence decisions about risk acceptability, a key one being benefits. If the benefits of any particular activity are perceived as being high, the perception of risk goes down and the willingness to accept the risk goes up. In terms of risk acceptability, perception is reality, and, as perception is often neither logical nor factual, this is one of the factors which makes communication so difficult.

What is the objective of risk communication? Some believe that it is to gain acceptability of the risk by an exchange of information, but Covello (1992) argues that, when trust and credibility are low, the objective is to establish trust and credibility, and only when this has been done can other objectives be achieved. Whether or not trust and credibility are established depends on four factors: caring, competence, honesty and dedication. Of the four, caring is the most important, with over half of an individual's credibility determined by whether there is a perception of being caring and empathetic. In other words, did the 'audience' perceive the communicator as a good listener, interested in their needs and concerned about their welfare. In most communication situations, a decision about caring and empathy is made in the first 30 seconds, and then is almost impossible to change.

Perceptions of competence and expertise are influenced largely by the professional background and behaviour of the communicator, and the reputation of the organization represented. Perceptions of honesty and openness mainly arise from non-verbal communications, such as body language, eye contact and physical barriers between communicator and audience, coupled with the style and clarity of responses to direct questions. Dedication and commitment are judged by whether the communicator is perceived to be hardworking, available and accessible when needed.

The issue of trust is also an important concern in risk communication, as results from persuasive communication studies show that the credibility of a communicator is critically dependent upon the trust placed in him or her (Lee 1986). If we do not trust the source, then we are unlikely to trust the message. Trust can be lost if precise predictions of risks are made by organizations, neglecting areas of uncertainty, which may, in the light of subsequent events, be interpreted as flaws in the risk assessment process. Similarly, trust may be lost following a serious incident, if the responsible bodies are not felt to be learning from and responding to the event openly. The use of credible third parties in risk communication can help, particularly in situations in which trust and credibility are low. In the areas of safety, health and the environment, it has been shown that credibility is highest for physicians working in the community, together with other health professionals, university professors, professional organizations, the media, non-profit voluntary health organizations and local knowledgeable citizens. Establishing relationships and sharing information with such third parties are an important part of successful risk communication.

In all risk communications, it is important to ensure that the terminology used has a common understanding between the parties involved. One of the continual confusions in day-to-day life is between hazard and risk, which are often used synonymously. However, the difference is important, and is worth re-emphasizing here. Hazard is the inherent potential of something to cause harm, whilst risk is the probability of that harm actually occurring in a given set of circumstances. This is a difficult concept to communicate to non-experts, but it is vital to do so. It is also important to remember that risk communication can raise several important dilemmas and paradoxes (Otway & Wynne 1989). For example, a message about the same activity may need to both reassure (the risk from such an activity is tolerable) and warn (but if, in the unlikely event that there is an emergency, the following action will be necessary). Otway and Wynne refer to this as the reassurance–arousal paradox.

As with all processes which are complex, planning and preparation are essential for good risk communication. It is most effective to have a proactive programme, well thought through in advance, with trained and practised communicators, although in some urgent circumstances time will not allow this, and crisis communications will be needed. This is a particularly demanding area of activity, and each organization would be well advised to maintain a cadre of experienced individuals for this possibility. In general, the more effort which is put into routine proactive risk communication, the better prepared the organization will be for any eventuality.

Developing the risk communication programme

Setting goals and objectives

The first step is always to define goals and objectives. These will reflect the nature of the risk issue under consideration, the stakeholder audiences, the timeframe of the activity and the resources available. The objective could be to provide information to the public, to meet the requirement of a particular regulation, to resolve conflict over alleged adverse impacts, to engage employees in safer working practices or to support a permit application; whatever the context, the end-point must be clarified. Once the end objective is set, goals should be mapped out along the way, a timeframe should be placed on these and responsibilities should be allocated to individuals. An assessment should be made of the level of trust and credibility opposite the stakeholder audiences and, if this is low, raising trust and credibility will almost certainly be the first goal.

At this stage, some critical success factors for the various goals should be worked out, and the types of measurement that will be needed to judge success should be defined. If these factors are not built into the programme from the start, they will be almost impossible to add later.

The team involved must have a clear and common understanding of the need for the risk communication programme, its objectives and goals, and their expected contribution. The objectives, goals and success factors should be recycled as necessary until everyone agrees.

Assessing target audiences

A knowledge of the prime target audiences should be available from the objective setting phase, but other stakeholder audiences should be considered. Within the various audiences, subgroups with special interests and needs should be examined. It must be recognized that the public have a legitimate interest in risks which affect them, even though they may not be directly involved. Likewise, employee groups have collective interests in risks in the workplace, even though they may not all be exposed to the same risk profiles. Regulatory agencies or organized bodies, such as trade unions, must not be forgotten; generally, the earlier they are involved, the more helpful they can be. Risk communication must focus and rigorously analyse the needs of each prospective audience at the onset of the risk communication process (Harrington *et al.* 1994).

Having identified all the stakeholders, it is important to assess what is known about their needs for the context in question. To understand the stakeholder audience in detail, it will be necessary to identify subgroups, such as health professionals, vulnerable groups, activists and emergency services, and pay attention to their needs. Assumptions should not be made about what people know, think or want doing. Often people in the community are more concerned about trust, credibility, voluntariness, fairness and equity than about quantitative risk assessment and statistical data. Techniques, such as interviews, surveys and focus groups, can all be helpful. If there is a community relations' panel in existence, it should be used. If not, consideration should be given to forming one. All interested parties must have an opportunity to participate, and attempts should be made to understand any underlying agendas or sociocultural, equity and broader community issues which may impact on the risk communication process.

Communication methods

It should be determined which channels are the most appropriate for reaching the target audiences. In general, face-to-face communications which establish dialogue are the most effective, but may not always be possible, and the various forms of the media may need to be used. The stakeholder audiences will usually have an expectation and it will establish credibility to meet this. For example, if the local community want to have an open dialogue with the factory manager, and a public relations' person is sent with a video, this will probably do more harm than good. It should be decided what formats will be most suited to the messages and chosen channels, e.g. videos, booklets, slide shows, personal presentations, public meetings, factory open days, press releases, radio or television. Well-produced booklets and leaflets can be very effective, and it is becoming common for industrial organizations to produce annual reports on their safety, health and environmental performance, and to send these to shareholders, customers, employees and other interested parties. These can be supplemented with brochures for local communities giving specific details of the local factory.

Once the method of communication and channels have been selected, the key stakeholder audiences should be asked whether or not this will meet their needs. Each risk communication opportunity should be used to build the relationship with the audience in order to establish an ongoing, routine, two-way dialogue.

Risk communicators and spokespersons should be chosen carefully, have excellent presentation and interactive skills, be able to listen and deal with emotions and be routinely trained. Anyone with these skills can be a good risk communicator, but the technical expert who has difficulty in delivering uncomplicated messages should be avoided. In the circumstance of community risk communication, the senior local line manager (e.g. factory manager) is the most appropriate person, supported by such technical experts as are relevant.

Role of the media

The media are the main disseminators of information and, for many members of society, represent the sole source of their communication on risk. It is important to realize and accept that the media have needs and, where possible, it is useful to help to meet them. As with all other areas of risk communication, it helps to build relationships with local reporters and editors which are based on trust and mutual respect. The provision of background information and historical data which facilitate the understanding of risk will be appreciated, as will being available to journalists and recognizing that they have copy deadlines to meet. Significant skill and competence are required for individuals who are to give interviews, particularly for radio and television, and appropriate training, development and practice should be undertaken.

Constructing communications

Language needs to be straightforward, avoiding technical jargon. Examples and images will help understanding and, in particular, there is a need to focus on what is being done to control risks rather than on the magnitude of the risks alone. For example, the details of how emissions are being controlled and reduced are likely to be of more interest than the probability of adverse effects resulting from the emissions.

Emotions, e.g. anger, fear, anxiety and outrage, must be recognized, acknowledged and responded to; it will be impossible to deal with any facts until the emotions are dealt with.

The values, credentials and background of the organization and the individual communicating should be stated, but trust cannot be asked or expected on this basis alone. Whatever risk information is available, with details of reliability, should be disclosed in a way which can be understood by everyone.

The use of risk comparisons to help put risks in perspective is a powerful tool, but needs to be employed cautiously. It is most effective in the context of an ongoing risk dialogue, where trust and credibility have been established. Any accurate risk comparison will be acceptable provided that it is seen to be relevant in the eyes of the stakeholder, and that it is clearly understood that the risk comparison is to help the stakeholder put the risk in perspective and not to determine acceptability *per se*. The detailed use of risk comparisons is beyond the scope of this chapter, but further guidance can be found in Covello *et al.* (1988).

The communication should be constructed so that it invites and encourages a discussion of the risks and the actions which are being taken to control them. Commitments to actions should be made which can be delivered, and it must be ensured that commitments are met. Commitments that cannot be achieved must be made clear. Once the communication is constructed, it should be tested with a target audience to assess understanding, recall, acceptability, format and willingness to engage in the process.

Legal requirements

The workplace

In virtually every jurisdiction, there is a requirement for routine risk communication to employees. This is usually based on a requirement for a structured risk assessment process, which includes the identification and assessment of hazards, the establishment and monitoring of controls, communication, audit and performance monitoring, corrective action and review. Whilst the details of the various regulatory frameworks vary, they all essentially require the correct identification of hazards, as discussed in Chapter 6, by labelling (with risk and safety phrases), by the provision of warning signs in specific risk areas, by the availability of materials safety data sheets and by the training of employees. The comprehensive availability of such risk information, in a language and format which are easily understandable by employees, is fundamental to the process of workplace risk management.

Products

The labelling of chemical products for transport and distribution and the provision of emergency transport information and materials safety data sheets are now required by virtually every country. The materials safety data sheets are of particular importance in underpinning the risk management process, as they are the basis for understanding the hazards of the product, and thus for being able to carry out a risk assessment. Labels and materials safety data sheets should be in the local language of the country, and this poses logistical problems when products pass through several countries during distribution. These problems can be overcome by the use of multiple language labels (where permitted by law) or by relabelling for local distribution and use.

Communities

Part of the increased interest in risk communication in recent years has been driven by the growing number of hazard communication and right-to-know laws relating particularly to chemical exposure. Legislation as a result of major accidents, such as the 1982 European Community Seveso Directive, has set specific requirements upon public bodies for information provision and preparedness in this respect. This type of legislation is not only leading to more openness in communicating with communities, but also to a more informed debate about risk between industry, regulators and the community (see Chapter 13). This movement is likely to continue and grow around the world, and it is sensible for industry to engage in the process early. Where legislation is already in place, managers should familiarize themselves with the requirements.

Implementing the programme

For those programmes in which there is a strong regulatory drive, it is important to ensure that specific requirements or rules are followed, e.g. format and content of labels and data sheets and submissions to regulatory bodies and community panels. However, it is necessary to be careful that compliance with the rules does not become the end in itself, and to ensure that risk communication does not stop at the provision of information but rather follows through into dialogue.

For all programmes, the implementation should be as planned, but a careful review should be maintained of key areas. Are the selected channels of communication actually working or are there barriers? Are the target audiences engaging and how are they reacting? Are there aspects of the programme which need to be improved/changed? Which aspects are having the most impact and how can these be built upon? These types of consideration should be in addition to the formal reviews of goals which have been planned, as they will give the earliest opportunities for enhancing the programme.

Evaluating the programme

The importance of evaluating risk communication programmes has been highlighted and discussed by several researchers (Kasperson & Palmlund 1987; Handmer & Penning-Rowsell 1990). Formal evaluation of risk communication programmes should be carried out with reference to the objectives, goals, critical success factors and review timetable established at the outset. In judging whether objectives and goals are being met, it is helpful to seek feedback and participation from the target audiences and any other observant third parties. If the risk communication programme has been effective, there will almost certainly be some observable changes, either in perception or behaviour, in the target audience. It will be useful for future programmes to understand how these changes relate to elements of the programme, so that success can be built upon.

Each stage of the programme should be assessed, paying particular attention to any changes made during implementation and whether or not these were ultimately helpful. The performance and behaviour of those involved should be carefully reviewed to identify weaknesses for further development and individual strengths to be built upon. This should include looking for ongoing partners within the target audiences and third parties, and then focusing to engage these in sustaining dialogue.

Records of programmes should be kept, with details of methods which have been found to be helpful and those which have not, with reasons. The communications team will change over time and it will be helpful to have a quick start.

Particularly with respect to communities, the evaluation should seek to identify the route to the establishment of a continuing dialogue and to the planning of a long-term, two-way, mutually satisfactory risk communication strategy. A very effective way to enhance skills in this area is to share the programme and evaluation with other organizations, and, by this benchmarking, to learn from each other.

Barriers to risk communication

The commonest barrier to effective risk communication is the failure to deal adequately with perceptions in the target audience. The understanding of the role of risk perception is dealt with in Chapter 14. It is essential to understand the target audience and, if necessary, to segment it on the basis of demographic, social, educational or other characteristics. The understanding of, and attitude to, science and technology have a marked effect on the perception of risk, as does familiarity with the particular technology/plant, e.g. amongst current and former employees and their families.

Another potential barrier occurs when the data for the risk assessment are inadequate or uncertain. In these circumstances, there is a heavy reliance on expert judgement, and this alone, or in combination with conflict between experts, can lead to an impasse. In this case, it is often helpful to involve the target audience in deciding what further data need to be generated.

Demands for 'zero risk' can be difficult to deal with, and it is important to understand why the demand is being made. There may be a need for a better understanding of the concept of risk. The response may be purely emotional. The response may be politically based. Whatever the reason, the solution will come from an understanding of why the demand is being made.

Language can clearly be a barrier, not just in terms of technical jargon, but also as a result of the different mother tongues and dialects in some territories. A clear understanding of the target audience will address this.

The most difficult barrier to address is that which is not risk based, but rather focused on other unrelated reasons, but risk communication is being used as the vehicle of expression, e.g. if there is fixed opposition to an industry generally or an individual plant specifically. In these circumstances, no activity will be acceptable irrespective of risk, and the only possible option is to attempt to address the underlying issue.

References

Covello, V.T. (1992) Trust and credibility in risk communication. *Health and Environmental Digest* 6 (1), 1–3.

Covello, V.T. & Allen, F. (1988) *Seven Cardinal Rules for Risk Communication*. US Environmental Protection Agency, Washington DC.

Covello, V.T., Sandman, P.M. & Slovic, P. (1988) *Risk Communication, Risk Statistics, and Risk Comparisons: A Manual for Plant Managers*. Chemical Manufacturers Association, Washington DC.

Handmer, J. & Penning-Rowsell, E.C. (1990) *Hazards and the Communication of Risk*. Gower, Aldershot.

Harrington, J.M., Rose, F.G. & Koh, D. (1994) Paint—health and environmental risk management. *Asia-Pacific Journal of Public Health* 7 (2), 115–118.

Kasperson, R.E. & Palmlund, I. (1987) Evaluating risk communication. In: *Effective Risk Communication: The Role and Responsibility of Government and Non-government Organisations* (eds. V.T. Covello, D.B. McCallum & M.T. Pavlova). Plenum, New York.

Kasperson, R.E. & Stallen, P.J.M. (eds.) (1991) *Communicating Risks to the Public*. Kluwer, Dordrecht.

Krimsky, S. & Plough, A. (1988) *Environmental Hazards: Communicating Risks as a Social Process*. Auburn, Dover, MA.
Lee, T.R. (1986) Effective communication of information about chemical hazards. *The Science of the Total Environment* **51**, 149–183.
NRC (1989) *Improving Risk Communication*. National Academy Press, Washington DC.
Otway, H.J. & Wynne, B. (1989) Risk communication: paradigm and paradox. *Risk Analysis* **9**, 141–145.

Chapter 16 Health surveillance

Tar-Ching Aw

Introduction

Surveillance refers to the 'vigilant supervision of individuals or certain groups of individuals'. Health surveillance refers to procedures for the supervision of health status and, in an occupational health context, has been defined as 'the periodic medicophysiological examination of exposed workers with the objective of protecting and preventing occupationally related diseases' (Notten *et al.* 1986). The examination includes clinical and/or physiological assessments of specific occupational groups to detect the early effects of exposure to occupational hazards. The term 'medical surveillance' refers to such procedures performed by, or under the supervision of, a physician. The rationale for health surveillance is to detect adverse health effects from occupational exposures at as early a stage as possible. This will enable appropriate preventive action to be taken before overt occupational disease results.

A wider definition of health surveillance refers to it as a generic term including 'any procedure undertaken in individuals or groups to review an employee's health, and assess any significant deviation from normality' (Bell *et al.* 1995). This broader definition includes medical assessments to detect occupational and non-occupational causes of ill health. Lifestyle health assessment programmes can also be provided at the workplace. These can include the evaluation of cardiovascular risk factors (smoking habits, alcohol consumption, exercise, stress), risk of sexually transmitted diseases and accidents during travel, sports and leisure at and away from work.

The UK Health and Safety Executive (HSE 1990) refers to health assessment prior to and during recruitment as part of the process of health surveillance. Strictly, preplacement assessment is not part of the regular process of supervision for exposure to workplace hazards. It provides baseline health information *prior to* exposure. For reference in this chapter to risk assessment in occupational health, the definition for health surveillance will be confined to surveillance for the detection of health effects from occupational exposures.

Health surveillance is part of secondary prevention, primary prevention being aimed at the elimination of noxious agents from the workplace. Health surveillance should be considered if exposure to a hazardous substance is unavoidable because its use is essential to the industrial process, and no other feasible alternatives are available. This may be because of some specific and/or unique chemical or physical property of the substance.

Health surveillance is useful as an additional tool for risk management. Where risks cannot be completely eliminated, measures to reduce or contain the risks can benefit from the addition of health surveillance procedures. These procedures can indicate the adequacy of control measures, help to identify individuals at increased risk, provide baseline medical data, set benchmarks for preventive action and can be used as an opportunity to provide health education. Health surveillance should be considered as a supplementary mechanism, and should not be used as the main or only approach for occupational risk management.

The rest of this chapter will cover:
- provisions for health surveillance;
- health surveillance procedures (including reference to biological monitoring and biological effect monitoring);
- requirements for health surveillance—legal and practical;
- health surveillance records—methods for keeping records, confidentiality of records and safe storage of records.

Provision of health surveillance

The extent of provisions for health surveillance in occupational health varies. A postal survey of 5000 employers in Great Britain showed that there was no consensus on the understanding of what is meant by health surveillance (Honey 1997). The survey also found that only a small proportion (less than one-third) of employers with staff exposed to workplace hazards had provisions for health surveillance. Even where surveillance was performed, record keeping was poor. This highlights the need for the better provision of information on the legal and occupational health requirements for health surveillance, and greater input by occupational health professionals in advising on the necessity for health surveillance, and on what should and can be included in an occupational health surveillance programme.

Health surveillance procedures

The procedures that can be included under health surveillance include:
- symptom review;
- clinical assessment;
- medical examination;
- special investigations and determination of immune status.

Biological monitoring and biological effect monitoring are strictly separate procedures from health surveillance, but these topics have been allocated separate sections as they can have a complementary role to health surveillance.

Review of symptoms

Symptom review is an integral part of clinical history taking. This procedure, when used for surveillance, requires the clinician (or other trained competent health professional) to enquire about relevant symptoms of exposure to specific occupational hazards. A clinical assessment is then made to decide whether these symptoms are likely to be due to workplace factors. The assessment includes the following.

1 A consideration of the nature and extent of exposure.

2 Other concomitant exposure to chemical, physical or biological hazards in the workplace, through hobbies or at home.

3 Findings on clinical examination.

4 The differential diagnosis. This refers to the consideration of other clinical conditions that can have similar manifestations. For example, occupational exposure to *n*-hexane can cause peripheral neuropathy, but in the general population diabetes mellitus is a much more likely cause of such neurological effects.

If the assessment suggests that the symptoms are due to workplace exposures, an investigation into the system of work is warranted. This can then lead to action to minimize exposure to the relevant hazards in the work area. If clinical assessment leads the clinician to conclude that the cause of the symptoms and signs is non-occupational, steps can be taken to ensure that further clinical investigation and treatment are performed. A diagnosis of non-occupational disease as opposed to occupational disease is more likely to warrant referral to other clinical specialists, as many instances of such diseases are amenable to specific treatment, whereas the scope for the specific treatment of occupational diseases is limited. For example, diabetes mellitus, if detected early, can be controlled by diet and/or medication, thereby reducing the risk of complications, such as vascular, neurological or visual effects; in contrast, neuropathy caused by *n*-hexane or methyl *n*-butyl ketone is unlikely to improve as there is no specific treatment available, and is likely to worsen if exposure continues.

It is important that the review of symptoms leads to the correct diagnosis, so that appropriate management of the individual can follow.

A different approach to symptom review is to provide a list of relevant symptoms to exposed individuals, and instruct them to report the experience of these symptoms for further clinical evaluation as described above. An example of this in occupational health practice is the reporting of symptoms by health care workers exposed to the risk of tuberculosis (TB). These workers include post-mortem room personnel and staff of infectious disease wards or chest clinics. Symptom reporting is also indicated for health care staff who intend to work with patients at risk, e.g. infants and children in paediatric or maternity wards and immunologically compromised patients, e.g. those suffering from acquired immunodeficiency syndrome (AIDS). The relevant symptoms to be reported to the occupational health department include unexplained fever, night sweats, prolonged cough, haemoptysis and other symptoms that suggest pulmonary TB. Clinical evaluation will lead to early investigation, treatment and further preventive measures if TB is confirmed.

Another example of the use of symptom review for health surveillance involves the review of respiratory symptoms for workers exposed to agents that cause asthma, e.g. isocyanates, complex platinum salts, glutaraldehyde, reactive dyes, tea dust and green coffee dust. Table 16.1 provides a fuller list of agents known to cause occupational asthma. This table is derived from the UK Industrial Injuries Advisory Council (1993), and has provisions for newly recognized sensitizing agents. The relevant symptoms are chest tightness, wheeze, breathlessness and nocturnal cough—symptoms consistent with obstruction of the airways.

Table 16.1 Agents recognized as causes of occupational asthma (list published by the Industrial Injuries Advisory Council for the purpose of obtaining benefits under the UK Prescribed Diseases system).

Isocyanates
Platinum salts
Fumes or dusts arising from the manufacture, transport or use of hardening agents (including epoxy resin curing agents) based on phthalic anhydride, tetrachlorophthalic anhydride, trimellitic anhydride or triethylenetetramine
Fumes arising from the use of rosin as a soldering flux
Proteolytic enzymes
Animals, including insects and other arthropods, used for the purpose of research or education or in laboratories
Dusts arising from the sowing, cultivation, harvesting, drying, handling, milling, transport or storage of barley, oats, rye, wheat or maize, or the handling, milling, transport or storage of meal or flour made therefrom
Antibiotics
Cimetidine
Wood dust
Ispaghula
Castor bean dust
Ipecacuanha
Azodicarbonamide
Animals, including insects and other arthropods, or their larval forms, used for the purposes of pest control or fruit cultivation, or the larval forms of animals used for the purposes of research, education or in laboratories
Glutaraldehyde
Persulphate salts or henna
Crustaceans or fish or products arising from these in the food processing industry
Reactive dyes
Soya bean
Tea dust
Green coffee dust
Fumes from stainless steel welding
Any other sensitizing agent

An alternative procedure for reviewing symptoms is to require the exposed individuals, e.g. health care workers in the above example on TB, to report to the occupational health department periodically, and for occupational health staff to enquire specifically about the experience of the relevant symptoms at each visit. The disadvantages of this approach are poor compliance with the required regular visits to the occupational health department, usually because individuals have forgotten the appointment dates for their regular visits, and the failure to report symptoms if they do not fall within the timeframe of a scheduled visit. The need to appear regularly for a brief review of the experience of symptoms can also be questioned justifiably by the workforce if they happen to be symptom free.

For symptom reporting to be effective as a means of health surveillance, those who are occupationally exposed to the hazard should be aware of the occupational activities that contribute to the risks, should be informed and reminded of the importance of early reporting and should be aware of the correct procedures for reporting.

Assessment by a health care professional

This includes limited examination by a trained health care professional, e.g. a nurse or a medical assistant. An example is the periodic examination of the skin and nose of workers exposed to chromic acid mist. The purpose is the early detection of skin ulceration or nasal septal ulceration or perforation, which, in turn, suggests excessive exposure to chromic acid mist. However, it would be easier and more practicable for the individual to examine his/her own skin and to be instructed to report any skin lesions early, so that the medical staff can institute diagnosis, treatment and follow-up, rather than to appoint a health care professional to perform this limited examination. Self-examination is relatively easy for the detection of skin lesions, especially if they occur on the hands. However, self-examination is difficult for the detection of abnormalities in the nose, e.g. nasal ulceration or perforation. For the detection of such lesions, a health professional able to recognize the pathology and relate it to relevant exposures is required.

Periodic examination of the scrotal skin of workers exposed to mineral oils for early malignant change is another example of where examinations are carried out by occupational health staff. The usefulness of this exercise can be questioned as the number of cases of early scrotal cancer detected by this process seems to be limited compared with the number and frequency of such examinations. In the UK, this procedure was established following a historic court decision in 1965 (*Stokes* v. *GKN*) (Howard 1998), where the courts held the company to be negligent for not instituting this health surveillance procedure which could have detected the effects of chronic occupational skin contact with mineral oil. Unfortunately, the low likelihood of detecting a case by this procedure was not taken into account by the courts, and the practice therefore continues in many UK workplaces where mineral oils are used.

Medical examination

This refers to examination by a physician. It has been suggested that regular medical examinations of the workforce, on some periodic basis, e.g. annually, would allow the detection of any clinical effects, whether work related or not. Regular medical examinations would be valuable only if there was a reasonable detection rate for abnormalities which could be treated effectively. This has been suggested for specific abnormalities, such as hypertension and glycosuria, which can be asymptomatic, yet have severe consequences if not detected and treated early. However, for occupational health surveillance, there is little justification for a full head-to-toe medical examination. If periodic medical examinations are warranted, they ought to be focused on target organ systems which can be affected by identified workplace exposures. Hence, for workers exposed to mercury, the medical examination should concentrate primarily on the central nervous system and the renal tract. For exposure to asbestos, the main target organs affected are the respiratory system (lung fibrosis, bronchogenic cancer, mesothelioma) and the skin (asbestos corns). For exposure to hand–arm vibration, regular examination should focus on neurological, vascular and musculoskeletal assessment of the hands.

Special investigations

Lung function tests

Periodic lung function tests have been used for the health surveillance of workers exposed to agents known to cause occupational asthma (see Table 16.1). These tests include the determination of the ratio of the forced expiratory volume in one second (FEV_1) to the forced vital capacity (FVC), and other parameters of spirometry (Fig. 16.1). For the comparison of spirometry tracings taken for an individual or group of workers over a period of time, several requirements must be met. These requirements have been recommended by international organizations, such as the European Respiratory Society, British Thoracic Society and American Thoracic Society, in order to harmonize the performance and interpretation of lung function tests (Quanjer *et al.* 1993; American Thoracic Society 1995; Cotes *et al.* 1997). The requirements are as follows.

1 The spirometer must be calibrated.

2 The tracing must be taken by a competent person, and the subject must be instructed adequately. A full and deep breath should be taken by the subject, who should then place his/her lips around the mouthpiece of the spirometer to form a tight seal, and exhale out as hard and as fast as possible, without stopping to re-inhale. The subject should be

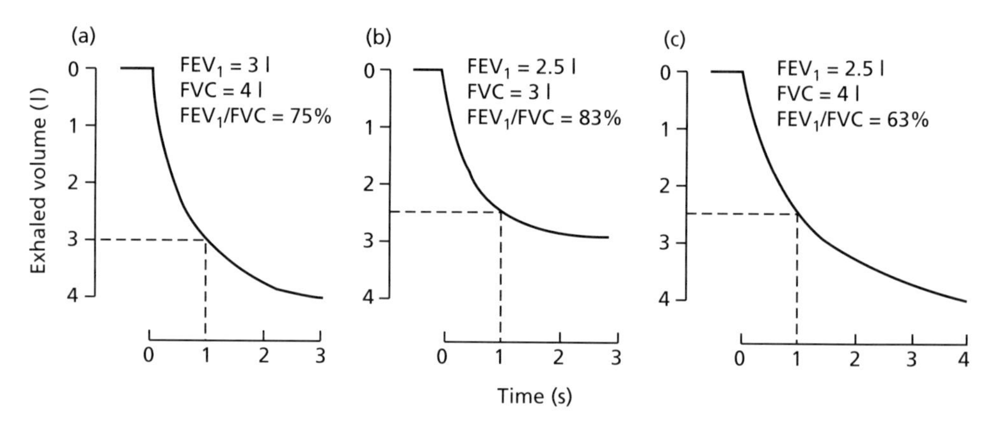

Figure 16.1 Spirometric tracings showing (a) normal, (b) restrictive and (c) obstructive disease of the airways. (From Levy & Wegman 1995.)

informed to stop breathing out only when told to do so by the person performing the test.

3 At least three valid tracings are needed on each occasion. A valid tracing is one which:

(a) has the start point for the stylus centred correctly on the recording sheet;

(b) has a steep initial rise (with maximum effort by the subject) leading to a plateau; the trace must continue until a definite plateau is reached;

(c) does not have any interruptions in the trace due to the subject coughing or stopping to re-inhale.

For a proper interpretation of a spirometric trace, the following items of information are needed:

- age, sex, ethnic group and height of the subject;
- the past medical history;
- whether the subject is currently taking medication, such as bronchodilators.

The trace is invalid if the subject has had a cigarette within an hour, a heavy meal within 2 h or a heavy cold within 3 weeks of the lung function test. The presence of these factors will require that the lung function test be performed on another occasion. Good quality data from correctly performed tests are essential if the results of lung function tests are to be meaningfully interpreted.

A limitation of this procedure for the health surveillance of workers exposed to asthmagens is that, because asthma presents as episodic, reversible obstruction of the airways, lung function tests can be normal in between asthmatic attacks, but there will be a decline in lung function tests during an asthmatic episode. In addition, those who are experiencing asthmatic symptoms, especially if they are severe, may not be well enough to present themselves to the occupational health department for health surveillance. Hence, periodic spirometry might show normal results in spite of the individual having occupational asthma.

Another method used for the assessment of lung function is serial peak flow readings (Fig. 16.2). This is done using a peak flow meter (e.g. Wright's peak flow meter). Portable versions of these devices enable them to be issued to workers by the occupational health department for the self-recording of lung function. In order to obtain reliable results, the individuals must be well instructed on how readings are to be taken and recorded. Readings are expressed in units of litres per minute and are taken at 2-h intervals (excepting the hours of sleep). The pattern of peak flow readings is evaluated to see whether there is any substantial deterioration in peak flow rate after exposure to the agent at the workplace. A difference of more than 15% between mean morning and evening values is clinically significant (Rees & Price 1989). The decline in peak flow rates in those with occupational asthma may occur soon after exposure to the causative agent, or there may be a delayed reaction where the respiratory effects occur after returning home from work. There is some subjectivity in the evaluation of a series of peak flow readings (Gannon & Burge 1997). What the clinician looks for is a pattern that indicates reversible obstruction of the airways. This is dependent, in part, on the number of readings and the duration of time over which the readings are taken. There have therefore been attempts to develop computer software programs to ensure consistency in the evaluation of serial peak flow results. The OASYS-2 program, developed at the Birmingham Heartlands Hospital in the UK, is an example of such a program (Gannon *et al.* 1996).

Audiometry

Periodic audiometry is frequently used for the health surveillance of workers exposed to noise. The principle is to detect any early loss of

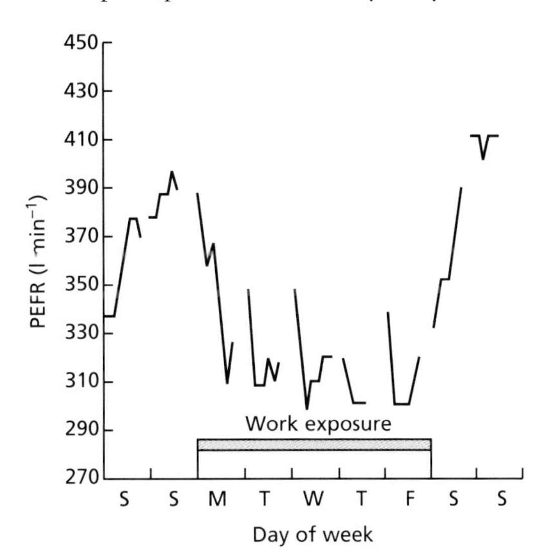

Figure 16.2 Serial peak expiratory flow rates (PEFRs) demonstrating reversible obstruction of the airways in a person before, during and after 1 week of exposure to glutaraldehyde. (Modified from Benson 1984.)

hearing, which will enable the affected individuals to be removed from further noise exposure, and to instigate the investigation of noise levels in the work area of the affected workers (as well as to consider exposure to non-occupational sources of noise). Several makes of audiometer are available for occupational health use. Those commonly used in the UK include the Peters or Kamplex models. These instruments must be calibrated before use. Quality control to obtain valid audiometric tracings (Fig. 16.3) also requires that these should be performed by trained health professionals using a sound-proof booth.

However, for the prevention of noise-induced deafness, the emphasis should be on periodic noise surveys to determine the extent of noise exposure and to map out noisy areas (more than 85 dBA) in the workplace, which can then be subject to noise reduction measures. At best, audiometry may detect a temporary threshold shift in those exposed to noise at work who do not resort to using ear defenders. When a temporary threshold shift is detected, removal of the individual from further noise exposure will allow some recovery of the hearing threshold. However, it is likely that, where workers are exposed to noise for prolonged periods of time, audiometry may confirm a permanent threshold shift. This is where the damage to hearing is irreversible, and therefore all that audiometry has succeeded in doing is to confirm noise-induced hearing loss. Audiometry during the preplacement assessment of workers at the start of a health surveillance programme can help to provide a baseline reading. The use of this is perhaps limited to medicolegal arguments about whether the individual suffered hearing loss from the present job, or whether there was pre-existing hearing loss before starting the job. A sensible approach would be to carry out periodic noise surveys and periodic audiometry as part of a hearing conservation programme.

Chest X-rays

Periodic chest X-rays have been advocated for workers exposed to:

• pulmonary carcinogens, e.g. asbestos fibres, bis-chloromethyl ether

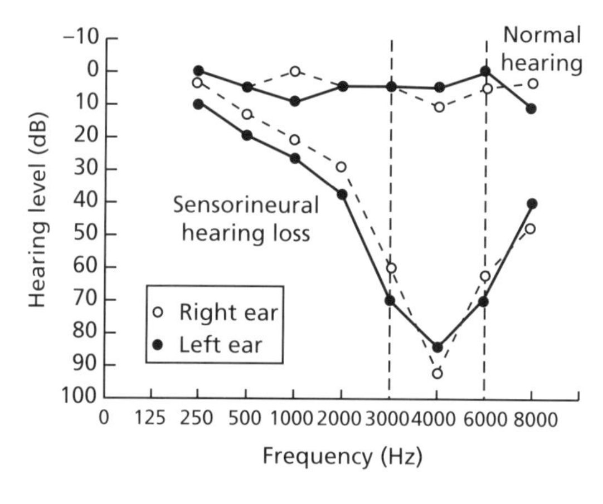

Figure 16.3 Audiometric tracing of an individual with normal hearing and an individual with sensorineural hearing loss from noise exposure. (From Croner Publications 1996.)

(BCME), beryllium and its compounds and some nickel and hexavalent chromium compounds; and

- workers exposed to fibrogenic dusts, such as silica and coal dust.

The basis for periodic X-rays for exposure to pulmonary carcinogens is that malignancies may be detected early, and surgical or other medical treatment may be carried out to effect a cure. Unfortunately, the ability to detect a tumour early by this method depends on the rate at which the tumour grows vs. the sensitivity, specificity and frequency of the X-rays. When chest X-rays are performed on an annual basis, it is still possible to miss a lung tumour that has had several months to develop. This is also true if the frequency of X-rays is increased to 8-month or 6-month intervals. With increasing frequency of X-rays, there is increasing exposure to radiation. The use of repeated exposure to radiation to detect lung cancer is questionable as radiation itself is a recognized cause of malignancy. There is also the difficulty of deciding whether an early 'shadow' on a chest X-ray is a small tumour which should be biopsied and surgically removed if possible, or whether it is just a radiological artefact. False positive readings in interpreting chest X-ray films will lead to unnecessary investigative procedures, such as bronchoscopy, biopsy and surgery—procedures which are uncomfortable and can cause undue concern in the individual. False negative readings, e.g. deciding that a shadow is possibly an artefact which need not be further investigated until the next chest X-ray, results in treatment delay if there is a malignant tumour. Evaluations of the effectiveness of periodic chest X-rays for the early detection of lung cancer in those occupationally exposed to hexavalent chromates have not demonstrated a conclusive benefit (Schilling & Schilling 1991).

One option in a health surveillance programme for exposure to pulmonary carcinogens is to institute periodic symptom review and symptom reporting and provide the full range of radiological and clinical investigations to those who are symptomatic. The limitation of this approach is that symptoms may be a late feature of the carcinogenic process. There are also similar considerations regarding false positives and false negatives in using the experience of symptoms as an initial step in screening for exposure to pulmonary carcinogens. Other measures that have been attempted include periodic sputum cytology. This procedure for health surveillance has yet to be evaluated fully.

It is probable that there are currently no effective periodic investigations that can be included in a health surveillance programme for lung carcinogens, and that the best effective means of prevention lies in the minimization of exposure and the reduction in concomitant exposure to other known pulmonary carcinogens, e.g. cigarette smoking, which may exert an additive (or even multiplicative) effect on the risk.

The limitations of periodic chest X-rays for the health surveillance of those exposed to occupational pulmonary carcinogens are also valid for exposure to fibrogenic dusts. All that periodic radiography will achieve at the moment is the early detection of lung fibrosis. There is no effective treatment for fibrosis and, even if the detection of fibrosis was used as an indication for the removal of workers from any further exposure, the fibrotic process may still continue. In any case, if the purpose of serial chest X-rays is to detect fibrosis, for exposure to silica dust and asbestos fibres, chest X-rays are not indicated for several years following initial exposure. For silica dust exposure, there is a latent period of 10–20 years after the initial exposure before fibrotic changes are detectable (Elmes 1994). Apart from the initial baseline chest X-ray on starting exposure, there is no good clinical reason for performing routine annual chest X-rays for the first 10 years of exposure to these fibrogenic dusts. It has been suggested that, for asbestos-exposed individuals, the detection of pulmonary fibrosis by chest X-rays can be used as an occasion to emphasize the importance of the cessation of cigarette smoking, as the pathological effects from asbestos exposure are multiplied with concomitant exposure to cigarette smoke. However, with the recognized synergistic effect between cigarette smoking and exposure to asbestos, and possibly for other pulmonary carcinogens, the advice to cease cigarette smoking should apply whether or not fibrogenic or other pathological changes in the lungs are detected.

Bladder cytology

Workers who have been exposed to known occupational bladder carcinogens, such as 2-naphthylamine in the rubber industry and 'aniline' dyes in the dyestuffs industry, have had health surveillance using periodic bladder cytology. This requires the collection and analysis of urine samples for the presence of malignant cells. Cells in urine specimens are stained using the Papanicolaou stain, which can help to indicate features of malignant change. This will act as a pointer for further clinical investigation. Periodic urine analysis for this group of workers can also include checking for microscopic haematuria. Microscopic and gross haematuria are early signs of bladder malignancy. In the UK, periodic cystoscopy as part of the health surveillance for this group of workers has been discontinued (Aw 1994) because of the discomfort of the procedure, poor compliance and a detection rate for bladder malignancy which has not been shown to be significantly better than that from periodic urinalysis.

Periodic eye tests

Tests for visual acuity on a periodic basis are required for some occupational groups, e.g. train and taxi drivers, airline pilots and ship navigators. Periodic vision testing may enable the detection of deteriorating vision which may be amenable to corrective action. However, this activity is not proposed for the detection of early effects on vision of occupational hazards. It is performed to detect defects in vision that may affect the safe performance of work. Examples of chemical agents that can cause damage to the optic nerve or alter colour perception are methanol (causes optic atrophy following ingestion) and styrene (causes distorted colour perception following inhalation of vapour). The incidences of such effects are rare, and periodic screening for visual effects from these chemical exposures are not warranted.

The traditional charts (e.g. Snellen's charts) used for distant vision, near vision and colour vision (Ishihara's charts) have been superceded by devices such as Keystone machines, which are able to test all these modalities of vision. Keystone machines are widely used in the UK for the periodic screening of the visual status of visual display unit (VDU) users. There is some debate over the usefulness of such regular visual tests for this category of workers. However, the Display Screen Equipment Regulations (1992) in the UK require that visual tests (eye checks) should be provided by employers for their VDU users if they request such tests.

Determination of immune status and antibody levels

Periodic checking of immune status has been suggested as a means of health surveillance for health care workers exposed to infectious agents. This would apply to certain groups of laboratory, pathology and clinical staff. Successful hepatitis B immunization of health care staff exposed to blood and body fluids results in adequate antibody levels. As these levels may decrease over time, periodic checking of antibody levels, followed by booster doses of vaccine, may be considered. The alternative is not to check the antibody levels, except once after an initial full course, and to provide a single booster dose of vaccine 5 years later. This is the current practice in most UK National Health Service (NHS) occupational health departments. The timing of the booster dose is debatable. In the USA, it has been suggested that a hepatitis B booster dose is probably not warranted until 7 years after the initial course. The regular checking of new groups of health care workers involved in exposure-prone procedures to ensure that they are protected against hepatitis B is an established part of the health surveillance programmes of occupational health departments for the health care industry.

Similarly, with the surveillance of workers exposed to the risk of TB, periodic tuberculin testing is used in the USA. Bacillus Calmette–Guérin (BCG) immunization is not offered routinely in the USA, and periodic chest X-rays for the detection of active TB are not performed. A strongly positive skin reaction to tuberculin is taken as an indication of likely infection, hence warranting clinical investigation and chemotherapy. In the UK, health care workers with no obvious scar showing previous BCG immunization are tuberculin tested using the Mantoux or Heaf test (Joint Tuberculosis Committee of the British Thoracic Society 1994). If tuberculin testing shows a lack of immunity to TB (Grade 1 reaction), BCG is administered. The health surveillance programme focuses on the reporting and investigation of symptoms suggesting active TB, rather than on the use of periodic checks of immune status by tuberculin testing.

Biological monitoring

Confusion over terminology (Zielhuis 1985) has led to biological monitoring occasionally being included as an activity under health surveillance. By definition, biological monitoring is not a clinical or physiological procedure to detect early health effects (Notten *et al.* 1986). It refers to the analysis of biological samples for the determination of the extent of exposure. However, the UK Control of Substances Hazardous to Health (COSHH) Regulations 1994 list biological monitoring as an option for health surveillance. This section is therefore included in this chapter, mainly for completeness, although there is likely to be continuing confusion and debate over the inclusion of biological monitoring as a health surveillance technique.

The biological samples commonly used in occupational health practice are blood and urine, and sometimes expired air samples. Biological samples, such as hair and nail, adipose tissue, sweat and faeces, could theoretically be used. However, these are of limited practical value in occupational health practice because of several factors.

1 The methods for analysis have not been developed sufficiently.

2 There are few laboratories with the experience or quality control procedures for such analysis.

3 The presence of contaminants and other factors can cause interference and error in the analysis.

4 It may be difficult to interpret the results once they have been obtained.

5 There are practical difficulties with the collection, storage, handling and dispatch of such samples.

Biological samples can be analysed for the presence of a chemical encountered in the workplace or its metabolite. There is variability in the clearance of systemically absorbed compounds, and there is also non-specificity for some substances, e.g. hippuric acid in urine can be an indicator of occupational exposure to toluene, but may also reflect the ingestion of benzoic acid which is used as a food preservative. Some organic compounds have several phases of clearance, and the biological half-life following systemic absorption can differ for various chemicals.

The principle behind the use of biological monitoring for risk assessment is similar to that for environmental monitoring. Biological monitoring provides an index of exposure and takes into account all routes of absorption. Environmental monitoring usually assesses exposure by the airborne route only, although an 'Sk' notation is used to indicate chemicals that can be systemically absorbed through the skin. In both environmental and biological monitoring, a means of interpreting the results obtained is essential. The American Conference of Governmental Industrial Hygienists (ACGIH) produces an annual handbook on threshold limit values (TLVs) for chemical substances and physical agents and biological exposure indices (BEIs) (ACGIH 1998). The BEIs are reference values that can be used to interpret the results of biological monitoring, and hence assist in the evaluation of exposure to potential health hazards. The UK HSE has started to publish reference values for biological monitoring. These values are now incorporated in *EH40*, a document containing occupational exposure limits, which is revised and updated annually (HSE 1998). Unlike BEIs, the UK biological monitoring guidance values are categorized into: (i) health guidance values (HGVs); and (ii) benchmark guidance values (BGVs).

Health guidance values are set at a level at which there is no evidence in the scientific literature that this would be harmful to health. Benchmark guidance values represent the 90th percentile of values taken from representative workplaces with good hygiene practice. The 1998 edition of *EH40* contains values for eight substances—five HGVs and three BGVs (HSE 1998). Table 16.2 provides examples of biological samples and the substances or metabolites that can be analysed for biological monitoring purposes.

Having established an indication for biological monitoring on the basis of legal requirements or from the risk assessment, there are several practical considerations which must be taken into account before starting a biological monitoring programme.

1 The type of biological sample to be collected, and how much will be required.

2 The timing of sample collection (in relation to the beginning and end of the shift or working week).

3 The type of special precautions to be taken with regard to the collection, storage, packing and dispatch of the sample to the laboratory.

4 The identification of an approved laboratory or one with the relevant experience to perform the analysis. The laboratory should have quality control mechanisms for the specific analysis.

5 The possibility that the sample may need to reach the laboratory soon after collection. This must be ensured if required.

6 The explanation to the subjects the reasons for the collection and analysis of the biological samples, and the provision of reassurance as

Table 16.2 Biological monitoring: substances and/or metabolites in biological samples.

Substance	Biological sample	Analyte
Inorganic lead	Blood	Lead
Organic lead	Urine	Lead
Mercury	Blood, urine	Mercury
Cadmium	Urine	Cadmium
Organophosphate pesticides	Urine	Dialkyl phosphates
Toluene	Urine	Hippuric acid
Xylene	Urine	Methyl hippuric acid
Styrene	Urine	Mandelic acid
	Urine	Phenylglyoxylic acid
Methyl ethyl ketone (MEK)	Urine	MEK
Perchloroethylene	Blood, expired air	Perchloroethylene
n-Hexane	Urine	2,5-Hexanedione

necessary that the samples will not be subject to other tests, e.g. for alcohol, drugs or human immunodeficiency virus (HIV) status.
7 The provision of feedback to the subjects when the results are available, including provisions for grouped data to be made available as required. Where biological monitoring is performed under specific regulations, there may be a requirement to report the findings to the regulatory authorities.
8 The safe storage of the data from biological monitoring in a system that also allows ease of data retrieval.

Biological effect monitoring

Unlike biological monitoring, which is a procedure primarily for the assessment of exposure to chemical agents, biological effect monitoring attempts to detect early effects from such exposure. The effects may be non-specific, and can often be difficult to interpret in terms of whether harm to health has resulted. As for biological monitoring, biological effect monitoring depends on the analysis of biological samples. While biological monitoring attempts to measure the amount of a chemical or its metabolite in the biological sample, biological effect monitoring often attempts to measure a certain biochemical parameter which is neither the chemical to which the worker is exposed nor its metabolite.

Examples of biological effects used for occupational health surveillance are given below.
1 *Free erythrocyte protoporphyrin (FEP) in blood and urinary δ-aminolaevulinic acid (d-ALA) levels for exposure to inorganic lead.* Elevated serum FEP and urinary d-ALA levels give an indication of a biochemical effect from the depression of enzymes involved in haem synthesis by inorganic lead. The affected enzymes include d-ALA dehydratase and haem synthetase. Depression of dehydratase activity leads to an increase in blood levels of the substrate d-ALA, which then appears in the urine.
2 *Serum cholinesterase levels.* Both serum and red blood cell cholinesterase can be depressed by exposure to organophosphate pesticides. The levels are reversible on cessation of exposure. Cholinesterase inactivates acetylcholine at nerve endings, and the depression of this enzyme leads to prolonged cholinergic activity such that, in organophosphate pesticide poisoning, the victims experience cholinergic effects, such as constriction of the pupils, blurred vision, tearing, chest tightness, wheeze, excessive salivation and sweating, weakness, slurred speech, vomiting, abdominal cramps and diarrhoea. The range of symptoms indicates the widespread effect on several target organ systems. The symptoms will depend on the extent of exposure and, where exposure is limited, there may be few symptoms accompanying the depression of serum cholinesterase. Exposure to pesticides belonging to the carbamate group will also produce similar effects.
3 *Detection of specific urinary proteins.* β_2-Microglobulin in urine

results from significant exposure to cadmium. The appearance of this low-molecular-weight protein in urine indicates proximal renal tubular dysfunction. The amounts detected in urine may be transient, suggesting a temporary reversible effect, or persistent, indicating possible long-term renal damage. In addition to causing β_2-microglobulin in urine, cadmium is also known to produce glycosuria, amino-aciduria and phosphaturia. A different protein—α_1-microglobulin—is also thought to be useful as an indicator of renal tubular dysfunction due to cadmium (Tohyama *et al.* 1986; Kido *et al.* 1995). Attempts have also been made to explore the use of various compounds in urine as a biological effect monitoring procedure for exposure to cadmium and other heavy metals. These include low-molecular-weight proteins, such as metallothionein and retinol binding protein (RBP), and enzymes, such as *N*-acetyl glucosaminidase (NAG) and β-galactosidase (Hoet & Haufroid 1997).

4 *Liver function tests.* Serum transpeptidase, transaminase and alkaline phosphatase levels can be used as indicators of possible liver cell damage. Serum γ-glutamyl transferase (γ-GT) is increased following chronic excessive alcohol consumption. The systemic absorption of chlorinated hydrocarbon solvents may have a similar effect. However, the elevation of these enzyme levels is often non-specific, and there is no consistent pattern to indicate a specific effect from occupational exposure. Hence, these indices of liver function are rarely used for the health surveillance of occupational groups. The determination of the clearance of bile acids shows some promise for the detection of an early liver effect from exposure to hepatotoxic chemicals.

5 *Other biological effects.* Several other biological effects associated with exposure to workplace hazards have been explored as possible biological effect monitoring procedures. These include the determination of DNA adducts in plasma or urine for workers exposed to carcinogens, and the detection of mutagenic activity in similar biological samples for workers exposed to cytotoxic agents (Hoet & Haufroid 1997). At present, such methods remain experimental, and further information is needed on the specificity, sensitivity and variability of these effects in relation to exposure, the background prevalence of such effects and the interpretation of different levels of these effects in relation to risk.

Requirements for health surveillance

Before starting a programme for the health surveillance of exposed workers, the following points must be considered.

Is there an indication for surveillance?

Health surveillance is indicated if there is continuing potential for occupational exposure to the agent concerned, and there is a valid method for surveillance with adequate means for interpreting the findings. It is especially relevant for exposure to chemical agents for which the relationship between dose and effect is not clear. Two examples are exposure to allergens and carcinogens. With exposure to respiratory sensitizers, there may be a threshold for sensitization, but, once an individual has been sensitized, very small exposures may be capable of triggering an asthmatic attack. In such instances, health surveillance by the use of periodic questionnaires, encouraging the reporting of respiratory symptoms for further evaluation, and lung function tests should be included. This will allow clinical effects to be detected for further occupational health management, whatever the extent of exposure. With occupational exposure to carcinogens, such as asbestos, small exposures may lead to an increased risk of malignancy. Hence, the inclusion of a procedure to detect early malignant changes in time for effective treatment is an attractive proposal. However, the number of effective procedures which can be incorporated into a health surveillance programme for occupational lung carcinogens is limited. As discussed earlier, periodic chest X-rays, symptom review, sputum cytology and bronchoscopy for the early detection of lung cancer all have their limitations.

Is health surveillance required by law?

Health surveillance for occupationally exposed groups of workers is required under specific health and safety legislation. Many countries require that workers exposed to inorganic lead and lead compounds should belong to a health surveillance scheme, e.g. the UK, USA, Germany, Malaysia and Singapore. In the UK, the Control of Lead at Work Regulations 1980 lay down specific intervals for blood lead determinations and clinical assessment, with recommendations for specific action, such as suspension from further lead exposure or increasing the frequency of blood lead analysis. Surveillance must be performed by medical advisers of the HSE (now termed medical inspectors), or by appointed doctors who are employed by firms with lead-exposed workers, according to the protocol specified by the HSE. The authority for appointing these doctors rests with the HSE, which is the UK agency within the Department of Environment, Trade and the Regions with responsibility for enforcing health and safety legislation. The appointments are reviewed periodically. In the USA, laboratories approved by the Occupational Safety and Health Administration (OSHA) must be used for blood lead determinations; OSHA is a federal agency similar to the HSE in the UK. It has responsibility in the USA for enforcing health and safety law, and is part of the Department of Labor. The National Institute for Occupational Safety and Health (NIOSH) in the USA is another organization that has a role in occupational health. It is part of the Centers for Disease Control and Prevention (CDC), an agency belonging to the Department of Health and Human Services. Within its health hazard evaluation programme, NIOSH officers may recommend health surveillance for groups of workers after worksite visits and risk assessment.

Under the UK COSHH Regulations 1994, medical surveillance is required for workers exposed to any of a list of chemical agents used in specified processes. Regulation 11(2)(a) and Schedule (5) in the COSHH Regulations provide a table listing the substances and the relevant processes (see Table 16.3).

The exact procedures required for surveillance are generally provided to the appointed doctors in notes of guidance from the HSE. Unfortunately, detailed guidance is not available for all the substances listed. For example, exposure to disulphur dichloride in the manufacture of indiarubber or indiarubber products is listed as requiring medical surveillance, but it is uncertain what specific procedures are needed. Disulphur dichloride (S_2Cl_2) is used for the cold vulcanization of indiarubber. It is corrosive and irritant to mucous membranes, such as the eyes, nose, throat and the respiratory tract. There are no reports of systemic toxicity in exposed workers in the UK, nor any recently

Table 16.3 Exposures requiring medical surveillance under the COSHH Regulations.

Substance	Process
Vinyl chloride monomer (VCM)	In manufacture, production, reclamation, storage, discharge, transport, use or polymerization
Nitro or amino derivatives of phenol and of benzene or its homologues	In the manufacture of nitro or amino derivatives of phenol and of benzene or its homologues and the making of explosives or the use of any of these substances
Potassium or sodium chromate or dichromate	In manufacture
1-Naphthylamine and its salts, *o*-toluidine and its salts, dianisidine and its salts, dichlorobenzidine and its salts	In manufacture, formation or use of these substances
Auramine, magenta	In manufacture
Carbon disulphide, disulphur dichloride, benzene, including benzol, carbon tetrachloride, trichloroethylene	Processes in which these substances are used, or given off as vapour, in the manufacture of indiarubber or of articles or goods made wholly or partially of indiarubber
Pitch	In manufacture of blocks of fuel consisting of coal, coal dust, coke or slurry with pitch as a binding substance

published reports of local irritant effects. From the properties of the chemical, the most relevant effects for medical surveillance would appear to be irritant effects on the skin and mucosae. These are probably best detected through self-reporting by the exposed workers, which can be followed by investigation and preventive action. Workers with a history of asthma may also need to be assessed before starting work with possible exposure to disulphur dichloride, as this may irritate mucous membranes and possibly trigger an asthmatic attack. However, if this is an acceptable basis for the requirement of health surveillance for disulphur dichloride exposure, it should apply equally to other chemicals which are strong irritants to the skin and mucous membranes, e.g. chlorine gas, hydrofluoric acid and other concentrated acids. The availability of detailed published guidance would ensure consistency in the method of surveillance for workers with similar occupational exposures.

The other chemicals listed under Schedule 5 of the COSHH Regulations (Table 16.3) include carcinogens and a few toxic compounds. The listed carcinogens include a liver carcinogen — vinyl chloride monomer — which causes angiosarcoma of the liver, a recognized occupational cause of leukaemia — benzene — used in indiarubber processes, and a number of occupational bladder carcinogens, e.g. auramine and magenta in manufacture and *o*-toluidine, dianisidine and dichlorobenzidene and their salts in manufacture, formation or use.

The toxic chemicals include carbon disulphide, carbon tetrachloride and trichloroethylene. Carbon disulphide is neurotoxic, hepatotoxic and nephrotoxic. Carbon tetrachloride and trichloroethylene are both hepatotoxic, and can also cause renal damage. The basis for health surveillance would be the early detection of such toxic effects. There are, however, many other neurotoxic, hepatotoxic and nephrotoxic agents which are not specifically included in Schedule 5 of the COSHH Regulations.

The Approved Code of Practice (ACOP) accompanying the COSHH Regulations contains additional guidance on surveillance. Reference is provided to typical procedures for the appropriate health surveillance of workers exposed to certain categories of substance or process. These are shown in Table 16.4.

The ACOP also states that the collection, maintenance and review of health records alone may suffice for surveillance. The examples given are for exposure to known or suspected carcinogens, man-made mineral fibres, dust and fume from rubber processes and leather dust in boot and shoe manufacture. This is likely to be because there are no readily identifiable early effects that can be detected by other means of medical surveillance for which early treatment can be effective, or because the purpose of surveillance in these examples is primarily epidemiological — to confirm that there is no added risk under current exposures, or that there is an excess risk which will warrant stricter control on exposure. The latter may benefit future groups that are likely to be exposed

Table 16.4 Substances/processes and typical health surveillance procedures.

Substance/process	Typical procedure
Recognized systemic toxicity	Appropriate clinical or laboratory investigations
Substances known to cause asthma	Enquiries seeking evidence of respiratory symptoms related to work
Substances known to cause severe dermatitis	Skin inspection by a responsible person
Electrolytic plating or oxidation of metal articles by use of an electrolyte containing chromic acid or other chromium compounds	Skin inspection by a responsible person
Contact with chrome solutions in dyeing processes using dichromate of potassium or sodium	Skin inspection by a responsible person
Contact with chrome solutions in processes of liming and tanning of raw hides and skins (including retanning of tanned hides or skins)	Skin inspection by a responsible person

at work, but will have no direct benefit for those under current surveillance.

Further details on the UK legal requirements for health surveillance at the workplace are well covered by various HSE publications (HSE 1990, 1997; Health and Safety Commission (HSC) 1996) and a comprehensive review by Deacon (1995).

Is the method appropriate? Is there a suitable method?

Whether or not the methods used for health surveillance are appropriate and suitable depends on their ability to detect early health effects. For example, in terms of the detection of early effects, the hierarchy of some of the procedures mentioned earlier would be as follows.

1 Biological monitoring (detects excess exposure before effects appear).

2 Biological effect monitoring (detects early effects, the clinical significance of which is uncertain).

3 Symptom review (detects symptoms that may precede or occur in established disease).

4 Signs on examination (detects gross clinical abnormalities indicating disease).

The choice of procedure will depend, in part, on availability, e.g. biological and biological effect monitoring vs. examination for symptoms and signs. A combination of procedures may also be considered, e.g. biological monitoring and symptom review for exposure to organic solvents.

Can any effective action be taken on the detection of effects?

An important consideration before advocating medical examinations as part of occupational health surveillance is whether anything effective can be done to treat the individual when clinical abnormalities are detected. If nothing can be done, the detection of abnormalities is of limited use, other than as a confirmation of exposure to a workplace hazard, and as an indication that the condition detected is progressive with no specific treatment available. This appears to be the case with the detection of lung malignancy in asbestos-exposed individuals and fibrotic lung changes in those exposed to silica dust. However, if specific effective treatment is available, as for early bladder cancer, periodic examinations are of value.

Which workers should be included in a health surveillance programme?

The major considerations in deciding who to include in a biological monitoring programme are as follows.

1 The extent of exposure to the hazard in the workplace.
2 The susceptibility of the exposed workers.
3 The requirements of health and safety law.

For example, where workers are exposed to metallic mercury in the repair of sphygmomanometers, and the work is performed on a daily basis with the potential for exposure which cannot be fully controlled, workers should be included. The extent of exposure can also be determined from any industrial hygiene monitoring results if available. However, if the work is performed intermittently, i.e. only a few hours are spent each time working on a limited number of sphygmomanometers, and the observation of the system of work suggests that significant exposure to mercury is unlikely, workers do not need health surveillance.

For nurses exposed to glutaraldehyde, which is an asthma-causing agent, in addition to considering the frequency, duration and intensity of exposure, health surveillance may be necessary for those with a past history of asthma, even if the individuals concerned do not work regularly with glutaraldehyde, but have occasion to use it sporadically.

For exposure to lead compounds, the requirements for health surveillance are clearly defined by the Control of Lead at Work Regulations 1980 (HSC 1985). In countries such as Germany (Wrbitzky *et al.* 1994), there are much more legally defined requirements for health surveillance with regard to exposure to a wide range of chemicals. In 1991, there were 43 separate directives for carrying out preventive medical examinations for those in hazardous jobs (Muller 1991). In other countries, the legal requirements may be limited to exposure to lead and ionizing radiation.

What can be done to ensure the continuation of health surveillance after the cessation of exposure?

A practical problem with health surveillance is that, for some substances, the effects of occupational exposure may occur after a long latent period. For example, for exposure to occupational carcinogens, such as asbestos and β-naphthylamine, 10–50 years may pass between the first exposure and the development of malignancy. Health surveillance systems may be in place whilst the individuals continue to be employed by the organizations involved. However, when individual workers leave to take up new jobs in other industries without exposure, or when they retire from employment, this may be the time when the need for health surveillance is greatest. This is usually because the latent period for the disease has been met, and health surveillance for the exposed worker is more likely to be effective. If the worker leaves the company where exposure occurred, it is not clear how health surveillance should continue. Various options are available for continuing health surveillance, each with certain limitations. For the UK, some of these options are as follows:

Giving the responsibility for continuing health surveillance to the new employer
This is impractical, because the new employer may not have the necessary resources, manpower or experience to carry out such surveillance.

Asking the worker to continue health surveillance through the previous employer
This can also be impractical if the worker moves to a different part of the country for a new job, and access to the facilities for health surveillance at the site of the previous job is difficult.

Asking the general practitioner (family physician) to continue health surveillance
This transfers the responsibility for surveillance from the employer to the general practitioner. While this is theoretically possible, the practical considerations include the transfer of records, the familiarity of the general practitioner with the exposure and what is required by way of surveillance and the availability of resources for continuing surveillance. Another limitation is the difficulty of ensuring consistency of health surveillance when different general practitioners, possibly in different parts of the country, are asked to carry out this procedure for a limited number of individual workers.

Giving the responsibility for continuing health surveillance to medical inspectors in the Employment Medical Advisory Service Section of the HSE
The occupational physicians and nurses in this organization will be able

to ensure that the procedures for surveillance are consistent, and they will also have access to health and safety and industrial hygiene data from their colleagues in the Factories Inspectorate if this is needed.

Giving the responsibility for continuing health surveillance to occupational health departments in the NHS
Every NHS hospital has access to an occupational health service, some of which are staffed by specialist occupational physicians, all with occupational health nurses, and a number with input from industrial hygienists and safety practitioners.

Health surveillance records

An essential requirement for an effective health surveillance programme is a system for good record keeping. One useful aspect of health surveillance is that it enables adequate data to be analysed for epidemiological purposes. This will facilitate the tracking of trends in disease occurrence, and will allow the early detection of an excess of specific diseases or conditions in defined occupational groups. Periodic analysis of such data can also help to identify clusters of cases. This can trigger investigations, leading to any necessary intervention to prevent further cases. The analysis of health surveillance records can confirm the adequacy of risk assessment conclusions, and give an indication of the effectiveness of control measures. It may also identify individual workers at higher risk of health effects as a result of genetic factors, increased susceptibility due to concomitant disease or the presence of other risk factors, such as atopy in those exposed to allergens.

Methods

There are different methods and requirements for keeping records on health surveillance. The form of health surveillance records may be specified by health and safety law. Data on hard copy can be filed within individual worker/patient files, and stored in alphabetical order, by unique identification number, such as the National Insurance or Social Security number, or by payroll number. Data in this form tend to be difficult to analyse epidemiologically, unless the information is first transferred to a summary sheet or onto a computer line listing or spreadsheet. It is also difficult to determine easily from individual paper records the number or proportion of workers with a specific feature, such as a blood lead level above a particular value or those whose lung function tests fall below a specified index. There are therefore advantages in storing such records on computer. This requires a good system of data entry and data retrieval. If data entry is performed manually, procedures must be in place to prevent transcription error. Such procedures can include the double entry of data, or the use of a scanner to transfer data from predesigned forms onto the computer hard disk.

All too often, data on health surveillance are collected and stored, but seldom analysed. Missing items of information, poorly collected data and data that are recorded incompletely all contribute to the limitation of the use of records for epidemiological analysis.

Confidentiality of health records

Medical information on individual workers pertaining to health surveillance should be kept confidential, in keeping with ethical and professional guidelines for medical records (Faculty of Occupational Medicine 1993; Medical Defence Union 1996). However, there is often a dilemma for occupational physicians and nurses in that, for effective preventive action to be taken with regard to occupational exposures, some information on health effects must be communicated to the appropriate managers. Otherwise, the managers will be unaware that ill health related to workplace factors has been detected, and will be unable to institute preventive measures. A compromise has been suggested where individual medical data remain confidential, but grouped data can be provided to third parties if there is a need for them to have this information, e.g. safety representatives, managers and union representatives. An example of grouped data includes the proportion of individuals in a specified group (either working in the same section or exposed to similar chemicals) with a particular health effect or with biological monitoring results above the BEI. The 'need to know' depends on a clearly defined role of the individuals receiving the grouped data in the institution of preventive measures at the workplace. The data provided should also be limited to essential information, and should exclude clinical details not relevant to occupational health. While there are usually no major concerns about revealing data from workplace exposure monitoring, there is often some reluctance in divulging data on biological monitoring. This is despite the fact that both forms of monitoring are used as indicators of exposure to chemical agents in the workplace. This may be because blood, urine and other biological samples may be used for the assessment of exposure when performing biological monitoring, but these samples are not needed for ambient air monitoring of workplace exposures. Individuals are often hesitant about releasing the results of their blood or urine tests to others, perhaps due to the mistaken belief that these could indicate that they have a specific disease which they would prefer to keep confidential. This misconception may be the result of a lack of understanding of what biological monitoring involves, and what its limitations are. This is an issue that occupational health practitioners must deal with, as it may affect the communication between practitioners and the workers participating in health surveillance. The provision of adequate information and explanation before biological monitoring would certainly help to reduce unwarranted concerns about what can and cannot be determined from such data.

Safe storage of records

Another aspect related to the confidentiality of health surveillance records is the safe storage of such information. Hard copy records should be kept secure, and only accessed by staff from the occupational health department. Computer records should be backed up, and protected by software security codes and hardware security devices.

Under the UK COSHH Regulations, records of health surveillance should be kept for at least 40 years. This is presumably to allow the epidemiological analysis of the data at some later date if required. It is uncertain how complete, how well collected and how useful such data sets, kept by many different employers, will be for epidemiological studies.

When a company with a health surveillance programme for its workforce goes out of business, there should be provisions for the safe and complete transfer of the records from such surveillance. If the stated purpose for keeping records of health surveillance is for future epidemiological analysis, the records should be transferred to a government agency with responsibility for occupational health and safety (such as the HSE in the UK) or to a research organization.

Conclusions

Health surveillance is a useful tool for assessing the extent of risk in occupationally exposed individuals. It enables an early investigation to be made of workplace exposures and systems of work, and facilitates the implementation of preventive measures. Health surveillance complements other methods for the assessment and management of occupational risks, such as workplace exposure measurements, evaluation of the system of work and epidemiological analysis of data on exposure and health effects. Effective occupational health surveillance depends on an understanding of the specificity and sensitivity of the chosen procedures and the advantages and limitations of each procedure. It is also essential that the data from health surveillance are integrated with information from other methods used in risk assessment and risk management to maximize the scope for prevention.

References

ACGIH (1998) *1998 TLVs and BEIs*. American Conference of Governmental Industrial Hygienists, Cincinnati, OH.

American Thoracic Society (1995) Standardisation of spirometry; 1994 update. *American Journal of Respiratory and Critical Care Medicine* **152**, 1107–1136.

Aw, T.C. (1994) Aromatic chemicals. In: *Hunter's Diseases of Occupations* (eds. P.A.B. Raffle, P.H. Adams, P.J. Baxter & W.R. Lee), 8th edn., pp. 191–212. Edward Arnold, London.

Bell, J.G., Bishop, C., Gann, M., *et al.* (1995) A systematic approach to

health surveillance in the workplace. *Occupational Medicine* **45** (6), 305–310.
Benson, W.G. (1984) Exposure to glutaraldehyde. *Journal of the Society of Occupational Medicine* **34**, 63–64.
Cotes, J.E., Chinn, D.J. & Reed, J.W. (1997) Lung function testing: methods and reference values for forced expiratory volume (FEV_1) and transfer factor (T_L). *Occupational and Environmental Medicine* **54**, 457–465.
Croner Publications (1996) *Croner's Management of Health Risks*. Croner Publications, Kingston upon Thames, Surrey.
Deacon, S. (1995) *Health Surveillance at Work*. Technical Communications (Publishing) Ltd., Hitchin, Hertfordshire.
Elmes, P.C. (1994) Inorganic dusts. In: *Hunter's Diseases of Occupations* (eds. P.A.B. Raffle, P.H. Adams, P.J. Baxter & W.R. Lee), 8th edn., pp. 410–457. Edward Arnold, London.
Faculty of Occupational Medicine (1993) *Guidelines on Ethics for Occupational Physicians*, 4th edn. Faculty of Occupational Medicine, Royal College of Physicians, London.
Gannon, P.F.G. & Burge, P.S. (1997) Serial peak expiratory flow measurement in the diagnosis of occupational asthma. *European Respiratory Journal* **10** (Suppl. 24), 57s–63s.
Gannon, P.F.G., Newton, D.T., Belcher, J., Pantin, C.F.A., Burge, P.S. & Coifman, R. (1996) The development of OASYS-2, a system for the analysis of measurements of peak respiratory flow in workers with suspected occupational asthma. *Thorax* **51**, 484–489.
Hoet, P. & Haufroid, V. (1997) Biological monitoring: state of the art. *Occupational and Environmental Medicine* **54**, 361–366.
Honey, S. (1997) Health surveillance in Great Britain. *Occupational Health Reviews* **September/October**, 14–18.
Howard, G. (1998) In: *Occupational Health: Pocket Consultant* (eds. J.M. Harrington, F.S. Gill, T.C. Aw & K. Gardiner), 4th edn. Blackwell Science Ltd, Oxford.
HSC (1985) *Approved Code of Practice: Control of Lead at Work*. HSE Books, Sheffield.
HSC (1996) *Approved Codes of Practice: General COSHH ACOP; Carcinogens ACOP; Biological Agents ACOP*. HSE Books, Sudbury.
HSE (1990) *Surveillance of People Exposed to Health Risks at Work*. HMSO, London.
HSE (1998) *EH40/98. Occupational Exposure Limits 1998*. HSE Books, Sudbury.
Industrial Injuries Advisory Council (1993) *Periodic Report 1993*. HMSO, London.
Joint Tuberculosis Committee of the British Thoracic Society (1994) Control and prevention of tuberculosis in the United Kingdom: code of practice 1994. *Thorax* **49**, 1193–1200.
Kido, T., Honda, R., Yamada, Y., Tsuritani, I., Ishizaki, M. & Nogawa, K. (1985) α_1-Microglobulin determination in urine for the early detection of renal tubular dysfunctions caused by exposure to cadmium. *Toxicology Letters* **24**, 195–201.
Levy, B.S. & Wegman, D.M. (eds) (1995) *Occupational Health—Recognizing and Preventing Work Related Disease*, 3rd edn. Little, Brown & Co., Boston, MA.

Medical Defence Union (1996) *Can I See The Records? Clinical Notes—Disclosure and Patient Access*. The Medical Defence Union Ltd., London.
Muller, R. (1991) Occupational health care in the Federal Republic of Germany. In: *Occupational Health Services in 6 Member States of the EC* (eds. P.J. Kroon & M.A. Overeynder), pp. 41–45. Hacquebard BV, Amsterdam.
Notten, W.R.F., Herber, R.F.M., Hunter, W.J., *et al.* (eds.) (1986) *Health Surveillance of Individual Workers Exposed to Chemical Agents*. Springer-Verlag, Berlin.
Quanjer, Ph.H., Tammeling, G.J., Cotes, J.E., Pedersen, O.F., Peslin, R. & Yernault, J.-C. (1993) Lung volumes and forced ventilatory flows: official statement of the European Respiratory Society. *European Respiratory Journal* **6** (Suppl. 16), 5–40.
Rees, J. & Price, J. (1989) *ABC of Asthma*, 2nd edn. British Medical Association, London.
Schilling, C.J. & Schilling, J.M. (1991) Chest X-ray screening for lung cancer at three British chromate plants from 1955 to 1989. *British Journal of Industrial Medicine* **48**, 476–479.
Tohyama, C., Kobayashi, E., Saito, H., *et al.* (1986) Urinary α-1 microglobulin as an indicator of renal tubular dysfunction caused by environmental cadmium exposure. *Journal of Applied Toxicology* **6** (3), 171–178.
Wrbitzky, R., Schaller, K.H. & Lehnert, G. (1994) The present state of occupational and environmental medicine in Germany. *International Archives of Occupational and Environmental Health* **66** (5), 289–294.
Zielhuis, R.L. (1985) Biological monitoring: confusion in terminology (editorial). *American Journal of Industrial Medicine* **8**, 515–516.

Chapter 17 Auditing risk assessment and management

Peter G. Nicoll

Introduction

This chapter briefly describes the importance of assurance processes in managing state-of-the-art occupational health programmes. It describes compliance audit and management systems assessments, discusses the main activities involved in carrying them out and provides practical advice on their implementation.

Background

Environmental, health and safety auditing activities in industry date back to the mid-1970s, when a handful of companies, working independently and on their own initiative, developed audit programmes as internal tools to review and evaluate environmental problems at the operating unit level.

Since that time, the discipline has experienced a significant degree of growth, and the sophistication of audit processes and programmes has undergone significant evolution. Today, several hundred companies in North America and Europe, and increasingly in other parts of the world, have established formal audit programmes designed to provide senior management with assurance that operations are being managed in accordance with established governmental standards and good industrial practices.

While concerns regarding environmental performance and compliance with regulatory safety requirements were the initial drivers for audit programmes, increasingly, occupational health concerns are the subject of audits. The rapid development of auditing as a management tool for occupational health and safety and the environment can be attributed to a number of pressures now placed upon companies. In many jurisdictions, regulatory requirements are becoming increasingly complex, and the penalties for non-compliance can be very significant. Fines resulting from violations of health and safety laws are no longer just a 'slap on the wrist', but can have a significant impact on the bottom line of an organization. In addition, officers of a company and its managers and employees can be held personally liable, and can and have faced fines and imprisonment for failing to manage the health and safety aspects of the business.

Boards of directors also face liability for poor health and safety performance in a business, and need to have some process to demonstrate that they have been diligent in the exercising of their responsibilities, often in operations that they may never have seen. Boards also need to respond to the increasing pressure from outside stakeholders in a company to be able to demonstrate that the company is responsible in the management of key aspects of business, such as occupational health. Leading companies are now very open with information regarding their health and safety performance, and often publicize this in annual reports or other special reports. In order to lend credence to the information being presented to shareholders, employees, regulators and the general public, audits are carried out, often by independent outside consulting organizations that have specialist audit skills.

Lastly, enlightened companies have come to the conclusion that it is important to manage effectively all hazards that can have an impact on public or employee health, safety or the environment, not just those that are subject to regulatory requirements. Audits are used as a key management tool in assessing the strengths and weaknesses of management systems for health and safety, in order to bring about a process of continuous improvement in performance.

Effective occupational health audit programmes can bring many benefits to an organization. They can:

- improve the public image of a company by demonstrating a commitment to continuous improvement;
- increase the awareness and understanding of health concerns by managers, employees and health professionals;
- assess the facility management's ability to achieve occupational health goals;
- reduce employee and community exposure to health hazards by identifying them, thus allowing early intervention;
- improve the level of compliance with regulatory requirements;
- reduce operating costs by reducing the financial and human impact of occupational disease;
- ensure that scarce occupational health resources are employed where they can be most effective and that the right blend of resources is available;
- protect a company from potential liability.

The term audit has been used to describe a broad range of assurance activities. A variety of names, such as audit, review, survey, surveillance, appraisal and assessment, have been used interchangeably.

Types of audit

A range of assurance processes are carried out by corporations. Effective assurance processes usually combine a number of types of audit at different levels through the organization.

- *Internal inspections*. These are usually carried out at the department or facility level by line managers and/or employees, often those who are members of joint health and safety committees. They will often be based on a simple checklist that ensures that a department is following facility rules, e.g. to ensure that employees are wearing the required personal protective equipment, eye-wash fountains and safety showers are maintained and functioning, appropriate hazard placarding is in place, etc.

- *Operational audits.* These are systematic checks carried out by a facility to ensure that operations are conforming to corporate requirements and are following the procedures laid out in the occupational health management system. They are typically carried out by site health and safety professionals to provide local assurance that the systems are functioning as designed.
- *Specialist audits.* These audits are usually conducted by corporate health and safety staff, and are focused on particular aspects of occupational health management. For example, assessments might target the maintenance of medical records and medical confidentiality, management of respiratory protection, audiometric techniques, etc.
- *Compliance audits.* These audits are usually instigated by a corporation to provide assurance that operations are complying with regulatory requirements. They can also be extended to assess compliance with general corporate policies or industry accepted standards. They are usually conducted by corporate health and safety professionals, corporate audit groups, external consulting companies, or a combination of these.
- *Management systems assessments.* Management systems are assessed by corporations to demonstrate diligence in the implementation of occupational health systems and to identify any gaps that may pose an unacceptable risk to employees, the corporation or other stakeholders. They can be conducted at the facility level or take an overview of corporate systems.
- *External inspections.* Inspections of facilities are periodically conducted by outside agencies, such as regulatory agencies or insurance companies.

In this chapter, two types of assurance process are addressed in some detail: occupational health compliance audits and occupational health management systems assessments.

Auditing is a methodological examination—involving analyses, tests and confirmations of local procedures and practices, and the reporting of findings—the objective of which is to verify whether a facility or organization is complying with regulatory or other legal requirements, internal company policies or procedures or other accepted practices. Auditing is a systematic process differing from less stringent assessment processes in that it is based on the collection and documentation of competent and sufficient evidence, rather than on an opinion based primarily on professional judgement.

An audit, in the true sense of the term, will generally only address non-conformances with established standards. It will not highlight 'good' or 'best' practices, nor will it provide recommendations for improvement. An audit will highlight non-conformances, but will not, in itself, provide an indication of the root causes, the failures of the management systems, that give rise to these non-conformances. Management systems assessments address the root causes of non-compliance situations and occupational health concerns.

An occupational health management system is part of an organization's overall management system, and includes the assessment, planning, implementation and review processes and the responsibilities, practices, procedures, processes and resources necessary for developing and maintaining an occupational health capability that is responsive to the needs of the stakeholders. Assessments of management systems depend on the professional judgement of an assessor of how well the various processes making up the system are working and delivering value.

Compliance auditing

Audit programme planning and considerations

Before committing resources to an audit initiative, it is most important to evaluate carefully the context in which the audit programme will be conducted. In order to make efficient use of resources, to ensure that effort is not wasted or misdirected and to avoid liability, there are some fundamental issues that must be resolved. There are six components to an audit programme (Fig. 17.1). These are, to a large extent, interdependent and changes to one component will have an influence on the others.

Objectives

The starting point in designing an occupational health audit programme is to understand fully the objectives of the audit, i.e. what the audit is expected to achieve or what questions it is intended to answer. The audit leader needs to know who are the principal clients of the audit

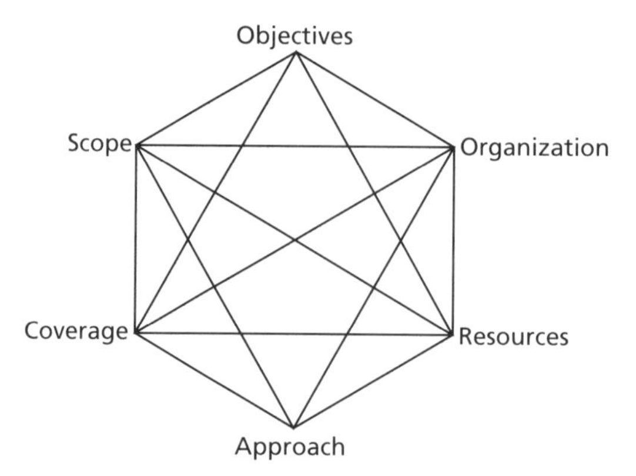

Figure 17.1 Components of an audit programme.

programme, and must ensure that their needs and expectations are considered. There may be multiple clients being served by an audit and their requirements may be very different. The needs of a facility manager, who is charged with the responsibility of complying with regulations and who will have to prioritize any corrective action requirements that come out of an audit, will be quite different from those of a board of directors. They will be more concerned with the general overall status of occupational health in the company, and will want to know of any liabilities that may affect the bottom line or reputation of the company. Occupational health managers need to know whether the resources made available for health management are effective in meeting the objectives set out for the occupational health programme, and whether the activities of the programme are aligned with business needs.

Audit programmes represent a significant investment for an organization, in terms of both financial and human resources. Not only is there a cost associated with fielding an audit team, but the audit process takes personnel in the operation being audited away from their primary responsibilities and this can have an impact on production. The responsible audit manager will therefore seek ways to maximize the return on the investment that is being made in the audit. The audit can be designed to meet its primary objectives and also to address special concerns of local facility management, thus providing 'added value'. It may provide a useful learning experience for audit team members or may be a means to transfer knowledge of how issues have been successfully resolved across the organization.

Scope

A key step in conducting an occupational health audit is to establish its scope and focus. This will, of course, be dependent on the reasons for carrying out the audit. It is most important that the scope and focus are clearly thought through before embarking on an audit programme. Are you attempting to address an identified concern, or is the intent to carry out a broad evaluation of occupational health issues across the organization? Who are the stakeholders in the audit? Is this a tool to assist management to address its local concerns, or a mechanism to allow the corporation to assess the effectiveness of its managers? Will the results be used internally, or are they to be presented to outside stakeholders? All these questions must be addressed in the design of the audit programme.

The scope and focus of an audit can be defined in terms of its geographical, organizational, locational, functional and jurisdictional contexts.

The *geographical scope* of the audit has important considerations in audit design. Regulatory requirements will vary between countries, states or provinces, and audit design may need to consider regional or international requirements. There are also the important logistical considerations of being able to gather and assess evidence in a foreign culture and operate in different languages.

The *organizational context* considers the business units, operations or departments that are to be included within the scope of the audit. These will be dependent on the original purpose for conducting the audit, the organizational structure of the company, corporate cultural considerations and the risk profile of the operations.

The *locational boundaries* address what specific area is covered by the audit. Is it to be confined to a facility fenceline or will it incorporate off-site facilities, such as satellite operations or off-site warehousing? Audits may be focused on the main occupier of a site or may extend to tenants located on plant property. Consideration must be given to whether the audit is focused on a particular operation or will extend upstream to suppliers and downstream to customers. Decisions will be needed on whether to include contractors or toll manufacturers.

The *functional scope* of an occupational health audit can be broad, encompassing all aspects of occupational health management, or can be narrowed, addressing only industrial hygiene, occupational health nursing, material hazard information systems, etc. Specialist audits may be very narrow, e.g. assessing a hygiene sampling technique, spirometric or audiometric practices or record keeping.

Finally, the *jurisdictional context* addresses the standards against which the operation is being assessed: regulatory requirements, company policies, local facility operational procedures, generally accepted industrial standards, such as the chemical industry's 'Responsible Care Codes of Practice', or international standards.

Coverage

The audit programme design must consider which facilities will be audited and the frequency with which they will undergo an audit. Criteria must be established on which these decisions will be made. Selection may be random, or a form of risk assessment may be employed for setting priorities or selecting facilities. Audit scheduling may be based on the performance of a facility in previous audits, or there may be other business considerations that dictate when an audit will be conducted. The audit manager needs to decide how much lead time is needed and how much advance notice will be given to a facility before an audit takes place. The lead time may be extensive, with some companies broadcasting their annual audit schedule across the organization. Others prefer to conduct 'surprise' audits to ensure that the audit findings are genuinely representative of the true state of health management, and that facilities have not specially prepared themselves to achieve a better showing in the audit.

Organization

In order to maintain the objectivity and independence of the audit process, the location at which the audit function is housed within the organization needs special consideration. Some companies establish specialist audit functions that are fully independent of the company occupational health, safety and environment departments, and which may even report to a subcommittee of the board of directors to guarantee their independence. More usually, it is the responsibility of the corporate occupational health department to manage the audit process for health service delivery across the company. Other organizations have no formal centre for the occupational health audit function, but rely on a co-ordinated approach to cross-facility auditing or self-audits.

Resources

Closely aligned with organizational considerations is the need to assess the resources required to carry out the audit. Many companies rely exclusively on specialist outside auditing firms to carry out audits that have a high degree of independence and thus credibility. Other organizations prefer to use internal teams, where the disadvantage of the loss of some independence is seen to be offset by the advantage of using people that are fully familiar with the company's operations, processes and culture. In addition, the cross-auditing of facilities allows for the exchange of ideas and sharing of solutions across the company. A powerful approach employed by some companies is to use mixed teams of professional external occupational health auditors and internal company resources. This retains a large measure of objectivity and provides a valuable training experience. The use of internal people working side by side with external consultants allows for a very efficient auditing process.

Consideration needs to be given to the necessary qualifications of auditors and how they will receive any required training. The roles and responsibilities of audit team members need to be carefully thought through and well communicated to all those involved in the auditing process.

Approach

The actual approach to be taken when conducting the audit must be considered. This involves the determination of exactly how the audit will be conducted, how long will be allowed for fieldwork, how the quality and consistency will be maintained and what audit guides will be used. At the pre-audit planning stage, it is also important to give some thought to how the findings of the audit will be recorded, and how and to whom they will be reported.

If sensitive findings are anticipated in carrying out an audit, or if there are other legal considerations, companies occasionally have the work carried out under '*solicitor/client privilege*'. Maintaining the confidentiality of audit findings by having the work carried out under a veil of legal privilege is not possible in all jurisdictions. Where this is a possible manoeuvre, it can only be done under strict guidelines, and will essentially require legal counsel to commission the audit. If such an approach or other safeguards on the confidentiality of findings are to be employed in carrying out occupational health audits, considerable thought needs to be given to this at an early stage in the planning process. It must always be ensured that there is agreement with facility management and occupational health professionals on the process for following up on any significant findings. Items of non-compliance that are left unaddressed and without an action plan to correct them can present a high degree of liability for an organization.

Characteristics of leading audit programmes

Well-established and effective audit programmes for assessing occupational health, safety and environmental performance tend to demonstrate a number of key common characteristics.

- *Independent corporate-level audit unit.* The organization has a specialist, professional audit function that is independent of the operations being evaluated. This unit has corporate support and a clear corporate mandate. While the audit function is a component of a comprehensive health and safety management programme, it is independent of operational and staff responsibilities.
- *Explicitly defined purpose and scope.* The purpose of the audit programme has been carefully decided upon to ensure that audits are fulfilling a useful function in furthering corporate needs. The scope and agreed purpose are clearly defined, and are well communicated throughout the organization, in order that the audit function is seen in a positive light and is regarded as adding value to the business and the operations being audited.
- *Well-defined audit protocols.* Audit protocols are prepared that clearly define the operating parameters of the audit programme and set out the framework for the specific audit steps to be used in conducting audits. The protocols are consistently applied to all audits, so that there is a basis of comparison of audit results between facilities and, for any given facility, between one audit and the next.
- *Staffing by professionals with considerable appropriate experience.* Audit programmes are staffed by health professionals with a strong understanding of audit procedures and techniques, and who have a working understanding of applicable regulatory standards and criteria. This ensures that important non-conformances are not likely to be overlooked and helps to build credibility for the audit process. It is helpful, although not essential, for members of the audit team to have a basic familiarity with the operations carried out at the facility being audited.
- *Sufficient resources and management support to achieve objectives.* A sufficient number of trained auditors is provided for each audit, and appropriately qualified personnel are selected to lead each audit team. An adequate budget is provided for the support of the audit programme, and a strong management commitment exists to support the audit activities and to resolve any conflicts that may arise.

- *Sound basis for selecting and scheduling audit locations.* The selection and scheduling of audits should reflect a proper assessment of inherent occupational health risk and exposure. Major higher risk facilities are audited frequently, while lower risk facilities receive attention less frequently.
- *Established reporting process.* The audit team provides dispassionate, accurate and informative written reports of audit findings that are seen by the audited facility as adding value and providing valued assistance. The reports provide a mechanism for initiating and managing follow-up, and periodic summaries of the audit programme status are provided to senior management.
- *Sufficient documentation.* Audit findings are well documented to clearly substantiate the results and any identified weaknesses in occupational health management in the audited facilities. Audits are carried out in accordance with specified field audit procedures with consistent administrative procedures.
- *Ongoing efforts to maintain and improve audit programme quality and effectiveness.* There is a strong quality approach that ensures the training and development of audit staff, the supervisory review of fieldwork and audit documentation and an ongoing evaluation of the effectiveness and efficiency of the audit programme.

Conducting audits

Figure 17.2 shows the steps involved in conducting a typical audit: pre-audit activities; the five steps involved in on-site activities; and the activities that must be completed when site work is complete.

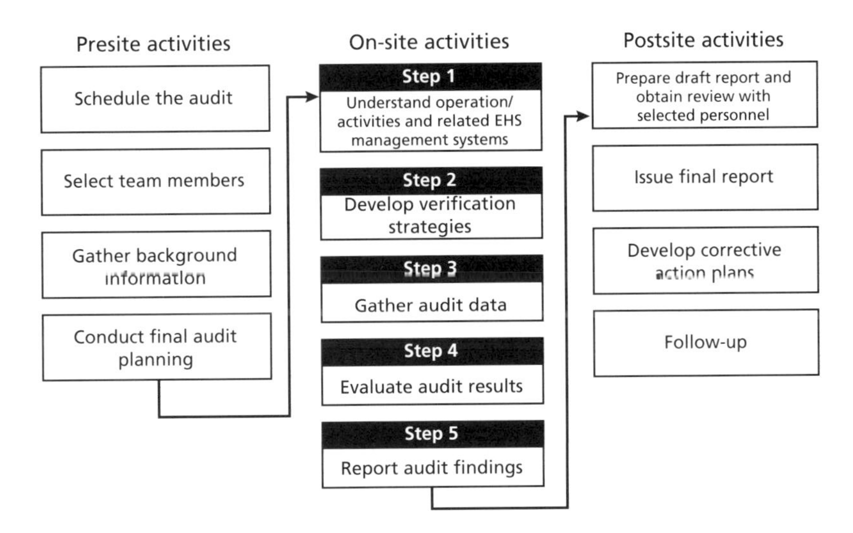

Figure 17.2 Steps in a typical audit process.

Pre-audit activities

The use of protocols. The definition of an audit includes the need for a systematic approach to the methodological examination of aspects of a facility's or company's activities. The need for a systematic approach to the audit and the importance of not overlooking any aspects of the activities being evaluated have driven the requirement for some form of written document to direct the activities of the audit team. These documents can range from simple checklists to detailed step-by-step auditing procedures. These documents are referred to by a number of terms, but a consensus is developing to denote them as *audit protocols.* Audit protocols may focus on regulatory requirements only, may include company policy or procedural requirements, or may even address accepted or 'best' industrial practice.

A well-designed audit protocol will list the step-by-step approach that should be taken to the audit. It will define each aspect of occupational health management that has to be assessed, and will give guidance to the auditor on the evidence to evaluate to effect the assessment. The protocol should reference the regulation, company standard or other code that applies to the audit step. An example of part of an audit protocol from a commercially available system is shown in Fig. 17.3. No matter how comprehensive or detailed a protocol may be, it must not be regarded as a rigid tool that cannot be deviated from. Every audit poses its own challenges, and the audit team should use the protocol as a guide and must be prepared to be flexible and use good judgement in determining the applicability of elements of the protocol in the execution of the audit. No audit protocol can be fully comprehensive and consider all local requirements, and therefore the audit team must be alert to important issues that are not addressed by the protocol.

All members of the audit team should be very familiar with the sections of the protocol for which they will be responsible before they go on site to commence the audit. Review before going on site allows the team members to seek additional advice or information when they are unclear of the intent of a protocol step or element, ensures that precious time on site is not wasted and allows the team to demonstrate professionalism and engender confidence in those being audited.

Pre-audit questionnaire

Audits can be very disruptive to plant operations, and can take away from other duties the highly qualified people who will execute them. It therefore makes good business sense to try to minimize, as much as possible, the time spent on site. One way of achieving this is to be well prepared before commencing the fieldwork. A pre-audit questionnaire can assist with this. The questionnaire should be sent to the site at least 2 weeks, preferably more, before commencing the audit.

It should request information on the organizational structure of the facility receiving the audit, who has responsibility for various aspects of

Employee Health and Medical Issues Audit Protocol	Auditor's comments	W.P. Ref.
Monitoring and Medical Surveillance Programmes		
24 Confirm that Medical Services staff are notified when new chemicals and processes are introduced into the workplace.		
25 Obtain a sample of employees who, based on exposure to hazardous materials, physical agents or job/task duties, should be included in a medical surveillance programme. Verify that these employees are included in the programme. In addition, confirm the following:		
a) Baseline measurements of employee exposures to air contaminants and physical agents have been made, and monitored exposure levels are within established limits for the following air contaminants and physical agents:		
1) Hazardous substances at or above the action level for a specific OSHA-regulated contaminant (e.g. asbestos, ethylene oxide, formaldehyde, arsenic, lead, benzene). (29 CFR 1910.1000-1910.1050)		
Note: *Refer to the Industrial Hygiene Audit Protocol Addenda for the medical monitoring requirements for formaldehyde, benzene, and lead in construction. For any other contaminant-specific OSHA-regulated substances, refer to the appropriate regulations. (29 CFR 1910.1000 through 1910.1050)*		
2) Hazardous substances that have company/ division/facility standards for medical surveillance.		
3) Noise exposure equal to or greater than 85 dBA (or less than 85 dBA if a company policy is more stringent). (29 CFR 1910.95)		
4) Other air contaminants or physical agents as a result of job task functions such as:		
a) Personnel who wear respirators (29 CFR 1910.134)		

Figure 17.3 A typical audit protocol.

occupational health management or programme delivery, the layout and nature of the operations carried out on site and any special hazards, such as asbestos, ionizing radiation, etc., that may be on site.

In addition to the information provided in the pre-audit questionnaire, the audit team may benefit by receiving other documents from the site being audited. Some of the pre-audit information requirements are presented in Table 17.1.

For complex facilities, or for those that have never received an audit before, the audit team leader may find it advisable to visit the site prior to the audit to assess the situation personally and to advise facility per-

Table 17.1 Pre-audit information requirements.

Recent regulatory agency inspection/enforcement correspondence, if any
Recent internal and intracompany audit reports
Occupational health policies and procedures
Current organizational chart for all departments
Facility plan(s) or map(s)
Safety statistics and serious incident reports
Description of operations, including safety and health control systems
Hazardous chemical inventory
List of primary contractors on site (including key contacts)

sonnel of what they can expect from the audit and what is expected of them.

Other pre-audit activities

There are a number of other tasks that the prudent audit team leader will ensure have been carried out before arriving on site.

- The most up-to-date regulations are available and have been considered in the audit protocol. The latest versions of corporate policies and procedures are available if these are within the scope of the audit.
- The audit team has been picked with the right blend of skills to get the job done efficiently and effectively. The audit team members will be available on the dates scheduled for the audit.
- An audit plan has been prepared that assigns responsibilities to audit team members so that everyone knows exactly what is expected of them. Time (and, if necessary, costs) should be budgeted for each task so that, as the audit progresses, it is clear whether things are on track or falling behind.
- The logistics of getting the team on site, accommodated while carrying out the work and home again have been checked and double checked. This is especially important if international travel is involved and if team members are congregating from different home locations. It does not get an audit off to a good start if, at the opening meeting, the audit team is still scattered across the country!

Planning and forethought can go a long way to making an audit a success and an experience that benefits all those involved.

On-site activities

The five-step approach to conducting environmental, safety and health audits, developed by the international consulting firm Arthur D. Little (Greeno *et al.* 1985, 1988), is described below. This approach has subsequently been adopted by the International Chamber of Commerce (ICC) and many leading companies internationally. Following on from the pre-audit activities already described, the five-step approach includes:

- step 1: the understanding of management systems;
- step 2: the assessment of internal controls;
- step 3: the gathering of audit evidence;

- step 4: the evaluation of audit evidence;
- step 5: the reporting of audit findings.

The principal activities and anticipated outcomes of each of these steps are shown in Table 17.2.

Step 1: the understanding of management systems

- *The opening meeting*. This is most important in setting the tone for the whole audit. The meeting affords the opportunity to introduce the audit team and explain the objectives of the audit. The scope and purpose should be very clearly defined so that there are no surprises for the auditees. The meeting also allows the audit team to become aware of any local concerns or sensitivities (e.g. labour relations' issues), and ensures that the team is fully advised of any safety rules or special hazards on site.

The other main purposes of the opening meeting are to schedule initial interviews, define documents that the audit team may wish to review and generally sort out the logistics and arrangements for the audit. During the meeting, the facility personnel and the audit team will be able to agree how the reporting of results will be handled, including end-of-day reviews.

Table 17.2 Audit steps.

Step	Principal activities	Outcome
Step 1. Understand management systems	Opening meeting Site tour Initial interviews Document review	Strong working knowledge of key systems on site Identification of key issues to review
Step 2. Assess strengths and weaknesses of internal controls	Review of step 1 information Audit team meetings	Develop verification strategies Reallocate audit resources, if required Identify risks and management system weaknesses
Step 3. Gather audit evidence	Physical inspections Focused interviews Data and record examination Verification testing	Analyse site programmes Develop evidence to substantiate findings Confirm status of compliance
Step 4. Evaluate audit findings	Review data collected Review factual accuracy of findings Analyse/integrate, as appropriate, findings of other team members	Prepare draft findings Confirm accuracy Identify potential root causes
Step 5. Report audit findings	Daily debriefing meetings Close-out meetings	Early, clear, consistent communication Understand facility concerns Prepare preliminary draft report

- *Site tour*. Following the opening meeting, it is usual, and most effective, to carry out a brief walk-through inspection of the facility. The purpose of this tour is to orientate the team to the layout of the facility and to gain an appreciation of the nature and organization of the work being carried out. One should resist the temptation to get into the audit proper at this stage, although, obviously, a note of any concerns identified should be made to be followed up later during the assessment stage of the audit.
- *Understanding of management systems*. The purpose of the understanding of occupational health management systems is to develop a grasp of the facility's overall approach to managing occupational health and its regulatory obligations. It is not the intent, in conducting this phase of an audit, to make an attempt to assess fully the effectiveness of occupational health management systems. Rather, after completing this phase of the audit, the auditor should understand:
  - how the facility has evaluated the applicability to facility operations of existing regulatory standards and other requirements;
  - the types of facility procedures that exist to implement compliance activities, and the general scope of such procedures;
  - the methods used by the facility to assist in the implementation of compliance programmes;
  - whether management roles and responsibilities are clearly understood;
  - the types of programme or activity engaged in to familiarize staff with employee occupational health information;
  - how the facility maintains and documents the effectiveness of its employee health programme activities.

Step 2: the assessment of internal controls. An assessment of the relative strengths and weaknesses of occupational health management systems allows the audit team to prioritize its activities to focus first on those inherently high-risk situations where the systems in place are least robust (Fig. 17.4). The initial focus should be on those high-risk situations where management systems are least effective.

Auditing includes two basic tasks: assessing information and verifying performance. Assessment, which constitutes step 2 of the audit process, relies on the expert judgement and/or opinion of the auditors

Strength of management system	Inherent risk: Low	Inherent risk: High
Weak	III	I
Strong	IV	II

Figure 17.4 Setting audit priorities.

on the hazards present in a facility, the risks they pose, the control measures in place and the effectiveness of management systems. This judgement is tested in step 3 by examining hard data, by the observation of activities, processes, tasks and equipment, by viewing documentation and by focused and probing interviews with key personnel.

Step 3: the gathering of audit evidence. The results of step 2 (i.e. setting the verification priorities by assessing the strengths and weaknesses of management systems) provide the basic framework for the auditor to develop a sound and defensible verification strategy. Once the audit team has determined where the audit priorities lie for the protocol assignment(s), a verification strategy is developed on the basis of the available resources, what needs to be done, how the information is to be gathered, where verification testing is to be applied and what sampling strategies are available to be employed. When gathering audit evidence, each auditor should ensure that the information evaluated is representative of the situation being assessed, and is sufficient to verify compliance or to substantiate non-compliance.

The auditor uses a range of techniques to verify information. Visual examination of the facility and its operations and the observation of aspects of occupational health management are often the starting points. The time spent observing operations in the facility will readily indicate whether proper warning signs and labels are in place, whether materials safety data sheets are available in the workplace, the state and functionality of eye-wash fountains, whether ventilation systems are functioning, etc.

Many aspects of occupational health programmes can effectively be assessed by inspecting documents, such as reports, records and the minutes of meetings. Industrial hygiene sampling strategies can be verified by looking at sampling reports; the minutes of health and safety committee meetings will reveal whether follow up to incidents and previous audit findings is taking place. The quality and completeness of medical surveillance programmes can be evaluated by inspecting health centre logs and medical records, taking necessary account of medical confidentiality.

With the mass of data accumulated in a modern occupational health programme and with the complexity of many facilities, it is clearly not possible to evaluate all relevant information. A strategy must be developed to allow a sample to be taken that is representative of the whole. A variety of methods are available to the auditor, e.g. the use of random number tables to select records for inspection or the choice of every fifth or tenth, etc., document for verification. As the intent in compliance auditing is to assess whether any non-conformances exist, it is perfectly acceptable to use non-random sampling strategies. The auditor can use professional judgement and experience to focus in on those situations that are likely to be out of compliance.

A very large amount of evidence comes from personal interviews with facility personnel. The audit team can expect to interview a broad range of site people, including management, safety and health professionals and personnel on the shop floor. Certainly, effective communication skills (and particularly listening skills) are one of the most important attributes of the successful auditor. The prime behavioural properties for gaining useful information from interviews are:

- *respect*: treat all interviewees with proper respect; be attentive to responses and ensure that a rapport is developed and maintained throughout the interview;
- *specificity of response*: focus on the adequacy of the data included in a response to the auditor's question, and ensure that the interviewee's answer is as concrete as necessary and conveys a properly understood meaning;
- *constructive probing*: resolve ambiguities or contradictions by means of follow-on questions.

Whenever meetings or interviews are being held with facility personnel, take time to make the environment as comfortable as circumstances will permit. Try to arrange the seating to provide a conversational environment and put the interviewee at ease by some polite small talk before probing for information. Never assume that the interviewee understands what the audit is about and how the results will be used. Even the most senior managers in a facility may be in the dark about what you are doing on site and why. If you are interviewing in an office where the telephone is constantly demanding attention and causing distraction, it might be a good idea to suggest a rescheduling of the interview for a time when the interviewee can give you undivided attention. At the end of the set of questions that you want to pose, it is good practice to relate briefly to the interviewee what you have learned from the interview. The interviewee should be given the opportunity to volunteer relevant information that has not been covered in the questioning.

Step 4: the evaluation of audit evidence. Throughout the audit process, it is most important to maintain contact with other members of the team to test ideas and seek the verification of findings based on their observations. As fieldwork is completed, the information gathered should be tested to ensure that it is sufficient to support the objectives of the audit and the conclusions that are reached. Evidence should be relevant, free from bias, objective and persuasive.

As the audit progresses, it may become apparent that not all of the work will be able to be completed in the time available. It is better to reduce the scope of the audit, perhaps cutting out the assessment of low-risk activities, rather than trying to cover the whole protocol in a less than rigorous manner. In particular, the temptation should be resisted to report findings on the basis of inadequate or incomplete evidence in an attempt to complete, or give the appearance of having completed, the assigned task. Any aspects of the protocol that have not been addressed thoroughly should be explained in discussing the scope of the audit in the report.

Step 5: the reporting of audit findings. To ensure the smooth and effective conduct of the audit, an ongoing dialogue with facility personnel should be maintained. End-of-day wrap-up meetings provide a very effective means of keeping management informed of the progress of the audit, and can prevent unpleasant and unnecessary surprises at the close-out meeting. The end-of-day meetings also help to keep the auditors on track, e.g. if the information received has been misinterpreted or the auditors have been talking to people who do not have the correct information. Audits are generally not pleasant experiences for an operation to undergo. The process can be made much smoother and more productive for all involved, auditors and auditees alike, if it is carried out in an open, co-operative manner with a strong emphasis on attempting to assist the facility to improve its performance, rather than to find its faults.

The close-out oral report of findings is an important meeting that will probably be well attended by representatives of the facility. Handled without empathy, close-out meetings can be very difficult indeed. It is the nature of compliance auditing that, generally what is reported are deficiencies or deviations from agreed standards, be they regulatory requirements, company policies or accepted industrial practices. It is very important that the audit team leader and team members are well prepared for the presentation of their findings and observations. In particular, all team members must be in agreement on the findings to be presented before the close-out meeting takes place. This is especially important where audit teams have not worked together before, or where they are made up of a mixture of corporate, facility and outside auditors. Few things are more damaging to the credibility of the audit process than dissension amongst the audit team in the close-out meeting. A balance must be struck in the close-out meeting between the presentation of sufficient evidence to demonstrably prove a point and the provision of long lists of trivial findings. However, some companies request that, in addition to non-conformances, the audit team should report on 'noteworthy efforts' or examples of good practices that have been observed by the audit team. Some audit programmes require that a full written report of findings be prepared before the audit team leaves the facility.

The close-out meeting should be viewed as a final opportunity for open dialogue between facility personnel and the audit team before the report is written. It provides an opportunity to test, one last time, the findings that have been made, and gives the facility the opportunity to ensure that the contexts of the findings have been properly understood by the auditors. Any disagreements in the 'facts' being reported should be noted, and every attempt to resolve them should be made. It is not uncommon for a disagreement to be not so much on the correctness of the finding, but rather on how it has been presented. In these circumstances, the audit team leader can agree to a modified wording for the finding that meets with the approval of the facility, but which retains the meaning that the auditor wishes to convey.

At the close-out meeting, it is appropriate to thank all facility personnel for their time and assistance throughout the audit. The subsequent steps and timetable in sending a draft written report to the facility, the facility review process and the issue of the final report should all be explained. If the audit team is aware of the consequent actions that will be placed on the management and occupational health professionals of the facility, e.g. the development of action plans, corrective actions, etc., these should also be described at this time.

Post-site activities

Audit papers. The notebooks used during the audit constitute an important record of the auditor's activities and findings while on site. Notes should be clearly written and pages dated and signed by the auditor. Notes taken in working papers should be fully factual accounts of what is done, the observations made and the facts verified. The language used in notes should be prudent and no editorial comments should be made. All exhibits should be numbered and referenced to notes in the working papers. As these records may be required at a later date, they should be carefully retained in secure storage.

The audit report. The structure and content of the report will vary depending on the nature of the audit, its scope and purpose and the client; for example, is the report intended to give advice and guidance to local facility personnel, is it part of a corporate overview process or is it intended to provide assurance to boards of directors and officers of a company that due diligence has been exercised in the management of health and safety? It is strongly recommended that the audit team leader has a clear conception of the purpose of the final report, and has a good appreciation of how it will be structured before embarking upon the audit. The audit report should be clear and concise, should provide the information needed by management to initiate corrective action and should describe a record of the conduct of the audit and its findings.

A typical audit report will have a structure similar to that described below.

- *Executive summary.* A report may include an executive summary that describes the most important findings in the audit report, particularly those that may present significant liability or are indicative of a serious failing in the management systems.
- *Introduction.* This should describe:
  - the purpose of the audit;
  - the scope of the audit;
  - the methodology employed, e.g. the protocols used, types of document reviewed, number of interviews conducted, etc.;

- any aspects included in the original scope of the audit that were not addressed, and the reasons why, e.g. a lack of time, key information not available, etc.
- *Findings*. Generally, it is helpful to clearly separate regulatory findings, findings of non-conformance to company policies, standards and procedures and situations in which there is a lack of adherence to generally accepted industrial standards or 'good practices'.

It is not usual to provide recommendations about regulatory findings. If the facility is not in compliance with the law, the recommendation is generally quite obvious—fix it! Laws and regulations are generally quite explicit. However, recommendations on how to address deficiencies in conformance to company expectations and generally accepted practice are useful, and are commonly included in audit reports.

Writing reports. Compliance audit reports should be thoroughly factual, not reflections of the auditors' opinions. They should be clear, concise and accurate.

Any statements in the report should be supported by evidence presented in the report, or should be readily defensible through reference to field notes. Wherever possible, specific information should be provided to put the finding in a proper context. For example, rather than making a generalized statement, such as 'many employees have not received refresher training in the use of respiratory protective equipment', a clearer representation of the seriousness of the deficiency and the statistical validity of the finding can be conveyed by more factual statements, such as 'a review of training records showed that six of 10 employees ...'.

Similarly, definitive statements should be avoided where the evidence has not been thoroughly tested. For example, statements such as 'the facility has not ...' should be avoided where the extent of the audit evaluation really only permits the auditor to say 'we were unable to confirm that the facility has ...' or 'facility personnel were unable to provide evidence that ...'.

Inflammatory or emotional words should be avoided in the report. The facts should be stated in a dispassionate manner, and expressions such as appalling, criminal, deliberately, fraudulent, negligent, incompetent, wilful misconduct, etc. should not be used. A well-written factual report should be able to make any concerns apparent to the reader without resorting to colourful language.

Finally, short phrases and common words should be used and deadwood should be cut out. Effective audit reports convey their message as economically as possible. Some commonly used auditing terms are presented in Table 17.3.

Distribution of reports. A concern for the auditor is how to handle the distribution of reports, particularly when they may contain information that is critical of performance or sensitive. A common concern that

Table 17.3 Some commonly used auditing terms.

Verify	To establish accuracy or reality
Confirm	To prove or establish actual facts or details
Review	To examine critically or deliberately
Examine	To inspect closely or enquire into carefully
Finding	The results of an examination or review
Exception	Not conforming to general requirements

many managers have with audits, and audit reports, is that, by disclosing deficiencies in a facility's programmes or reporting items of non-compliance with regulatory requirements, individuals or the company may be put at risk or incur liability. These concerns, while real, are not sufficient reasons for a prudent employer not to attempt to determine the status of occupational health or safety performance by means of a well-managed audit programme. Liability can be minimized by a strong commitment by the corporation to address any issues of non-compliance in a forthright way, and to put in place corrective actions when deficiencies are observed and reported. A corporate policy which requires that an audit report will automatically trigger the process for the review of deficiencies and the initiation of corrective action will greatly reduce liability. In some circumstances, solicitor/client privilege may protect the confidentiality of audit findings, but this cannot be relied upon. The careful preparation of findings and prompt action to address deficiencies are by far the best protection and the most responsive approach.

It is important to ensure that reports are not distributed too widely; the audit programme manager and audit leaders must be very clear in their minds who is the client, and must take direction from the client in the distribution of reports. In many circumstances, it will not be the auditee who is the client who commissioned the audit and who is therefore the owner of the report.

Compliance audits can be very powerful tools in highlighting deficiencies in aspects of occupational health and safety in a facility. Well-conducted audits, carried out by experienced auditors, may also provide useful information on aspects of health and safety management that are weak and are the cause of the deficiencies noted. However, compliance audits are not designed to determine the root causes of deficiencies.

To evaluate the underlying failures or weaknesses of occupational health and safety management systems, it is necessary to conduct a management systems assessment.

Management systems assessment

Compliance audits are generally facility-focused, bottom-up assessments of conformance to established performance criteria. They are compliance driven, and the assessment process is one of fact finding and verification. To be effective, the audit process must be very rigidly structured and the findings are primarily based on exceptions to, or deviations from, the established operating criteria. By contrast, management systems assessments are systems orientated and are top-down assessments. While management systems assessments can be focused on the evaluation of management processes in a facility, or even a department, they are equally applicable to the evaluation of corporate occupational health and safety management.

Management systems assessments are concerned with the quality of system design, the effectiveness of the implementation of health programmes and the competence and adequacy of resources. Generally, the assessment will also consider how well the management systems are integrated into, or aligned with, other broader business processes. The focus of the assessment is to identify the underlying weaknesses, the root causes, that can present an unacceptable level of risk to an organization. While reporting recommendations is optional in compliance auditing, the presentation of recommendations to correct deficiencies is the primary purpose of an assessment of management systems.

While there are a number of parallels between the performance of compliance audits and the evaluation of management systems, management systems assessments require their own special methodology.

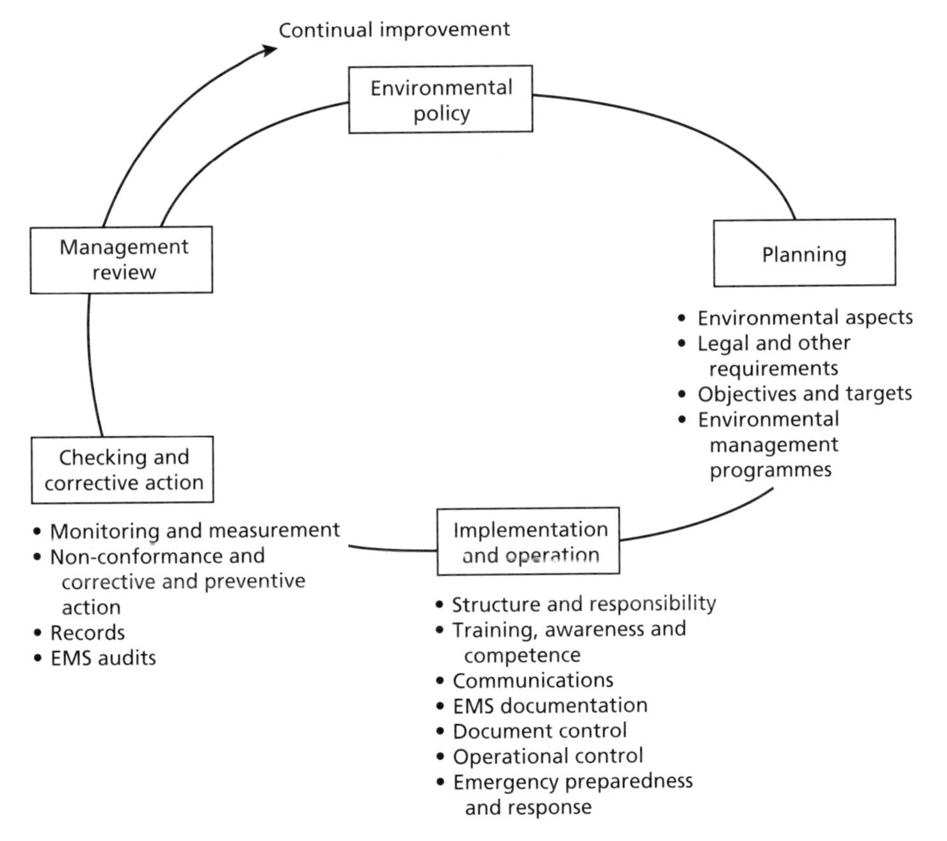

Figure 17.5 ISO 14001 standard for environmental management.

The emphasis is far less on the application of tests of conformance to elements of technical programmes set out in protocols and relies much more on professional judgement, based on experience.

Management systems can be broken down into a number of modules or elements, but they all follow the basic organization of 'plan, do, check'.

The International Standards Organization (ISO), which has pioneered quality management systems, has recently introduced ISO 14001 (ISO 1996), an environmental management system. This defines a management system as: '... the organizational structure, planning activities, responsibilities, practices, procedures, processes and resources for developing, implementing, achieving, reviewing and maintaining the ... policy'.

ISO 14001

Figure 17.5 shows the ISO 14001 model for environmental management. Discussion is continuing on whether a similar standard will be developed by the International Standards Organization for Health and Safety Management. The approach and structure of ISO 14001 are almost entirely compatible with those needed for occupational health management

A typical model of a management system for occupational health is presented in Fig. 17.6. This incorporates management processes under four key management actions: the assessment of needs; the planning of activities to address the identified needs; the implementation of the system; and an assurance process to review the continuing effectiveness and relevance of the system. The four key management activities are supported by the cross-cutting processes of training and awareness, and the documentation and management of information.

As with compliance auditing, the management systems assessment relies on three principal means of data collection:

- personal interviews;
- physical observations;
- document reviews.

However, as shown in Fig. 17.7, the amount of time spent on these activities is quite different between a compliance audit and the assessment of management systems. In carrying out a management systems assessment, considerably more time is spent on interviewing personnel throughout the organization, and the analysis of findings and observations takes almost as much time as the fieldwork. This information is derived from the opinions of experienced auditors on the typical time breakout for conducting audits and assessments.

The assessor must evaluate not only what the management system requires, but how well expectations have been communicated throughout the organization, how well these requirements are understood and the level to which they are actually implemented. Management systems

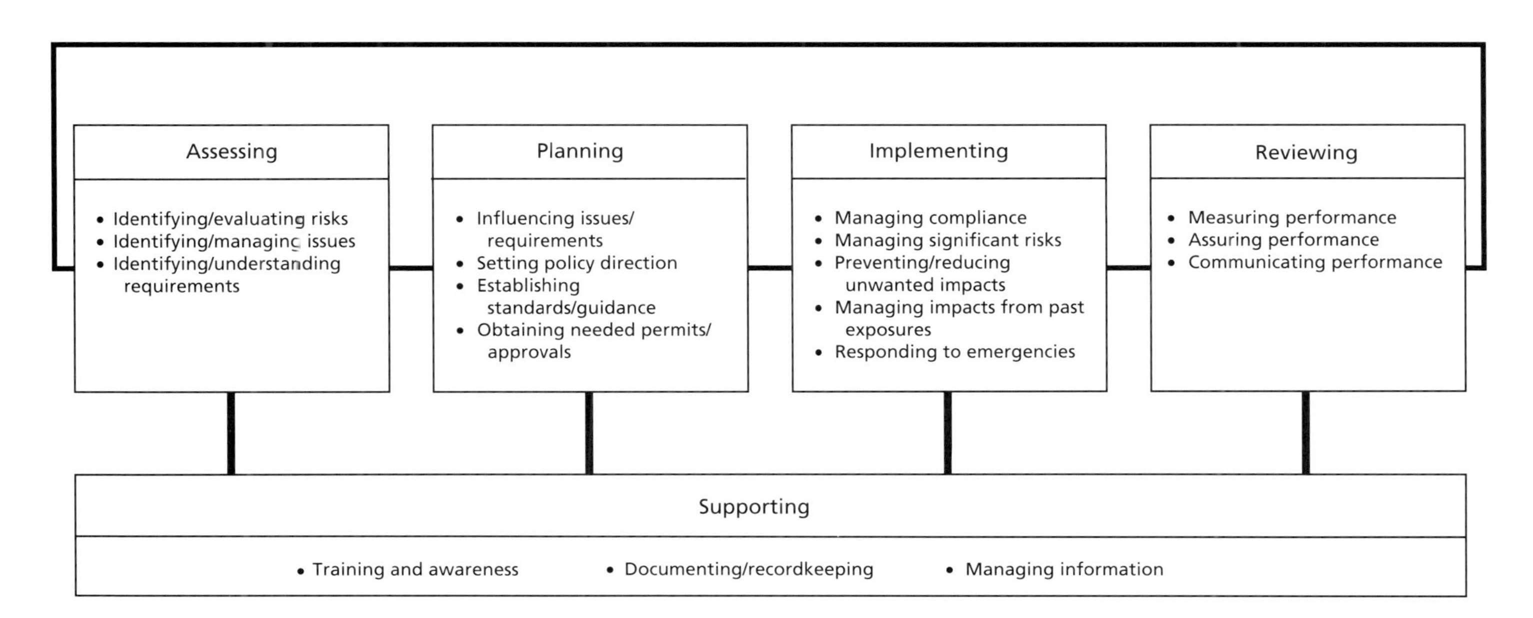

Figure 17.6 Model of a management system for occupational health.

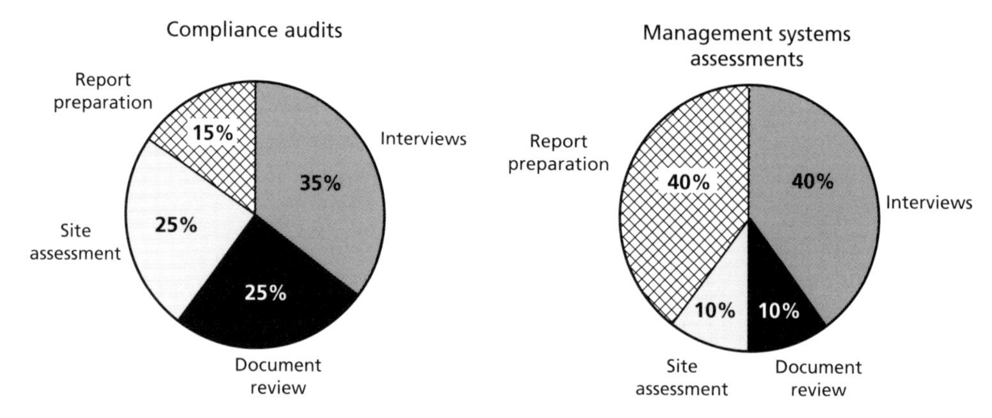

Figure 17.7 Relative time spent on audit tasks.

assessments are very much orientated towards an attempt to uncover the root causes of occupational health programme deficiencies. These root causes may relate to weaknesses of fundamental management processes as described below.

- *A lack of clear policy or expectations.* Policies do not relate to the issues of importance on site, and no clear indication is provided of what top management regards as acceptable practice.
- *Insufficient commitment on the part of management.* If management is not truly committed to, and supportive of, occupational health activities, practices will not be applied uniformly across a facility and performance will not be sustainable.
- *Lack of line management accountability.* The line organization does not take responsibility for aspects of occupational health management that are under its control, and senior management fails to hold the line accountable.
- *Inappropriate occupational health organization.* Occupational health services are not properly aligned with the general organization of the facility or workplace they are serving. The mix of skills is not appropriate for the type of issues that need to be managed.
- *Confused roles and responsibilities.* Are the respective responsibilities of line supervision, top management and specialist occupational health resources properly understood by all involved? Is there inefficiency through duplication or a danger of issues 'falling between the cracks'?
- *Inadequate resources, including staff, budget and equipment.* Are there sufficient resources to manage the occupational health risks on site properly? Are these resources of the necessary calibre and equipped with the necessary skills?
- *Occupational health activities out of alignment with business needs.* This often reflects a failure to assess properly the needs of the various stakeholders in the effectiveness of the occupational health programme, legislative and other requirements or the true risks posed by the activities of the organization. The assessor should look for evid-

ence that the occupational health team properly understand the strategic direction of the organization, and have a thorough appreciation of how their activities can support this. Similarly, can line managers articulate what their needs are and their expectations of the occupational health function?

- *Ineffective programmes for employee training and awareness.* Well thought through programmes and procedures have been designed, but have been inadequately communicated to the people on the shop floor who must use them. Often, occupational health professionals will put together guidelines and processes that are so technical and comprehensive that they are unusable and/or unsustainable. Procedures must be written that reflect the realities of the workplace. The most elegantly written occupational health programme is useless if it is of no value to those who must use it and if it does not therefore leave the bookshelf.
- *Lack of usable programme and/or procedural guidance.* Programme guidelines and procedures are not written in the language of the workplace and do not relate to the other business processes in the organization.
- *Failure to measure and periodically check performance and take appropriate corrective action.* No situation is static. There is a need to check constantly the continuing effectiveness of the implementation of health programmes to ensure that they remain relevant and bring about the desired outcomes.

Management systems assessments assess the quality of management process design and the effectiveness of management process implementation. As will be appreciated, these are very subjective assessments, and impressions must be tested thoroughly by interviewing representatives of all levels of management and staff of a facility or organization.

Some of the subjectivity involved in assessing the robustness of management processes can be removed by assigning clear criteria to the characteristics required of each process if a management system is to be effective. As an example, let us consider the management process 'managing compliance'. Figure 17.8 shows the various attributes that make up the management process and, for each attribute, criteria have been developed which describe what would need to be in place to consider the strength or weakness of the attributes in supporting the management system.

Management systems assessment reports

Assessment reports are designed to provide the senior management of a business, facility or occupational health service with the information it needs to ensure that occupational health services are efficient and effective and are meeting business needs. To be effective, findings need to be crisp, to the point, clearly framed and expressed in terms that are meaningful to the management. Recommendations should add value by

Management process
Managing compliance

Process attribute	Needs improvement (1)	(2)	Meets threshold expectations (3)	(4)	Significant strength (5)
Appropriate scope, coverage	Some, not all applicable legal requirements		All applicable legal requirements		Applicable legal, company requirements, voluntary standards
Clear ownership, assignment of responsibilities	SHER staff-driven		Line management accountable		Line management-driven
Reliability, reproducibility of results	Uneven, hit-or-miss compliance		Essentially in compliance		Compliance routinely achieved, strong systems in place
Utility, value of results	Typically not measured, managed		Routinely measured, low management value		Measured, managed, drive continuous improvement
Efficiency, cost-effectiveness	Heavy SHER staff use, every time non-routine		Subprocesses defined, performance improvements possible with fewer resources devoted		Subprocesses streamlined, operations staff well-leveraged
Flexibility in identifying, handling exceptions	Lax inspection, spotty follow-up		Effective inspection, persistent exceptions		Strong find-and-fix, treat root causes
					Overall rating

Figure 17.8 Management process criteria for 'managing compliance'.

providing a practical and implementable solution to a real problem. To be effective in bringing about sustainable improvement, they must target the root cause of a deficiency, not address the symptoms of ineffective processes.

In getting the message across to those who have the responsibility to act on assessment recommendations, it is important to frame findings and recommendations clearly using non-technical jargon. It should be ensured that recommendations target deficiencies in the *management system* and do not 'shoot the *manager*'. To be of value to managers, the recommendations need to be expressed in 'action' terms, and must be readily assignable or capable of being delegated.

The auditor can never expect to know the business being assessed as well as the management team responsible for the facility or operation. Recommendations should therefore be directional rather than firm, and should focus on what needs to be done, rather than providing advice on how to achieve it.

As far as possible, the auditor should be sensitive to any implementation considerations, such as cultural issues, the state and direction of the business and any barriers to implementation.

The assessment report must be concise, designed to be read by top management and in a suitable format for personal presentation. It is helpful if the recommendations can be placed in context and supported by examples. The focus should be on the benefits that will ensue from implementation. An example of part of a typical management systems report is shown in Fig. 17.9.

Stage 1	Stage 2	Stage 3
●		

Process Identifying/managing issues

There is no clear process for the management of safety
However, the follow-up to incidents is

Strength	Areas for
→ An effective process for learning from losses and potential losses has been put in place. ‰ Accident and incident investigation processes are very strong and root causes of incidents are evaluated.	‰ Management of health-related issues is not conducted in a consistent manner across the departments of the mill. ‰ There are no clearly defined roles or responsibilities for the management of occupational health issues that could impact mill operations. ‰ Group data generated by periodic health assessments are not analyzed to identify trends or potential areas of concern (e.g. noise monitoring data and audiometric testing results are not sufficiently analyzed to identify potential future liabilities).

Recommendation:
- *Establish a safety management system which includes procedures to be followed across the mill and which defines roles*
- *Link and analyze occupational medical and hygiene data to permit assessment of the incidence of chronic health effects such as noise-hearing loss or respirator*

Figure 17.9 Typical management systems assessment report.

Conclusions

A systematic approach to the management of health issues in industry is essential in today's complex operating environment, and assurance processes are fundamental to the effective implementation of an occupational health management system.

In this chapter, the types of audit that are used to assess aspects of occupational health management have been described, and practical advice on the implementation of audits and audit programmes has been provided.

Well-designed audits can provide many benefits to those who have a key stake in the effective management of occupational and environmental health. Audits can provide assurance that health services are competently resourced and that their focus is appropriate to the risks and issues faced by employees, customers and the public. A periodic review of health services is essential in ensuring that they remain relevant and that their performance is sustainable. Audits provide assurance to managers and officers of a company that facilities are operating within the law and that health risks are being managed.

To boards of directors, audits are an important means of demonstrating 'due diligence' and, to potential investors, insurers and lending institutions, they provide a level of comfort that health issues are being managed well and reduce the likelihood of surprises.

There are many secondary advantages that can accrue from a well-managed audit programme. Audits afford important training opportunities, and are a powerful means of raising the awareness of managers and employees of the importance that a corporation places on health and safety. Audits can also be effective mechanisms for passing on good practices from one facility to another, thereby raising the level of the performance of the organization as a whole.

Most importantly, effective audits and assessments can assist management and health professionals to ensure that health services are well aligned with the businesses they serve.

Audits can drive the process of continuous improvement that is so essential in ensuring that health services remain attuned to the needs of their client groups and continue to add value.

The science and art of auditing have developed tremendously over the past decade. It is clear that assurance processes are going to be fundamental to professional occupational health management in the future. The number of companies and organizations that have formal audit programmes is expected to increase, and the scope of audits is anticipated to become broader. Perhaps the most significant change in the years ahead will be an increase in the depth and rigour of review. More and more companies will shift from informal inspection processes to compliance verification, and from compliance verification to a full assessment of their management systems. Furthermore, the development of international standards is likely to bring about a higher level of consistency and rigour in the approach taken to assessment and assurance.

Auditing came late to the management of occupational health, but audit and assessment processes are emerging as powerful tools in assisting occupational health managers to take a more professional, quality-driven approach to satisfying the needs of their customers, the stakeholders in a healthy workplace.

References

Greeno, J.L., Hedstrom, G. & DiBerto, M. (1985) *Environmental Auditing—Fundamentals and Techniques*. Arthur D. Little, Cambridge, MA.

Greeno, J.L., Hedstrom, G. & DiBerto, M. (1988) *The Environmental, Health and Safety Auditior's Handbook*. Arthur D. Little, Cambridge, MA.

ISO (1996) *Environmental Management Systems—Specification with Guidance for Use*. ISO 14001. International Organization for Standardization, Geneva.

Chapter 18 Demonstrating compliance with the law

Linda Goldman and Gillian S. Howard

Introduction

Standards of occupational health vary in accordance with the degree of national economic development and the strength of both the legislature and the enforcement authorities. Effective criminal sanctions depend on the weight of state power. The pursuit of civil liability is only practicable in jurisdictions in which the legal system is accessible through sophisticated litigation support for the impecunious victims of accidents. In the specialized legal area of occupational health, the modern ethos of prevention through risk assessment procedures is central to the law of negligence, whilst also being supported by well-enforced criminal sanctions within Europe, Australia, New Zealand and North America. Through a combination of variability of enforcement and weak legislation, the working population of the Third World remains vulnerable despite the universal awareness of risk.

The USA has been the forerunner of changes in workplace health and safety on four principal levels. Firstly, by state legislation for the protection of the health of employees in the workplace. Secondly, by establishing risk-funded civil litigation, whereby lawyers take on civil cases on a no-win, no-fee basis, bringing the hope of achieving compensation for injury to those who might not otherwise have been able to fund their own cases. Thirdly, the Americans have led equal opportunities legislation (Americans with Disabilities Act, Equal Employment Opportunities Act), bringing the disabled and the disadvantaged into the workplace where, supported by occupational health professionals, they are able to become functional and independent in society (now reflected in the UK Disability Discrimination Act 1995). Fourthly, the integration of risk assessment and supervised return-to-work procedures is bringing injured employees back to work, thereby reducing compensation claims [1].

Despite this progress, now being repeated in many countries, the compliance with equal opportunities and occupational health legislation is perceived worldwide as being expensive and unprofitable. As multinational corporations bear at least the moral burden of following the high standards of the parent country in places where occupational health is less of a priority, it is all the more important for norms to be set. This chapter gives principal consideration to the UK legal systems (there are three: England and Wales, Scotland, Northern Ireland) affecting occupational health, both criminal and civil. Not only are they broad-based, effective and readily accessible but, being the product of homogenization within European health and safety legislation, they reflect the development of common standards of decency which need not be enclosed by national borders. It is to be hoped that these standards will be emulated abroad within the goals envisaged by the International Labour Organization (ILO), so that occupational health services are developed and accessible to all workers in all workplaces.

Broad-reaching UK law

The Health and Safety at Work, etc. Act (HASWA) 1974 is a UK statute with counterparts throughout Europe, and is arguably a model of its kind. Carrying the weight of criminal law, it applies to all workplaces, all workers and non-working visitors. Reasonably practicable steps are required to be taken to protect health and safety, subject to a cost–benefit ratio. What is reasonably practicable is not a static concept, and is dependent on current knowledge, combined with the resources and stature of the organization. Subordinate legislation, giving effect to European Union directives, sets out detailed parameters of control. It contains unique provisions enabling the enforcement agency, the Health and Safety Executive (HSE), to require immediate improvements or closure of dangerous workplaces, thus ensuring the rapid cessation of risk. The breach of enforcement notices is a criminal offence, carrying a fine or sentence of imprisonment or both.

It is the European pattern that, employers who send their staff to work on the premises of others, whether or not those premises are the employees' own homes, should not assume that they can delegate their health and safety responsibilities. Failure to assess for risk carries criminal penalties, ranging from fines to imprisonment, while civil damages are as high as necessary to compensate for the injuries suffered. Most statutory provisions are subject to the test of what is reasonably practicable. This is set out in *Edwards* v. *National Coal Board* [1949] 1 KB 704 as being basically a cost–benefit equation. However, the argument that a company is small and cannot afford the burden of compliance with health and safety law will generally be given short shrift.

General principles

The criminal law should set out to punish, and by punishment deter those who would otherwise take the short cuts which are injurious to health. Its precepts should be easy to understand and enforce. The importance of HASWA is that it changed the emphasis from punishment and penalties for injurious incidents in the workplace to prohibition and prevention. It is implicit that compliance with the provisions of the Act requires an assessment of risk, so as to be able to take appropriate steps to secure health and safety in the workplace in general. Regulations, such as the Control of Substances Hazardous to Health (COSHH) Regulations 1994 (SI 1994 No. 3246, updating 1988 COSHH Regulations SI 1988 No. 1657 and intervening updates), carry their own risk assessment requirements specific to the nature of the operation or the materials used. The year 1993 began with the biggest revision of general health and safety law since HASWA came into force, with the introduction of six sets of regulations which have come to be known collectively as 'the six-pack'. These refer to different aspects of the entire spectrum of working activities. (The following are not mentioned specifically in this chapter: Personal Protective Equipment at Work Regulations 1992 (SI 1992 No. 2966); Provision and Use of Work Equipment Regulations 1992 (SI 1992 No. 2932); Manual Handling Operations Regulations 1992 (SI 1992 No. 2793); Workplace (Health, Safety and Welfare) Regulations 1992 (SI 1992 No. 3004).) The core of the six-pack is formed by the Management of Health and Safety at Work Regulations (MHSWR) 1992 (SI 1992 No. 2051) (updated on the 1st December 1994 (SI 1994 No. 2865) to take into account the Pregnant Workers' Directive 92/85/EEC), which implements the European Council of Ministers Framework Directive on the Introduction of Measures to Encourage Improvements in the Safety and Health of Workers at Work, 98/391/EEC. The assessment of risk is the central theme and, where risks are identified, taking the appropriate measures to reduce and control them. The most recent major development is the implementation into UK law of the European Working Time Directive 93/104/EC which has the broad effect of limiting weekly working hours of day workers to a maximum of 48 hours and restricting night shifts to 8 hours (Working Time Regulations 1998 (SI 1998 No. 1833)).

The arrival of the six-pack provoked inordinate concern, particularly about the expense of carrying out suitable and sufficient assessments and taking reasonable steps to reduce risk. Many organizations expressed concern about the cost-effectiveness of conformity with the law. In the early days of getting to grips with the new regulatory infrastructure, London employers were lukewarm. The Industrial Society's (1994) 'London safety survey' [2] showed that, whereas most respondent organizations had a safety policy, 45% had not updated it in the previous 6 months. Only half of those surveyed had written policies on risk assessments. There were serious shortfalls in the implementation of training programmes required by the new regulations and, where training was provided, only 30% was in risk assessment. On the plus side, 75% had new safety policies on display screen equipment, with roughly the same proportion having a smoking policy.

The Chartered Institute of Management Accountants' 1994 survey [3] revealed a general perception (nearly 70%) among financial directors and controllers that health and safety costs had risen faster than other costs over the preceding year. A sizeable proportion (nearly

20%) of those questioned believed that the cost of compliance with health and safety regulations was putting their business at a disadvantage. Most respondents saw the costs as a hindrance to recovery from the recession.

With the advent of the technology revolution, flexible times and places of work have become commonplace. Contracts of employment now provide for employees to work from home and, indeed, from any form of transport, so that the employer now needs to extend the concept of a safe place and safe systems of work. Although the traditional boundaries of the shop floor are no longer fixed, protection is afforded to distant and teleworkers by the new assessment provisions. Where accidents occur, the Reporting of Injuries, Diseases and Dangerous Occurrences Regulations (RIDDOR) 1995 (SI 1995 No. 3163) provide information for measuring the consequences of failing to assess.

For all the anxieties about its introduction, the six-pack of regulations is not isolated, but is closely connected to other legislation. Examples of interactive regulations include the Control of Industrial Major Accident Hazards Regulations 1984 (SI 1984 No. 1902, regularly amended); of criminal statutes, the Environment Act 1995; and of civil legislation, the Occupiers' Liability Acts of 1957 and 1984. Furthermore, statutory duties are complemented by the common law duty requiring employers to take care of the health and safety of their employees. This duty has long encompassed an assessment of risks (*Thompson, Gray, Nicholson* v. *Smiths' Shiprepairers (North Shields) Ltd.* [1984] IRLR 93).

Insurers have traditionally picked up the bills for compensation. Between 1989 and 1993, employer's liability insurers paid out £2.8 billion for claims for work-related accidents and ill health [4]. That was during the time of unlimited cover, which came to an end on 1st January 1995, when a £10 million limit of indemnity for single claims under employer's liability insurance (as required by the Employer's Liability (Compulsory Insurance) Act 1969) came into effect. The notion of direct responsibility may freshen up attitudes to the improvement of health and safety through risk assessment. A separate aspect of insurance is that which covers legal expenses: this neither covers fines nor time lost from work to appear as a defendant, nor 'hidden costs', such as witness time off work, cost of training replacement staff, re-equipping, etc.

Crime and punishment

Breaches of the main provisions of HASWA are punishable by fines, with a maximum of £20 000 in the Magistrates' Court and at large in the Crown Court. The criminal courts may also award compensation to victims who retain the right to seek further damages in the civil courts. An example of a relatively high fine is that which was meted out in 1995 at Mold Crown Court, when Nuclear Electric were fined

£250 000 with costs of £138 000 for breach of Section 2(1): 'failing to take all reasonably practicable steps to ensure danger was averted when a meltdown was narrowly avoided' [5]. Fortunately, no one was hurt, but the high level of fine was imposed to underline public insistence on safety in the nuclear industry.

Whereas companies can only be punished by fines or brought to a standstill by a Prohibition Notice, individual wrongdoers may also be subject to custodial or non-custodial sentences on conviction. Two company directors were each sentenced to 4 months' imprisonment in 1996 at Bradford Crown Court for breaching a Prohibition Notice forbidding the use of a dangerous machine. The Prohibition Notice was issued after an employee lost an arm in a textile garnetting machine when helping others to clean it. The directors pleaded guilty to offences which included the continued use of the garnetting machine and a similar one which was in use on other premises belonging to the company [6]. In an earlier case based on two breaches of a Prohibition Notice, a Glasgow director was sentenced to 240 hours of community service and fined £2500 for having failed to ensure that highly flammable liquids were stored safely [7].

Breaches of regulations are generally subject to a £5000 maximum fine, but some regulations, such as the COSHH Regulations, carry a higher level (£20 000) of fine. Fines imposed on the company can be supplemented by fines on individuals and/or other punishments. Breach of the Asbestos (Licensing) Regulations 1983 (SI 1983 No. 1649) and the Control of Asbestos at Work Regulations 1987 (SI 1987 No. 2115) led to the first jail sentence to be meted out in the UK, when Roy Hill was sentenced to 3 months' imprisonment at Bristol Crown Court in 1995 [8]. On his behalf, it was said that he 'behaved with ignorance, even crass ignorance'. The judge stated, 'The courts cannot and will not tolerate ignorance of the dangers on which you were convicted', and ordered Mr Hill to pay £4000 of the HSE's £11 000 costs in addition to the prison sentence. If the prosecution was right when it said that it was 'inconceivable' that the accused could have been unaware of the risk, had a risk assessment been carried out, knowledge could have been acquired.

The operation of HASWA is now closely linked to MHSWR, as seen by the requirement for risk assessments to be carried out by competent personnel, so that steps may be taken to reduce risks in the workplace. Risk assessments should be carried out or planned by those with appropriate expertise, particularly in specialized situations (such as those that arise in the use of visual display units, as prescribed by the Health and Safety (Display Screen Equipment) Regulations 1992 (SI 1992 No. 2792)). Failure to carry out risk assessments is, in itself, an offence, carrying a fine of up to £5000, and a conviction or the fact of failure, where no prosecution has been brought, may also be used as evidence of negligence in any civil action which may arise where an injury has occurred.

HASWA in action

The ethos of HASWA is set out in Section 2, the 'catch-all'. (Note that MHSWR extends these health and safety duties to temporary workers, as well as to trainees, whether or not on a fixed-term contract.) It requires 'every employer to ensure, so far as is reasonably practicable, the health, safety and welfare of all his employees' across the entire spectrum of work activities. The employer must provide and maintain safe plant and work systems, ensure safe handling, storage and transport of articles, provide adequate training and supervision and ensure safe access to and egress from the workplace. Most prosecutions commence under Section 2, with other charges being brought under other sections or regulations as appropriate. A series of examples illustrates the effect of combined charges.

- The occupier of the site where work is carried out has overall responsibility for health and safety. In 1982, Swan Hunter was convicted under Sections 2(1) and 2(2)(c) of HASWA: failing to 'inform, instruct, train and supervise' contractors' employees who worked on their premises (*R* v. *Swan Hunter Shipbuilders Ltd.* [1982] 1 All ER 264). The duty under Section 2(2)(c) is expressly imposed on employers with regard to their own staff on matters of health and safety, but the Court of Appeal held that these duties extend to contractors' employees whose work activities could affect the health and safety of the main employment force. It was not 'an intolerable burden' on all contractors and subcontractors working in shipyards to provide health and safety information and instruction as to potential dangers to persons other than the employer's own employees. The requirement to instruct employees in matters of health and safety extends to employees of other undertakings where there is a vast conglomeration of tradesmen working together.
- In 1993, Van Heyningen Brothers Ltd. were fined £1000 plus costs of £5000 under Section 2(1) on the HSE's appeal against the dismissal of charges by Sittingbourne Magistrates [9]. An employee fell through the roof of a horticultural glasshouse and was injured. Section 40 of HASWA required the company to prove that it was not reasonably practicable to do more than it had done to ensure a safe system of work. The company had failed to discharge its duty under Section 40, and the magistrates were wrong to find that it was not reasonably practicable for the company to provide a safer system than that which was in operation. This case was brought before the introduction of MHSWR. It would nowadays require a risk assessment to avoid further prosecution under Regulation 3.
- In 1995, Severn Water were fined £50 000 under Section 2(1) and £50 000 under Section 4(1) with costs of £8111.76 at Leicester Crown Court [10]. The company had been warned of the dangers of overhead powerlines a week before a subcontractor was electrocuted after his lorry came into contact with the cables on a site which was

under their control. The company failed to identify the hazard of delivering materials where lorries might come into contact with the lines. The accident could have been prevented by replacing a support timber which had been removed, causing wooden 'goalposts' (designed to limit the height of vehicles entering sites where there are powerlines) to collapse.

- In 1996, Earls Sandwich Shop in Windsor was fined £9700 under Sections 2(2)(a) and 2(3) and under Regulation 3(1) of MHSWR after an employee's finger was badly injured in an accident involving an unguarded slicer. The managing director was fined a further £4700 for the same offence [11].

Other people's places and employees

Persons not in the employment of an employer, but who may be affected by the activities in a workplace, are protected by Section 3(1) of HASWA. Persons working on the premises of an employer who are not his/her employees, nor in a contractual relationship with him/her, such as subcontractors, independent contractors and their employees, must be provided with information and training. Section 3(2) places duties on self-employed contractors in respect of other self-employed persons and of employees who are not their own, thereby linking the chain of liability from building owners and occupiers to main contractors.

For the purposes of Section 3, an employer is deemed to have control over an operation conducted within the general umbrella of his/her business even if the work has been subcontracted to a competent contractor. This is illustrated in *R* v. *Associated Octel Company Ltd.* [1996] 1 WLR 1543, a prosecution arising out of a chemical explosion which occurred during the routine maintenance of one of Associated Octel's chlorine storage tanks. Resin Glass Producers (RGP) were subcontracted to clean the tank. Their employee was badly burned when his lamp broke and ignited flammable vapour from the cleaning material which he was using. The Court of Appeal made it clear that Section 3(1) is intended to protect persons not employed by the defendant from risks to their health and safety caused by the conduct of the undertaking. The duty could not be delegated by Associated Octel to RGP, the independent contractor. The cleaning, maintenance and repair of buildings or plant which are part of the nature of the activities of an organization are part of the 'undertaking', whosoever carries out those activities.

Section 4 of HASWA deals with the control of premises. Any person having control to any extent of premises must take reasonably practicable steps to safeguard the health and safety of persons working there who are not employees. In *Moualem* v. *Carlisle City Council* (*The Times* 8/7/94, QBD), a play centre was held to be 'non-domestic premises' and equipment in it was 'plant', thereby establishing that children, as lawful visitors to the play centre, were entitled to the protection of the Act.

Section 4(3) applies to those in control of premises. Control of rented premises usually lies with the person or entity responsible for maintenance of the premises. In the case of *Westminster City Council* v. *Select Managements Ltd.* [1985] 1 WLR 576, it was held that common parts of a block of flats are premises; they are not domestic, because they are used by all the occupants of the group of private dwellings which comprise the block of flats. That includes residents and workmen who visit the site to carry out maintenance and repairs.

A defence arises to a charge under Section 4 where premises are not used for the designated purpose. In *Mailer* v. *Austin Rover Group* [1989] 2 All ER 1087, an employee of a contractor was killed whilst cleaning a sump. He flouted instructions which he and others had been given, namely: not to use Austin Rover's paint thinners from a certain projecting pipe; not to enter the sump when other cleaning operations were being carried out above; to use an approved safety lamp. He was killed in a flash fire which was caused by his failure to adhere to instructions. Austin Rover were charged under Section 4(2) as they were in control of all aspects of operation of the Cowley works, including plant isolation procedures and use of the ventilation equipment. Their conviction was overturned by the House of Lords on the basis that they could not have reasonably foreseen the wrongful use of their premises which caused the fatal accident.

Sections 7 and 8 impose duties on employees while at work to take care of themselves and others who may be affected by their activities. In general, the HSE is perceived to be reluctant to prosecute individuals, but prosecutions do occur and punishments are heavy. The manager of a site at which flats were being constructed in north London was fined £3500 for a breach of Section 7 ('failure to take reasonable care of his employees') in *HSE* v. *Wimpey Homes (Holdings) Ltd. and Briden* [12], when he permitted his staff to install lintels which had been wrongly delivered and which were not in accordance with specifications. When they started to bow, he told the men to carry on working with them, but to prop them up with scaffolding boards. This weakened the structure so that the floor and one corner of the building collapsed, bringing down another wall against which employees were standing, injuring them. The prosecution said that there should have been a system for assessing the risk associated with changes in design, and that the manager should have stopped the work. Wimpey were fined £10 000 under Section 3(1) of HASWA.

Sections 36 and 37 impose personal liability on a director, manager or secretary if an offence has been committed with their consent or connivance. This liability may be in addition to that of the company. In 1993, the managing director of a Blackpool car parts' firm was found guilty by magistrates under Section 37 of HASWA, and fined £300 plus £1000 costs (*HSE* v. *Watson*) [13]. The company was served with an Improvement Notice which the director passed on to two senior managers, but did not ensure that they complied with it. His conviction was in addition to two convictions against the company for failing to provide proper training for workers exposed to hazardous substances (under COSHH Regulations 1988, Regulation 12) and failing to comply with the Improvement Notice contrary to Section 21 of HASWA. The company was fined £4000 plus £750 prosecution costs.

Foreseeability

Occupiers are expected to take reasonable measures to ensure the safety of their premises in the light of their knowledge of the use to which the premises are to be put and the extent of their control. They cannot therefore be liable for unforeseeable events. Section 3(1) was analysed in *R* v. *Board of Trustees of the Science Museum* [1993] 1 WLR 1171. The museum's air-conditioning tower was found to contain *Legionella* bacteria on a routine inspection by the HSE. At trial for breach of Section 3, the Board argued that there was no case to answer as no actual risk to the public had been proved. The Court of Appeal held that it was sufficient to prove 'risk' for the prosecution to prove that members of the public were exposed to the possibility of danger; proof of actual harm was unnecessary.

Employer cannot delegate responsibility under Section 3

In *R* v. *British Steel plc* [1995] ICR 588, the Court of Appeal held that corporate liability under Section 3 of HASWA could not be delegated to the contractor or subcontractor. Subject to the statutory defence of reasonable practicability, Section 3(1) imposes absolute criminal liability. Thus, a corporate employer was not able to avoid liability under Section 3 on the basis that the company at 'directing mind' or 'senior management level' was not involved, having taken all reasonable steps to delegate supervision.

The facts were that British Steel commissioned subcontractors to reposition a steel platform. The subcontractors provided two men on a labour-only basis to be supervised by a British Steel employee. The subcontractors failed to secure the platform, which fell upon one of their men working beneath it, killing him. The defence of proper delegation did not arise as: 'Section 3(1) ... is cast in absolute terms. The words "so far as is reasonably practicable" ... are simply referable to measures necessary to avert the risk ... the defence (to a prosecution under Section 3(1)) is a narrow one ... which simply comprehends the idea of measures necessary to avert the risks to health and safety.'

Thus, criminal liability cannot be avoided simply because responsibility for the act or omission accrues to a person who is not the directing mind of the company. Persons not employed by the occupier of the site or operator of the main undertaking must not be exposed to risks to their health and safety by the conduct of the undertaking.

Application of civil law

The occupier of premises, whether or not the employer, is under a duty of care to visitors, both at common law and under the Occupiers' Liability Act 1957. The Occupiers' Liability Act 1984 gives protection to trespassers. It is arguable that the fleeing shoplifter could sue the management of shop premises if the floor is not kept safe, level and free from obstruction if he/she trips and is injured during flight!

The general health and safety requirements are listed in *Wilsons & Clyde Coal Company Ltd.* v. *English* [1938] AC 57, closely mirroring the standards of criminal law:

- competent and safety conscious personnel;
- safe appliances, equipment and plant for doing the work (and maintain them);
- safe system and safe place of work.

The duty to protect the health and safety of employees cannot be delegated, so that employers are liable for the acts of third parties to whom they entrust their employees (*McDermid* v. *Nash Dredging and Reclamation Co. Ltd.* [1987] AC 906). However, where the employee is sent abroad to work, there is no general duty of care on the part of the employer to protect the employee's economic welfare by insurance against special risks or by advising the employee to insure himself. In *Reid* v. *Rush & Tomkins Group plc* [1989] 3 All ER 228, the employee was injured in a road accident which was the fault of an uninsured driver. He failed in his attempt to claim his losses from his employer on the grounds that they should have advised him to insure himself.

The purpose of the assessment of risk in the workplace is to identify and avoid not only physical, but psychological, hazards [14]. An employer is under an implied contractual duty not to injure the health of an employee. This duty may extend to employees seconded to others or to employees of others who are required to work on site. The employer may not put employees' health at risk by requiring them to work such long hours as may injure them, notwithstanding a contractual term that employees make themselves available for prolonged periods of overtime. That was decided in the case of *Johnstone* v. *Bloomsbury Health Authority* [1992] QB 333, where a junior doctor sought the right to claim damages for ill health suffered by having to work onerous hours of overtime. His case settled out of court in 1996. Since then, there have been increasing claims for damages for work-related stress-induced diseases, and it is now settled law that risk to the health of the employee covers mental health. In *Walker* v. *Northumberland County Council* [1995] ICR 702, a social worker suffered a stress-related illness after having worked through demanding conditions imposed by his employer. His claim was settled in 1996 for £175 000, which covered the pain, suffering and loss of amenity of a nervous breakdown as well as his loss of income incurred by being unable to continue his chosen career as a social worker. At the hearing on liability, the court held that it was not foreseeable that he would have suffered his first breakdown because of his initial workload. However, on his return to work, his employer imposed an intolerable workload on him, failing to take account of his vulnerability to stress, and was therefore liable for the second breakdown which rendered him unfit for work. Again, risk assessment could nowadays pinpoint the danger areas of the development of this situation.

The *Walker* v. *Northumberland County Council* case should be compared with *Petch* v. *Customs and Excise* [1993] ICR 789, where there was no liability for the nervous breakdown which the employee suffered as he had not been exhibiting any signs that the illness threatened, his workload was not such as would carry a real risk of stress-induced illness and his employer had tried to persuade him not to return to work after an episode of mental illness. Despite the finding on specific liability, the court held that a duty of care is owed by the employer in relation to the mental as well as physical health of his/her employees. Causation was acknowledged to be more difficult to establish in mental illness.

Employees who are injured when working at sites distant from the home site may find it difficult to fix their employer with liability. The principles which guide the courts are set out in *Square D Ltd. and others* v. *Cook* [1992] ICR 262, a case in which an employee was injured while commissioning computer control systems in offices in Saudi Arabia. The Court of Appeal held that it was casting too high a responsibility on the home-based employers to hold them liable for the daily events of a site in Saudi Arabia occupied by a third party. Where an employee is injured on premises in the occupation of a third party, the extent of the employer's responsibility depends on what is reasonable in the circumstances based on the following matters:

- place where work is to be done;
- nature of any building or site concerned;
- experience of employee dispatched to the site;
- nature of work he/she is expected to do;
- degree of control employer can reasonably be expected to exercise;
- employer's knowledge of the defective state of the premises.

In *Square D Ltd. and others* v. *Cook*, there was no evidence to show that the accident was caused by the employer's breach of duty. The Court of Appeal was satisfied that the site occupiers and the general contractors were both reliable companies. The plaintiff's problem was the fact that the occupier of the site was abroad. Had the accident happened in the UK, a claim would have been made against the occupier as well as the employer, and the principal employer would have been expected to have had some knowledge of the state of the premises to which the employee was to be sent. The window cleaning company in *General Cleaning Contractors Ltd.* v. *Christmas* [1953] AC 180 was held liable in negligence for not checking the state of repair of the windows before sending staff to work on a site; in modern terms, for failing to assess the risk to which it was subjecting its employees. The risk of defective windows was a special risk incident to the calling of a window cleaner. Therefore the employer of the cleaner must take care for his/her employee or subcontractor, and not rely on the occupier of the premises (a club in this case) to know or warn of risk. Here, no inspection or repairs had been carried out to a defective window which fell and injured the cleaner's hand. There was no cause of action against the Club, as the inviter's liability only extends to unusual hazards, and this was not an unusual hazard.

Risk assessment and repetitive strain injury (RSI)

The chicken pluckers' case, *Mountenay (Hazzard) and others* v. *Bernard Matthews plc* [1994] 5 Med LR 293, illustrates what a court requires employers to have done in order for them to show that they took reasonably practicable preventive steps to protect the health and safety of their employees. At the head of the list is the duty to warn in a situation where risk arises, now amply covered by MHSWR. Where there is a risk, the courts then consider whether there is a causal link between the risk factor, the acts or omissions which could have prevented the harm and the harm which in fact happened. The protection of employees at risk of tenosynovitis can be covered by the following steps:

- warn of the risk;
- enable employees to make an informed choice as to whether they will take the risk;
- advise employees to take medical advice at the first sign of aching wrists or hands;
- provide mechanical assistance for squeezing movements;
- gradual introduction of new employees to repetitive working movements;
- rotate duties.

Because the company did not take these steps, it was liable for the injuries suffered by its employees. Some of the 'RSI' cases present salutary lessons in the advisability of following risk assessment procedures.

The British Telecom operators in the case of *McSherry and Lodge* v. *British Telecommunications plc* [1992] 3 Med LR 129 were awarded £6000 general damages for pain, suffering and loss of amenity resulting from their condition, in addition to their claim for loss of earnings. In *Sketchley* v. *Cradley Print Ltd.* [15] damages were agreed at an amount of £64 224 for an employee whose job was designated as 'table hand'. She had developed tenosynovitis in 1990 while carrying out her work, which involved picking up sections of magazines, thereby straining her wrists. She is now able to carry out office work and has been redeployed within the company. *Harris* v. *Inland Revenue*, reported in *The Times* (19 January 1994), settled out of court for £79 000. The plaintiff, who had been employed for 15 years as a typist, developed pain in her right arm in 1990, which was diagnosed as epicondylitis. By 1993, she was obliged to retire 12 years early on the grounds of ill health. Her case reflected her loss of future earnings at £11 000 per annum. Her workstation details are a lesson in themselves: she had an incorrectly positioned desk and chair, and she worked 7.5 h each day with a single half-hour break for lunch. She regularly typed between 13 000 and 16 000 keystrokes per hour.

The future

Harmony in health and safety matters is increasing through the activities of the World Health Organization, whose plenary meeting in May 1996 endorsed a global strategy for occupational health. Article 3 of the International Labour Organization's Convention 161 requires that: 'Each member undertakes to develop ... occupational health services for all workers ... in all branches of economic activity and all undertakings'. Until that occupational health Utopia is established, individual countries will continue to set their own standards, balancing moral duties, the cost of law enforcement and encouragement of high standards through the development of occupational medicine. One intermediate solution could be the development of greater occupational health awareness amongst general practitioners, with increased efficacy of referral systems for advice from appropriately trained professionals. The external occupational health team requires a broad range of skills, but need not be medically qualified [16].

Where prevention fails, redress must be sought. It is arguable that improvements could be made to the present system so that an element of punishment could be introduced into civil claims, thereby bringing deterrence into the armoury of persuasion for improvement in working conditions. In January 1994, a Consultative Paper was published in England entitled: 'Aggravated, exemplary and restitutionary damages'. It is recommended that, under certain defined circumstances, employers should pay punitive damages for deliberate breaches of health and safety law and for negligence. At present, damages are only awarded to redress the balance, and any punitive element is taken care of by criminal sanctions where appropriate. If such a proposal was accepted, there would be a great increase in the level of awards. The deterrent aspect might be offset by a greater tendency for employers to fight rather than settle a claim, so that legal and preparatory costs would tend to spiral.

Prevention, as always, is better and probably cheaper than cure, and is the backbone of risk assessment. The future should contain a developing awareness that the short-term cost of reducing workplace dangers will be offset by the increased productivity of a healthy workforce.

References

1 Silverstein, B.A., Hays, J.R. & Kalat, J. (1996) Returning workers with

musculoskeletal disorders to work—the role of ergonomics programmes. In: *ICOH (International Conference on Occupational Health) 96, Book of Abstracts*, Vol. 2, p.40.

2 Industrial Society (1994) London safety survey. In: *Health and Safety Information Bulletin*. Public Industrial Relations Services, London.
3 Chartered Institute of Management Accountants (1994) *Costs of Business Survey: June 1994*. CIMA, London.
4 Association of British Insurers (1994) *1994 Report*.
5 *Health and Safety at Work Act Newsletter* (1995) 44,1. British Safety Council, London.
6 *Health and Safety at Work Act Newsletter* (1996): Vol. 2, No.2, 1.
7 *Health and Safety at Work Act Newsletter* (1994): 28, 1.
8 *Health and Safety at Work Act Newsletter* (1996): 49, 1.
9 *Health and Safety at Work Act Newsletter* (1993): 18, 2.
10 *Health and Safety at Work Act Newsletter* (1995): 37, 1.
11 *Health and Safety at Work Act Newsletter* (1996): Vol. 2, No. 5, 2.
12 *Health and Safety at Work Act Newsletter* (1995): 37, 2.
13 *Health and Safety at Work Act Newsletter* (1993): 13, 1.
14 Levi, L. & Lunde-Jensen, P. (1996) *A Model for Assessing the Costs of Stressors at National Level: Socio-economic Costs of Work Stress in Two EU Member States*. Office for the Official Publications of the European Communities, Luxembourg.
15 *Health and Safety Information Bulletin* 1994.
16 Ballard, J. (1997) Editorial. *Occupational Health Review* 66, 1.

Section 4 Applications of risk assessment and management in industry: case studies

Chapter 19 Agriculture (pesticides)

Ian Brown

Introduction

The agricultural industry and farming practices in the UK and European Union are highly mechanized. There are usually less than five workers per farm, compared with the labour intensive practices before the Second World War. This is in contrast with other regions of the globe, where labour is relatively inexpensive compared with the capital cost of farm machinery.

The greatest risk to life and limb on the farm is physical trauma, and approximately one person per week loses his/her life on the farm in the UK (Baxter 1992). In this chapter, the prevention of serious, traumatic injury is not discussed; instead, the much more emotive and potentially complex subject of risk assessment for those workers handling and applying agricultural pesticides is examined.

Defining the problem

Occupationally related, acute pesticide poisoning is unusual in the UK but, in many other regions in the world, the situation is very different. Koh and Jeyaratnam (1996) have estimated that many millions of agricultural workers in the Third World experience an episode of pesticide poisoning each year.

As a broad generalization, the more specific and targeted the pesticide, the less likely it is to be acutely toxic to humans. This is especially so with herbicides, and a good example involves a comparison of the quaternary nitrogen herbicide, paraquat, with the triazine group. Paraquat is essentially a totally non-specific contact herbicide that rapidly destroys green plant tissue regardless of species. By a somewhat similar biochemical action, it also produces multisystem organ failure and pulmonary fibrosis in any animal ingesting it. The adult lethal dose is between 3 and 6 g. Triazines are much more specific in their activity: they inhibit chloroplast biochemistry, which is quite plant specific. The triazines therefore show low acute toxicity, and there has never been any substantiated case of acute poisoning with any member of this group.

Similar parallels may be drawn from the more commonly used insecticides, and again the toxicity may be reduced by specific biochemical targeting. The majority of insecticides invoke their action by disturbing the normal function of the nervous system, and the organophosphate (OP) group exerts its acute effects by mimicking the naturally occurring and widely distributed neurotransmitter acetylcholine. Once absorbed in sufficient doses, OP insecticides successfully compete for the active site on the enzyme that destroys acetylcholine (acetylcholinesterase) and, once *in situ*, will phosphorylate the usually acetylated enzyme (Figs 19.1 & 19.2). Phosphorylation causes a much firmer bond to be established between enzyme and substrate, and therefore the enzyme is

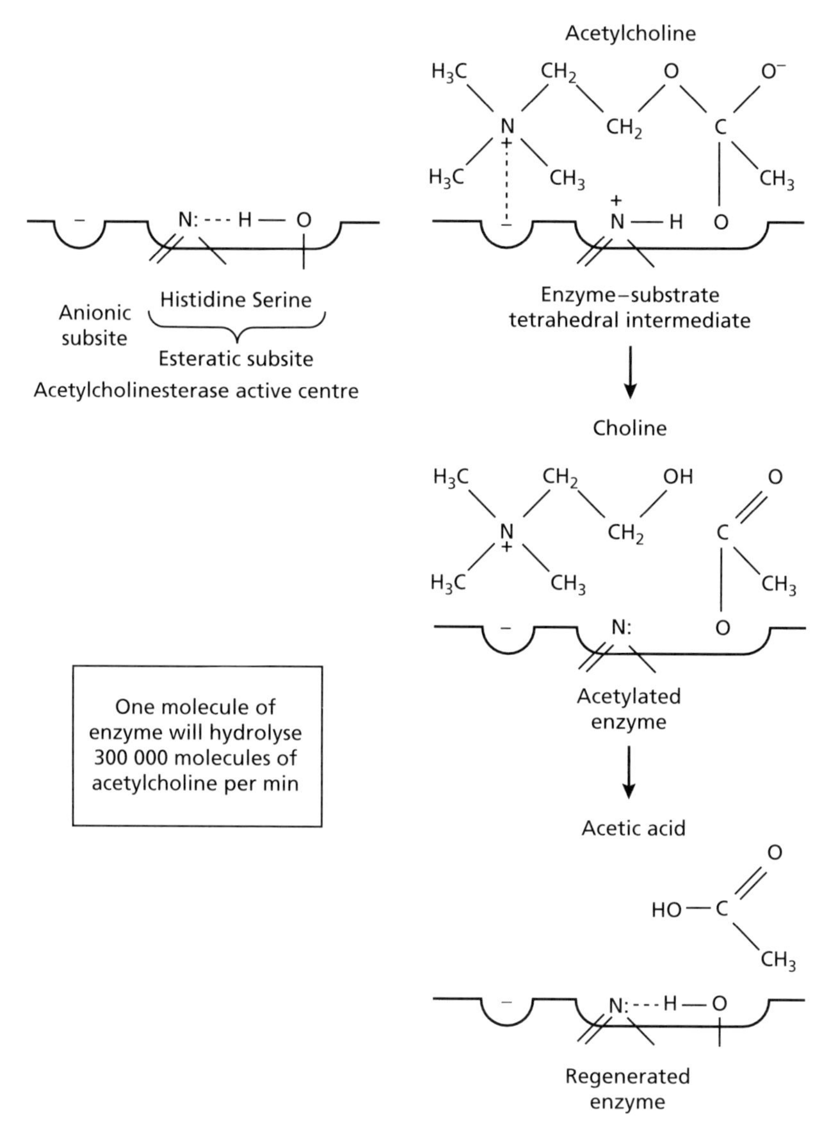

Figure 19.1 Under normal circumstances, acetylcholine, a chemical neurotransmitter, is broken down by the enzyme acetylcholinesterase. Accumulation of acetylcholine is thus prevented.

One molecule of enzyme will hydrolyse 0.008 molecules of organophosphate per min

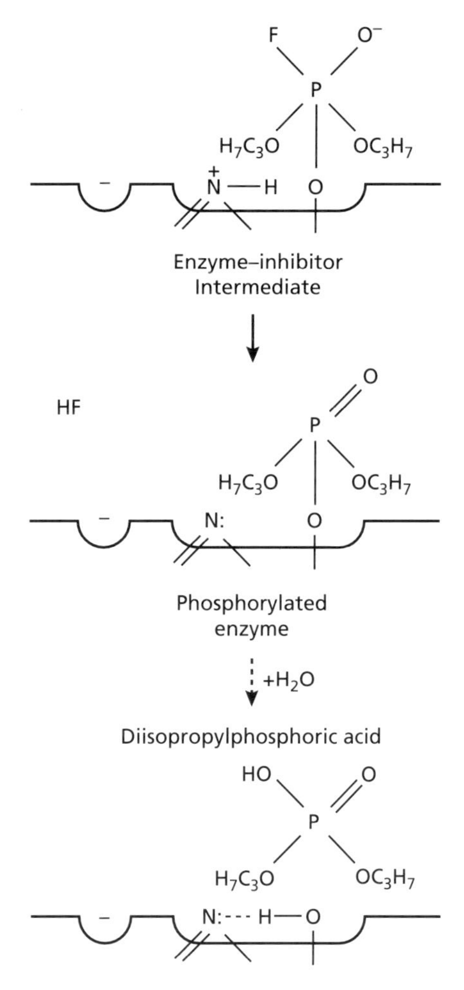

Figure 19.2 Organophosphate insecticides can phosphorylate the active site on the acetylcholinesterase enzyme, preventing it from breaking down acetylcholine.

effectively rendered useless. The end result will be an excessive accumulation of acetylcholine and, in due course, a totally refractory depolarized post-synaptic membrane or muscle endplate and death by respiratory arrest and pulmonary oedema. As acetylcholine is a common neurotransmitter to virtually all biological systems, OPs are as toxic to insects as they are to mammals once absorbed. Of course, if the rate of absorption could be modified, the toxicity could be changed as dose is very important (Paracelsus 1499–1541). There are now novel ways of doing just this, and considerable work is presently being undertaken on new delivery systems such that 'slow release' formulations will deliver a constant small dose of insecticide to the critical site of activity. This has a double benefit for the user—it allows persistence of activity to occur without bioaccumulation and results in very low toxicity to humans as the delivered dose over time is so slow (even when ingested). Despite this, OPs are still intrinsically toxic, and especially so when compared with the synthetic pyrethroids (the main constituents of fly spray) which, in general, are of very low toxicity to humans. This is by virtue of their stereospecificity and the ability of mammals to hydrolyse pyrethroids rapidly to their inactive acid and alcohol components. These insecticides again affect the nervous system and are sodium channel toxins. The flux of sodium into and out of nervous tissue is critical to membrane potentials and the passage of nervous impulses. These channels can be blocked by chemicals of highly specific shape (stereospecificity), and the shape of the insect channel is different from that of mammal's. Therefore, biochemical specificity allows the pyrethroids to be used with relative safety, whilst still maintaining a significant insecticidal action.

Hazard identification

The agricultural worker will obtain hazard identification information from the pesticide product label, supplied by the manufacturer on the container. The direct supervisor of the worker will also have the benefit of a materials safety data sheet, also supplied by the manufacturer, and this will provide further information and address environmental and disposal concerns.

Product labels are printed in the local language and fulfil the statutory labelling regulations of the user country. In the UK, there will be appropriate international symbols for harmful, poisonous, corrosive, etc., and a clear description will follow of the statutory conditions relating to use and essential precautions. There will also be an emergency telephone number should a problem or query arise, and most major pesticide manufacturers provide a 24-h helpline.

Exposure assessment

There are hundreds of pesticides registered for use throughout the world, but one of the commonest classes of highly effective, yet potentially acutely toxic, substances is the OPs. The biochemistry of these chemicals was discussed in the section on 'Defining the problem', and this pesticide will make a good specific example for 'exposure assessment'.

Exposure will occur when the worker is handling and using the pesticide product, especially in its concentrated form. The assessment of exposure will therefore involve two inter-related activities: (i) observation of the worker during product and equipment handling; and (ii) biological monitoring. Exposure potential will be apparent during mixing, loading, applying (spraying) and equipment cleaning. This will be limited by personal protective equipment, careful handling and sensible personal hygiene. Biological monitoring will then reveal the effectiveness of protective equipment and worker compliance with recommended safety practices.

Biological monitoring of OP exposure is undertaken indirectly as 'biological effect monitoring' (see Chapter 16), and venous blood is taken from the employee at regular intervals after potential OP exposure to measure the inhibition of the enzyme cholinesterase (red blood cell acetylcholinesterase, plasma cholinesterase, or both). The mechanism of this effect is illustrated in Figs 19.1 and 19.2. The greater the inhibition, the greater the absorption of OP. The problem here is that cholinesterase levels are highly variable in the population, and can also vary by as much as 32% in some individuals (plus or minus 16% with a coefficient of variation between 7.6% and 11.3%; Callaway *et al.* 1951; Kane 1958; Gage 1967; Brown 1993). It is therefore essential to establish the normal, unexposed mean cholinesterase level of an individual worker, and understand how any specific measurement will vary around that mean. Small decreases in cholinesterase may indicate OP exposure, but may also be part of the individual's normal biological variation. In the case of a worker for whom a mean cholinesterase level has not been established, it will only be possible to compare that individual's results with the normal range supplied by the laboratory. This will only give an indication of significant poisoning (which will probably be obvious clinically!), and will not provide any information on subclinical cholinesterase reduction. Small changes in cholinesterase will be hidden within the normal biovariability of this enzyme, and a true reduction will only become obvious when the range of biovariability is understood for an individual worker. For workers regularly exposed to OPs, a flow chart needs to be established, preferably some weeks before exposure occurs. By using a suitable computer program, a graphical relationship can be achieved between cholinesterase level and time, with upper and lower parameters of normal variation. These so-called 'upper and lower control limits' are, in fact, the calculated 'normal' (Gaussian) distribution of that individual's results, and a drop below the lower control limit (lcl) is a true depression of cholinesterase (see Fig. 19.3). If such a drop were to occur, the case must be investigated thoroughly, and the worker possibly withdrawn from exposure until the enzyme returns to the individual's normal range.

Risk characterization and health surveillance

The risk will be quantitatively and qualitatively characterized as negligible, acceptable or unacceptable. If the risk is considered to be unacceptable, improved control of exposure will need to be implemented, and this can be achieved by substitution, separation or improved personal protective equipment. In the case of OP exposure, the risk would be acceptable if cholinesterase depression rarely occurred below the lower control limit and the individual did not demonstrate clinical signs or symptoms. An unacceptable risk would be the occurrence of clinical signs or symptoms at any time following exposure, and/or frequent excursions below the lower control limit.

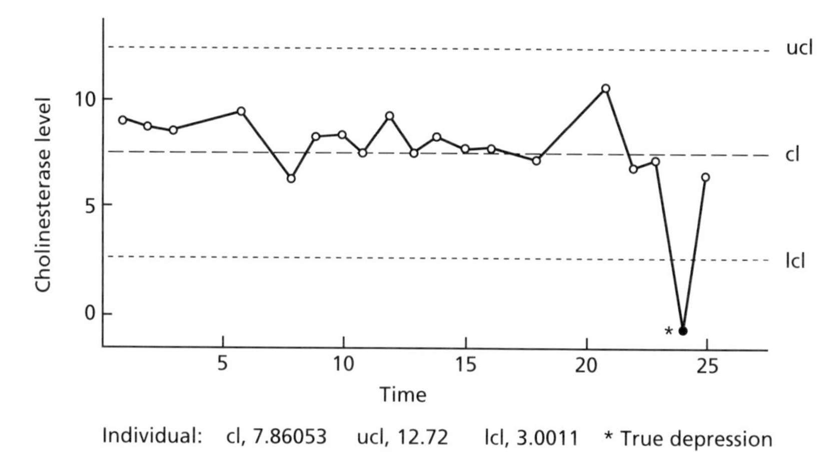

Figure 19.3 Individual exposure flow chart: 'ucl' and 'lcl' are the upper and lower control limits, respectively.

Health surveillance is part of the risk characterization programme, and will consist of targeted medical examinations and specific, periodic biological monitoring for cholinesterase. Targeted medical examinations will be periodic and will concentrate on potential target organ damage. Chronic organ damage in the case of OP exposure is presently speculative, and a general health questionnaire is probably all that is required in the first instance. The questionnaire should be biased towards chronic neurological and psychological enquiry (chronic fatigue syndrome), as much of the speculation is in these areas of disability, although there is presently no firm evidence to support the association.

Prevention and control

The most profound method of prevention is to substitute the OP with an alternative pesticide formulation that is equally effective, but has a better health hazard profile. This is often impossible or not at the discretion of the worker. Other more practical measures are listed below.

- Activity risk analysis of the work practices to minimize the contact of the worker with the active substance.
- Reassessment of personal protective equipment to ensure that it is comfortable, of appropriate impermeable material and ergonomically efficient.
- Technical assessment of packaging, physical state of substance (granular, liquid, powder) and delivery system to ensure optimum design characteristics.

Risk communication, training and information

In the UK, the whole area of risk communication, training and information is addressed by the Health and Safety at Work, etc. Act 1974, and is more specifically defined in the Control of Substances Hazardous to Health (COSHH) Regulations 1988 and 1994. The COSHH Regulations ensure that a suitable and sufficient assessment of health risk must be undertaken before the pesticide is used, and that prevention and control of exposure to the pesticide should be employed. In addition, Regulation 12 states that: 'information, instruction and training for persons who may be exposed to substances hazardous to health must be undertaken'. This whole area of legislation is understandably explained in the Ministry of Agriculture, Fisheries and Food (MAFF) publication, *Pesticides: Code of Practice for the Safe Use of Pesticides on Farms and Holdings* (MAFF 1990). As part of the COSHH Regulations, the user of the pesticide has to undergo training in the safe use of the product, and most users must also hold a 'Certificate of Competence' recognized by UK Ministers of the Crown for the purpose of the Control of Pesticide Regulations 1986 (a part of the Food and Environment Protection Act 1985). A valid certificate comprises at least two parts: a foundation module, which tests safety knowledge, and one or more application modules, which test practical skills.

Similar regulatory measures operate throughout the world, but, in remote regions of the globe, risk communication and training are poorly organized locally and there is very little enforcement of regulations. This is recognized by most of the ethical major pesticide manufacturers, and they usually provide an extensive and well-funded product stewardship programme (to ensure at least the safe use of their product). Enforcement is more difficult and worker compliance is usually inadequate where economic circumstances are poor and where the climate does not encourage pesticide users to wear hot, uncomfortable, protective equipment. This is a subject that is presently being tackled by international agencies, such as the World Health Organization and The International Centre for Pesticide Safety in Milan.

Conclusions

The risk assessment and management of pesticide exposure in the agricultural industry are extensively regulated throughout the European Union and in many other regions of the globe, but policing and enforcement are patchy. This is because of the nature of the job, which often involves enormous numbers of employees globally who often work in isolated circumstances. The only solution is a highly efficient programme of risk communication and training. This must be aimed specifically at the culture and population in question, and should be continuously reinforced by local government and the pesticide manufacturer working together. Before the product reaches the end user, the manufacturer can do much to ensure 'intrinsic' product safety by the use of a sensible physical form (no powders) and slow release formulations. This must be supplemented by ergonomically efficient packaging and the safe disposal of used containers.

As with most risk management strategies, the key factors involved are hazard minimization, clear risk communication and full co-operation and compliance by the potentially exposed worker. The handling of pesticides by agricultural workers is no exception.

References

Baxter, P. (1992) Health and safety on the farm. *British Medical Journal* 305, 6–7.

Brown, I. (1993) The measurement and assessment of plasma and erythrocyte cholinesterase following potential low dose exposure to the organophosphate chlorpyifos. Abstract. *Proceedings of the 24th Congress of the International Commission on Occupational Health, Nice.*

Callaway, S., Davies, D.R. & Rutland, J.P. (1951) Blood cholinesterase levels and range of personal variation in a healthy adult population. *British Medical Journal* 2, 812–816.

Gage, J.C. (1967) The significance of blood cholinesterase activity measurements. *Residue Review* 18, 159–173.

Kane, P.F. (1958) *The Normal Variation in the Interpretation of Blood Cholinesterase Activity.* Report No. 2662. Chemagro Corporation Research Department. (Cited by Gage 1967.)

Koh, D. & Jeyaratnam, J. (1996) Pesticide hazards in developing countries. *Science of the Total Environment* 188, 78–85.

MAFF (1990) *Pesticides: Code of Practice for the Safe Use of Pesticides on Farms and Holdings.* HMSO, London.

Paracelsus (1499–1541) *All Substances are Poisons: There is None Which is Not a Poison. The Right Dose Differentiates a Poison and a Remedy.*

Chapter 20

Assessment of exposure to isocyanates

Iain MacKenzie

Introduction

This case study is concerned with the use of isocyanates in the automotive component industry, and with the provision of an appropriate system for the management of their use, so that the risks involved are brought within acceptable limits.

The isocyanates are a class of low-molecular-weight chemicals containing a highly reactive isocyanate (NCO) group. The NCO group is attached to an organic radical that can be aliphatic, aromatic or cycloaliphatic. The production of polyurethane polymers requires at least two NCO groups in the molecule (diisocyanates). The methods of use vary, the essential process being the combination with polyols so that an exothermic reaction occurs between them (Fig. 20.1). The reaction creates durable polyurethane foams, elastomers, paints or adhesives. The most important compound is toluene diisocyanate (TDI), which is highly volatile at room temperature and exists in two isomeric forms, the 2,4- and 2,6-isomers (shown in Fig. 20.1), usually in a ratio of 80:20. Approximately 95% of all polyurethanes are based on TDI and methylenediphenylisocyanate (MDI) (Vandenplas *et al.* 1993).

Unfortunately, although diisocyanates are incredibly useful, their use carries a potential disadvantage, as they are known to have a number of negative effects on health, many of which are both serious and permanent. Acute or chronic exposure to high concentrations of isocyanates can result in respiratory health effects through a direct irritant action (Davies 1984). Isocyanates are of special interest, however, because, in some exposed workers, they can cause occupational asthma through a sensitizing mechanism (Mapp *et al.* 1994). Indeed, exposure to diisocyanates is now recognized to be the leading cause of occupational asthma (Chan-Yeung & Malo 1994). It is generally accepted that 5% of exposed subjects develop occupational asthma after exposure to TDI (Butcher *et al.* 1977), but estimates as high as 15% have been proposed (Peters & Wegman 1975).

Extended exposure to isocyanate vapour at barely measurable levels can cause asthma or asthma-like conditions in some individuals. Alternatively, a single event involving a high exposure may have similar effects. The susceptibility to these effects seems to vary from individual to individual, for a variety of reasons, some perhaps genetic and some related to general health or lifestyle factors. Also relevant are previous exposures to similar substances.

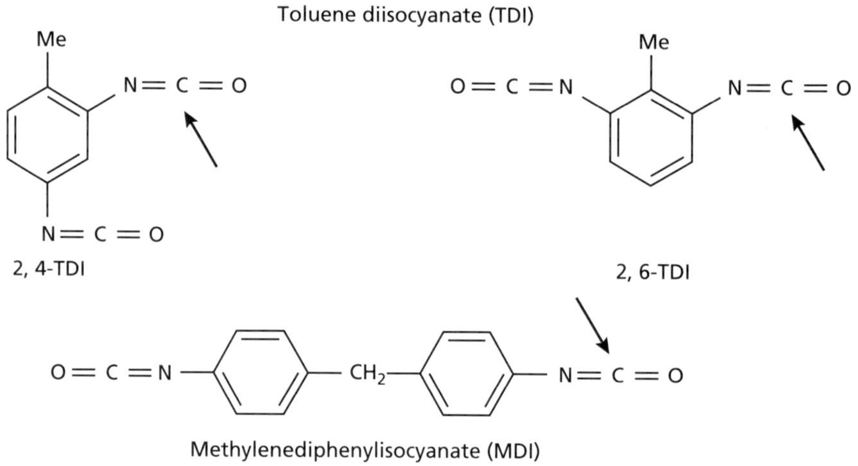
Toluene diisocyanate (TDI)
Me
N=C=O
O=C=N
2, 4-TDI
2, 6-TDI
CH2
Methylenediphenylisocyanate (MDI)

(a) Monomers of aromatic diisocyanates

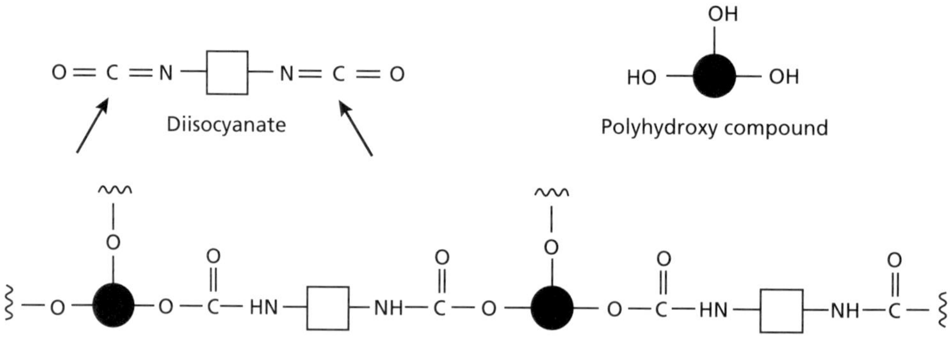
O=C=N
N=C=O
Diisocyanate
OH
HO
Polyhydroxy compound
O
C
HN
NH

(b) Addition reaction between an isocyanate (NCO) and a hydroxyl (OH) group to give a urethane linkage. This is the basic mechanism for the production of polyurethanes

Figure 20.1 Diisocyanates—structures of aromatic monomers and formation of polyurethane.

The use of isocyanates in the automotive industry is widespread: in paints, adhesives and as foams. Indeed, it is difficult to see how the modern car industry could survive without them. This study confines itself to the description of how one particular plant managed the risks to health arising from the use of isocyanates in one particular application.

Defining the problem

The plant in question produced internal trim for motor vehicles, i.e. car dashboards, internal door cappings and other internal panels. The products produced by the factory essentially consisted of wood fibre mouldings, the outer surfaces of which were covered by a flexible plastic skin.

The elements of the process that caused concern were those connected with the gluing of the plastic cover material onto the mouldings. Two-part polyester adhesives using TDI had been specified for these operations.

Ideally, TDI would not have been used as it is a known problem substance. It is the most volatile of the common isocyanates (vapour pressure *c.* 0.00009 mmHg at 25°C) and, at room temperature, will give off more vapour than the other common isocyanates, such as MDI. It is therefore more likely to be inhaled, and is correspondingly more likely to cause harm to health.

However, only TDI-based adhesives were identified as meeting both the necessary stringent product quality standards for durability and strength of adhesion and the production requirements for curing time. Its use meant that there was a significant potential for the causation of sensitization and occupational asthma.

The use of various formulations of these adhesives had taken place over a number of years, during which time comparatively little had been done to assess accurately the risks involved or to ensure that control measures were adequate. Although there were some control measures in place (e.g. spray booths and personal protective equipment (PPE)), their effectiveness was not monitored. The effects on the health of employees during this period were difficult to quantify, partly because of the high turnover of employees and partly due to a lack of regular health monitoring. However, a number of civil legal claims were made against the company in respect of occupational asthma during this period.

Description of process

The facility operated a wood pulping plant which fed pulp to a moulding process; this formed the basic structure for the products. The outer surfaces of the mouldings were then covered by the plastic materials that most of us are familiar with in our vehicles. There were a number of steps involved in the process.

- *Step 1.* Softwood logs were broken down into pulp and were mixed with waxes and resins.
- *Step 2.* The pulp was fed to a moulding press which formed a wet, 'felt' moulding.
- *Step 3.* The 'felt' was 'cooked' in heated press tools to convert it into a hard moulding.
- *Step 4.* The outer surface of the moulding was sprayed with an adhesive containing TDI (either by robot spraying arms or by manual sprayers in extracted spray booths).
- *Step 5.* The sprayed moulding was placed in a vacuum forming machine and was heated to reactivate the adhesive. A plastic sheet was clamped above it, and air suction was used to pull the sheet down so that it formed itself onto the moulding.
- *Step 6.* The majority of the excess material around the rim of the

moulding was trimmed away manually using knives. Adhesive was applied to the remaining loose edges. The edges were tucked over the rim of the moulding and were fixed to its rear so as to form a neat edge. This manual process was known as 'turning in'.

- *Step 7*. Further fitments, such as handles and decorative strips, were added to complete the product.

This case study is principally concerned with potential exposures to TDI vapour arising from the 'turning in' phase of production, although it also touches on other potential exposures.

Hazard identification

Turning in

The turning in process involved close manual work on the mouldings. This included hand application of small quantities of adhesive, which were taken from small pots on the workbench. Hand-held heat guns (similar to those used for paint stripping) were used to reactivate the adhesive, and to enable the loose edges of the plastic cover material to be stuck down. Individual operators adopted different stances and positions when doing this work, and some brought their faces close to the workpiece during some of the operations described.

At the time of the *initial* investigation, neither extraction ventilation nor respiratory protective equipment (RPE) was provided for this process. No efforts were being made to increase dilution ventilation by means of overhead or bench-mounted fans.

Risk characterization

Isocyanates are covered by a maximum exposure limit (MEL) as published in the UK Health and Safety Executive (HSE) *Guidance Note EH40* (updated every year). The current limits for all isocyanates are $0.02\,mg\,m^{-3}$ (8 h) and $0.07\,mg\,m^{-3}$ (15 min). These values refer to exposures and concentrations of isocyanates in air, and are limits which must not be exceeded for the two reference periods. There is also a legal requirement to reduce exposures to as low as reasonably practicable.

Clearly, an exposure which exceeds the MEL is unacceptable and represents a high risk. However, exposures that are below the MEL can also represent high risks (see Chapter 7). The MEL does not represent a guaranteed frontier between high and low risks. Furthermore, the role of intermittent, short peaks of exposure to isocyanates is not catered for by the time-weighted nature of the MELs.

Due to the complexities of the sensitization process and the potential means of exposure, it was felt to be inappropriate to relate directly risk factors to specified measured concentrations in air. Instead, a more flexible, subjective assessment of risk was made, taking into account the measured concentrations, but also health surveillance results and direct observation of the process. The categories of risk used were high, medium, low and negligible.

Prior to this particular assessment programme, the following guidelines had been created to judge what category the health risks fell into:

- *high*—reasonably foreseeable risk of either death or permanent serious ill health to one or more people, or permanent, minor ill health to several people;
- *medium*—reasonably foreseeable risk of permanent, minor ill health to one or more people, temporary, serious illness to several people, or temporary, minor illness to large numbers of people;
- *low*—reasonably foreseeable risk of temporary, minor illness to one or more people;
- *negligible*—no readily foreseeable risk of causing ill health.

In due course, the above guidelines were felt to be inappropriate for the assessment of the risks arising from the use of isocyanates. New guidelines were developed:

- *high*—any exposures approaching or exceeding the MEL, or any detectable exposures (even at low levels) combined with clear evidence of the deterioration of lung function in the exposed population;
- *medium*—occasional, detectable exposures (well below the MEL) with no apparent deterioration in lung function;
- *low*—theoretical exposure to isocyanates, but with no detectable exposure and no deterioration in lung function;
- *negligible*—no exposure to isocyanates.

Exposure assessment (atmospheric monitoring and health surveillance)

Work processes involving the use of isocyanates were assessed informally when experienced health and safety personnel joined the company. Formal assessment and atmospheric monitoring followed a little later.

Certain practices involving TDI adhesive (such as operators sometimes spraying adhesive without wearing RPE) were clamped down upon immediately, as were lax cleaning regimes for spray booths. These factors were obviously giving rise to unacceptable risks, and could be dealt with without delay. Other risks, however, such as those arising from the vacuum forming and turning in operations, were not so easy to assess, and more detailed investigations were required.

Health surveillance was critical in assessing the level of risk to health involved. The section on health surveillance in the UK HSE *Guidance Note MS25* was taken into account when devising the surveillance programme. An occupational physician was engaged to provide additional advice on the structure of the surveillance programme, to review the results obtained and to investigate suspected cases of occupational asthma

All unexplained sickness absence was tracked (particularly where individuals worked with isocyanates), although the close nature of the rest of the surveillance programme meant that this was of peripheral value. All complaints from the workforce which might be related to isocyanate exposure and respiratory problems were investigated.

An occupational health nurse carried out a programme of lung function testing (including forced expiratory volume in 1 s (FEV_1) and forced vital capacity (FVC)) for all employees on the site, initially establishing benchmark readings, and then continuing with ongoing tests so as to detect any patterns of deteriorating lung function in the workforce.

Some of the benchmark readings were of concern. A number of individuals who had worked with isocyanates in preceding years displayed lung functions that were certainly poorer than the average that might have been expected, allowing for their age and height. However, there was no conclusive evidence that this was due to isocyanate exposure, as other factors could have been involved. Some of these other factors, e.g. histories of smoking, were identified by means of a respiratory questionnaire (originating from the Medical Research Council in the UK), and the information obtained was used to try to clarify the lung function data.

The individuals with apparently depressed lung functions were observed further to determine whether they had symptoms that could be tied into their exposures at work. When the flow of information from repeat tests began to come through, it became possible to put the readings in context. Readings from individuals varied over time. Some of these variations could have been related to infections or to allergies, such as hay fever, that individuals were known to suffer from, but others had no apparent cause. However, over a period of time, attention began to focus on the readings of several employees who worked on the turning in process.

From the outset of the assessment programme, and before formal health surveillance began, the turning in process had been regarded with suspicion. The adhesive used for gluing the edges of the mouldings was the same as that employed in spraying. The amounts used, however, were small. An operator would use perhaps 250 ml in a shift, this being applied by a small hand brush. Periodically, additional heat was provided by means of a hand-held heat gun, so as to help the glue to bond.

Personal monitoring was undertaken to determine what the exposures were likely to be. Ten minute pumped samples using colorimetric paper tape were taken from sample numbers of 'turners in'. Operators were fitted with a precalibrated pump which pulled a measured air sample through a test card holding the reactive tape, mounted near the operators' breathing zone. The presence of TDI caused the tape to turn pink, the strength of the colour indicating the concentration of TDI. The manufacturers claimed that as little as 0.0034 mg m^{-3} of TDI (expressed as NCO) could be measured by this technique.

This round of monitoring indicated that there had been isocyanate exposures (in some cases), although these were well below the MEL.

Some samples had not recorded isocyanates at all. A further round of monitoring confirmed this pattern.

It appeared that there was a risk, but its severity was difficult to quantify. At this stage, however, it was tentatively assessed as being a *medium* risk. Options for control were reviewed, and a decision was made to use dilution ventilation to reduce exposures. This was a low-cost option which involved mounting overhead fans above each of the turning in workstations (and ensuring that they were used). After installation, further rounds of monitoring indicated that exposures had fallen further, but that some individuals still had detectable exposures. The action taken had not been sufficient to lower the risk rating to *low*.

With the dilution ventilation in place, the results of lung function testing continued to cause concern. The lung function of some 'turners in' had declined since their benchmark readings had been made. Further investigation was deemed to be necessary, and several individuals agreed to co-operate by carrying and using portable peak flow meters at 4-h intervals over an extended period of 2 weeks or more. This would cover periods both inside and outside work. The individuals would keep records of their own readings. It was hoped that it might be possible to either relate the individuals' readings to potential exposures at work, or to rule out any such relationship. In practice, this proved to be difficult to achieve, as even the best intentioned individuals had difficulty in remembering to use the meters at regular intervals, and the data obtained proved to be rather erratic and non-conclusive. However, more extensive use of the lung function programme revealed that several 'turners in' displayed better lung functions on a Monday morning than they had on the previous Friday. This was more obviously the case when individuals returned from leave, and their before and after lung function data were compared. The indications were that work exposures *were* having an effect on lung function.

As a consequence of the lung function test results and various symptoms noted, e.g. rhinitis, for precautionary reasons, several employees were removed from the turning in process.

Reassessment of risk

The health surveillance programme had brought into question the original assessment of the risk based upon the observation of the process and short-term personal sampling. If a more accurate assessment of the risk was to be obtained, further investigations were necessary.

The use of passive sampling techniques introduced more flexibility into the monitoring process. More frequent and less intrusive monitoring could be implemented. Again, colorimetric paper tape was used but, rather than taking short-term, pumped samples, passive, 8-h samples were taken using TDI badges. Over an 8-h period, the badges were claimed by the manufacturer to be capable of measuring as little as

0.0043 mg m^{-3}. The data that resulted showed that, although many readings remained low or non-detectable, periodically a badge would reveal a higher reading, approaching or even exceeding the MEL. The smaller numbers of samples taken previously had not detected this.

The combination of health surveillance and the renewed personal monitoring programme made it apparent that, notwithstanding the introduction of dilution ventilation, adequate control of the risk had not been achieved. The risk was now identified as being *medium/high*. Further (or alternative) control measures were required.

Prevention and control

Once it was recognized that there was a significant risk to be dealt with, all practicable solutions had to be considered. Those at least initially considered were the following.

1 The substitution of TDI by a less hazardous alternative.
2 The automation of the turning in process.
3 The provision and use of local exhaust ventilation.
4 The reduction of exposure time.
5 The provision and use of PPE.
6 The provision of procedures, information and training.

Investigations were made into the viability of each of these approaches, and the following conclusions were drawn.

The possibility of replacing TDI in the adhesive formula was reconsidered, and alternative formulations were sought. This had become complicated by the fact that, due to environmental considerations, the company was committed to removing organic solvents from its spraying processes, and to ensuring that the adhesives would become water based. The adhesive suppliers were unable to develop water-based, non-isocyanate adhesives that would meet the adhesion, durability and setting time requirements Therefore, TDI still had to remain a part of the formulation.

If the use of a less hazardous replacement was not viable, then neither was it possible to remove operators from the vicinity of the process. Equipment designs had been prepared to enable 'turning in' to be automated, but these designs were not felt to be viable and development had to be discontinued.

The reduction of the exposure time was not a viable option for several reasons. Firstly, the demands of a 'just in time' production system meant that flexible working was necessary, and the hours required to be worked could vary greatly. Furthermore, job rotation was limited by the availability of skilled operators. More importantly, it was possible that the duration of exposure might not be the critical factor; rather, occasional peak exposures could be the source of the problem. The reduction of the exposure time would not therefore have guaranteed a significant reduction of risk.

The provision of PPE, such as positive pressure full facemasks fed from the compressed air system, was considered, but was regarded as a solution of last resort.

The drawing up of a revised procedure for turning in was clearly not a viable response, unless other control measures were also put in place.

It appeared therefore that the best option for control would be local exhaust ventilation. Various designs of equipment were considered with some designs being tried; a downdraught workbench with a mesh top was finally selected. The manufacture and installation of each workbench cost £3000. A number of workbenches were required. With the benches in use, the measured exposures were significantly reduced and, in most cases, were non-detectable. A programme of regular testing of the extracted benches was put in place, so as to ensure that they were functioning correctly and to their intended performance specifications.

Information, instruction and training

From the outset of the programme of assessment and control, information on the risks involved was being passed to the employees. This transmission of information regarding risks was a requirement of the company safety policy and, specifically, the section on isocyanates.

The transfer of information on health risks by means of formal training sessions or the distribution of literature was not felt to be necessary. Instead, the regular programme of lung function tests provided the opportunity for the transmission of information and advice on a one-to-one basis. Additionally, the team meetings held by each of the production areas, and attended by shop floor employees, were used as forums for the open discussion of these issues.

With regard to operational matters, integrated production procedures covering operational needs, quality and health and safety requirements were produced for the turning in process and, having been agreed by the relevant personnel, were introduced by the line supervisors via the team meetings.

Periodic auditing of all aspects of these arrangements was put in place so as to ensure that they were functioning and remained appropriate.

Review

Since the introduction of the downdraught benches (plus integrated working procedures), personal dose measurements of free isocyanates have indicated that exposures have generally fallen and are now rarely detectable. However, on rare occasions, higher readings still emerge for no apparent reason. Consequently, despite the attention given to this process, there remains a residual, although much reduced, risk.

Health surveillance testing has continued, and the lung functions of the 'turners in' have apparently ceased to deteriorate (other than the deterioration expected due to the ageing process).

Management has benefited in that disruptions to production lines no longer occur due to the redeployment of employees caused by health concerns.

This is a circumstance in which the risk was originally identified as being '*medium*'. The information provided by the monitoring and health surveillance programmes gradually made it apparent that this assessment was incorrect, and that the risk was considerably higher. The first attempt to control the risk (dilution ventilation) proved to be of slight efficacy, and it was only when local exhaust ventilation of a suitable design was introduced that broadly acceptable levels of control were achieved.

The current assessment of the situation is that the risk is *low* to *medium* and that further risk reduction measures should be implemented as they become available. The removal of TDI from the adhesive is the long-term aim, with automation of the process being the second favourite option.

References

Butcher, B.T., Jones, R.N., O'Neil, C.E., *et al.* (1977) Longitudinal study of workers employed in the manufacture of toluene diisocyanate. *American Review of Respiratory Disease* **116**, 411–421.

Chan-Yeung, M. & Malo, J.L. (1994) Aetiological agents in occupational asthma. *European Respiration Journal* 7, 346–371.

Davies, R.J. (1984) Respiratory hypersensitivity to diisocyanates. *Clinical Immunology and Allergy* **4**, 103–124.

Mapp, C.E., Saetta, M., Maestrelli, P., *et al.* (1994) Mechanism and pathology of occupational asthma. *European Respiration Journal* 7, 544–554.

Peters, J.M. & Wegman, D.H. (1975) Epidemiology and toluene diisocyanate (TDI) induced respiratory disease. *Environmental Health Perspectives* 11, 97–100.

Vandenplas, O., Malo, J.L., Saetta, M., *et al.* (1993) Occupational asthma and extrinsic alveolitis due to isocyanates: current status and perspectives. *British Journal of Industrial Medicine* 50, 213–228.

Chapter 21 Vibration

Ian J. Lawson

Introduction

This case study concerns the application of a risk assessment and management approach to the control of hand-transmitted vibration (HTV). This is a localized physical hazard arising when the hand is held directly in contact with a vibrating surface, as found in the use of hand-held vibrating tools or workpieces. Prolonged exposure to HTV can lead to a variety of effects, including those on the peripheral circulation, peripheral nerves and musculoskeletal system. The now generally accepted terminology in the UK for these effects is hand–arm vibration syndrome (HAVS) (Faculty of Occupational Medicine of the Royal College of Physicians 1993). There are numerous accounts in the literature (Griffin 1990) of the principal component: the episodic blanching of the fingers, often referred to as vibration-induced white finger (VWF). Epidemiological data presented following a workshop held in Stockholm in 1986 led to the recognition that symptoms of numbness, tingling and reduced tactile discrimination constituted a separate sensorineural component of this syndrome (Brammer *et al.* 1987). Although the vascular and sensorineural components can develop independently, more often they present and progress together. The vascular effects of HTV have been recognized since the beginning of the century, following research by Loriga (1911) and Hamilton (1918) on rock drillers and stone cutters, respectively. As a forerunner to modern day risk assessment, Hamilton (1918) referred to 'long continued muscular contractions of the fingers ... vibration of the tool ... gripping the tool too tightly ... using a worn loose air hammer ... and cold in the workplace' as contributing to the cause of this condition. Despite a number of international conferences in the last 20 years, there is still a 'lack of fundamental epidemiological data and insufficient pathophysiological knowledge' (Pelmear 1995) (... on which to base reliable quantitative risk assessments). At a more pragmatic level, these limitations need to be translated into a workable model that fulfils the requirements of the Management of Health and Safety at Work Regulations 1992 (Health and Safety Executive (HSE) 1992). This case study outlines how this translation was applied to a precision casting foundry manufacturing turbine blades for aero engines.

Defining the problem

It had been accepted for a number of years that the nature of the work in the cut-off area of the Rolls-Royce foundry in Derby had the potential to cause what was colloquially known as 'white finger'. Some employees had received disability pensions under industrial injuries provision as a prescribed disease, and some were pursuing civil litigation against the company. No formal health surveillance had been undertaken, and there had been no measure of the prevalence of cases. Furthermore, there had been no formal assessment of exposures. A decision was made to formulate a company policy that would cover issues of identification, assessment, health surveillance, case management and redeployment, information, instruction and training and exposure controls. In the first instance, this would have to be accepted by the management and employees before any further action could be taken. This was done in the form of separate management briefings and employee education. Before introducing any form of health surveillance, agreement was sought from legal, employee relations' and employee representatives on how individual cases would be managed, including the use of the company's redeployment policy for more severe cases. Exposure assessment and health surveillance in isolation may lead to a conflict in employees, who become fearful of their future employability on the one hand and the search for compensation on the other.

Description of the precision casting process

The precision casting foundry is a modern facility which uses a technique that is some 4000 years old, known as the 'ancient lost wax' process. The process is designed to manufacture hollow nickel alloy turbine blades that, when in use, operate at a higher temperature than the melting point of the alloy. The casting process has to be extremely precise, with the inclusion of hollow cores and fine holes to allow air flow and blade cooling. There are six steps to the process.

- *Step 1*. Hot wax is injected into a metal dye to form a disposable pattern. These moulds have ceramic cores which are held in place by platinum pins that will subsequently melt and form part of the alloy of the blade.
- *Step 2*. The pattern is assembled and attached to a central wax runner and base to form a cluster or assembly.
- *Step 3*. A ceramic shell is then formed around the wax pattern by dipping the assembly into a ceramic slurry and then sprinkling with refractory grain to form a ceramic-type stucco.
- *Step 4*. The wax is then melted and drained from the ceramic core by a steam autoclave to leave a cavity to subsequently receive the molten metal.
- *Step 5*. The shells are then preheated before being delivered to a

vacuum furnace where the molten metal is delivered to the shell cavity.

- *Step 6*. After cooling, the remains of the ceramic shell are 'knocked out', and each individual casting is cut from its adjacent runner by an abrasive disc; any ceramic cores are dissolved away by strong acid.

Subsequent stages include the electrical discharge machining of air flow holes, polishing, quality checks with X-ray and non-destructive testing. The vibration hazard is associated with the knock-out, cut-off and grind and subsequent polishing stages. This case study concentrates on the knock-out and cut-off and grind.

Hazard identification

Knock-out

This is carried out by a foot-operated, enclosed knock-out device and a hand-held percussive hammer (Fig. 21.1). Several moulds are knocked out during the day. In addition to the vibration hazard, there are associated hazards of noise and dust from the ceramic shell.

Cut-off and grind

The separate blades are cut from the assembly by a bench-mounted hard grind wheel, and then the individual blades are ground (Fig. 21.2). As a result of the force required to complete the task, it was common practice for a piece of wood to be used to push the blade against the grind wheel. Again, apart from the vibration, there are the associated hazards of noise, dust, wheel breakage and injury. In the absence of formal exposure levels or index cases suggesting injury, a rule of thumb

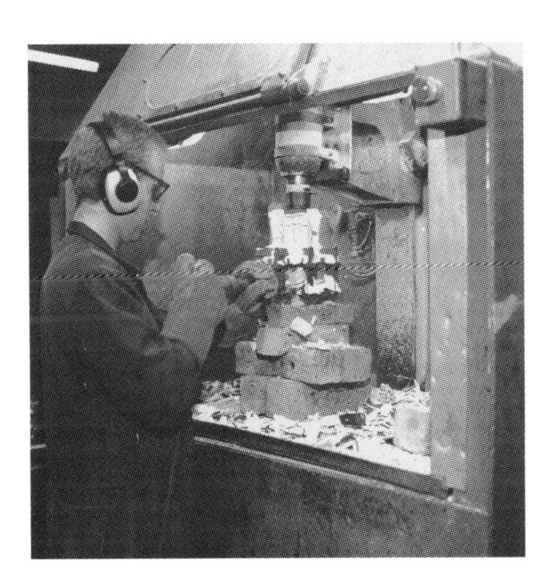

Figure 21.1 The knock-out process.

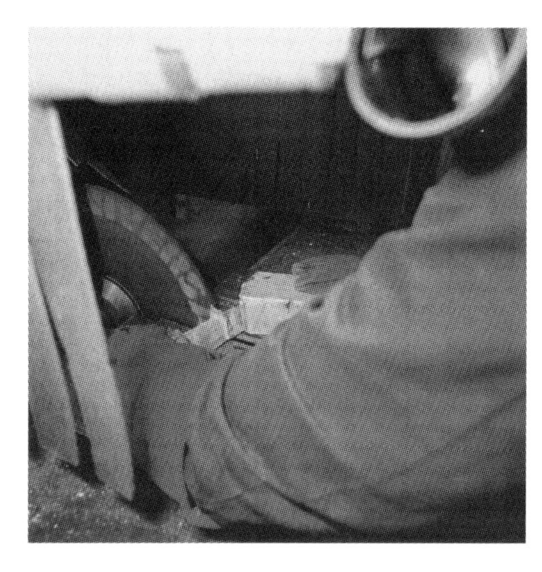

Figure 21.2 Bench-mounted hard grind wheel—cut-off process.

is to suspect any tool or machine if the employee experiences tingling or numbness after 5–10 min of continuous use (HSE 1994a). At this initial hazard identification stage, it is also important to be aware of contributory factors which may have an effect on the transmission of vibration at the hand–arm interface. These include:

- gripping forces;
- push forces;
- length and frequency of work;
- intermittency of exposure;
- posture adopted by the employee;
- local environmental conditions.

In the knock-out task, the employees were leading with the left hand on the piston end of the tool in most cases. From the postures adopted in the cut-off and grind activity, it was clear that considerable forces and awkward postures were being used. The workplace was also described as being cold by the employees during the winter months.

In addition, supplier's data on vibration magnitudes for the older equipment were unavailable.

Exposure assessment

Although a number of methods have been developed to measure the vibration magnitude, it was decided to perform measurements in accordance with British Standard recommendations (BS 6842) (British Standards Institution (BSI) 1987), and make an assessment of the average (root-mean-square, RMS) frequency-weighted acceleration ($a_{h,w}$). The most hazardous frequencies are thought to be between 5 and 20 Hz, yet those outside 2 and 1500 Hz may also be damaging. The measuring device, an accelerometer (Bruel & Kjaer type 4374), was housed in either a hand or handle adaptor (types UA 0891 and UA 0894, respectively), and allowed the measurement of the three orthogonal axes as described in BS 6842. A calculation of the vector sum was performed (unless the vibration in one axis was twice the value of the other two axes, in which case the dominant axis was taken). Having identified the tasks for each work cycle, the vibration magnitude was measured for between 5 and 15 min. Daily exposure times were measured for each of the discrete tasks, allowing partial vibration exposure to be calculated, i.e. $A_i(8)$, and then an overall 8-h value $A(8)$. The partial vibration exposure magnitude for the knock-out and cut-off tasks was calculated using $A_i(8) = a_{h,w}\sqrt{t/8}$, where t is the partial exposure time in hours. The 8-h vibration exposure magnitude was calculated using $A(8) = \sqrt{A_1(8)^2 + A_2(8)^2 + A_3(8)^2}$, where $A_1(8)$, $A_2(8)$ and $A_3(8)$ represent the partial vibration exposures. Normograms to facilitate the calculation of this daily vibration exposure have been produced (HSE 1994a). The results for the knock-out and cut-off and grind operations are shown in Table 21.1.

Risk characterization

Action levels have been recommended by the HSE (HSE 1994a), although there is no specific occupational exposure standard. Preventive programmes are recommended, including health surveillance, if the $A(8)$ value regularly exceeds 2.8 m s^{-2}. The BSI (BSI 1987) has attempted to quantify the risk in terms of the time required for 10% of the exposed population to develop finger blanching. In an attempt to produce a qualitative risk evaluation, this time period was halved and doubled to obtain high-, medium- and low-risk categories (Table 21.2). This made the operation of the knock-out and cut-off machines medium risk and the chipping hammer knock-out high risk. The overall time

Table 21.1 Daily vibration exposures.

Tasks monitored and equipment details	$a_{h,w}$(m s^{-2}) (vector sum)	Actual exposure time per shift (h)	No. of employees	$A_i(8)$ (m s^{-2})	$A(8)$ (m s^{-2})	HSE action level (h per day)
Knock-out						
Operating knock-out machine	10	1.5	15	4.3		
Pneumatic chipping hammer	30	1.5	15	13	14	0.3
Cut-off machine	6.0	3	15	3.7		

Table 21.2 Risk rating

Risk	Vibration magnitude $A(8)$ ($m\,s^{-2}$)
High	5.6
Medium	2.8
Low	>1.4

required to reach the HSE 'action level' was just 19 min per day. The application of this risk rating does not take account of gripping forces, push forces, individual factors and overtime patterns. Putting this aside, however, the overall risk of developing symptoms of HAVS was clearly high.

Health surveillance

Although a rudimentary questionnaire had been performed for some years prior to the formal assessment of exposure, and there were index cases, no systematic health surveillance had been applied. A more detailed questionnaire was introduced, including symptoms, past medical history, vibration exposure and simple screening tests. A modified form of this questionnaire was eventually adopted and published in the Faculty of Occupational Medicine Working Party Report (Aw *et al.* 1993). Vascular and sensorineural symptoms were graded in accordance with the Stockholm classification, and the results are shown in Table 21.3. All cases had some neurological symptoms, with 67% reporting finger blanching. This contrasted with the mean prevalence of 18% blanching experienced by 672 employees exposed to HTV screened that year across all Rolls-Royce sites in Derby. In 1996, objective testing was introduced, including cold provocation testing, vibrotactile thresholds, thermal aesthesiometry, two point discrimination and grip strength (Lawson & Nevell 1997). These tests supported the level and degree of symptoms experienced by the employees in the foundry. The mean latency for the onset of symptoms was 2.4 years. The surveillance regime was extended to include pre-employment or initial assessment for transferred employees, six monthly assessment in the first year and annual assessment thereafter.

Prevention and control

Having characterized the risk as significant, a programme of preventive measures was introduced. Initial discussions with management centred

Table 21.3 Stockholm classification: cut-off and knock-out employees.

	Stockholm sensorineural stage			Stockholm vascular stage		
Number at risk	1	2	3	1	2	3
15	8	7		3	7	

on the practicality of using traditional occupational hygiene control measures, such as elimination, substitution, minimization and reduction of exposure. All potential solutions had to be assessed in terms of practicality and cost implications. The review undertaken considered the following control measures.

1 Elimination of the hazard by automation or robotization.
2 Substitution by lower vibration processes and antivibration tools.
3 Minimization of vibration transmitted to the hand–arm system.
4 A reduction in exposure time.
5 Information, instruction and training on the correct operating procedures.
6 Regular planned maintenance.
7 Purchase specification for new tools and equipment.

Ideally, the responsible manager, engineering manager, design department and purchasing department should be involved in discussions, although this was found to be difficult to achieve in practice.

Where it was problematic to eliminate completely or substitute for a low-vibration process, consideration was given to the design of the metal dyes and clusters for the wax mould in an attempt to avoid the need for metal removal later in the process. This was quickly discarded as an idea, because of the specialized nature of the process and customer specifications. Concentration was then turned to processes of greatest risk as a priority. Enquiries to trade associations and manufacturers of low-vibration equipment identified a 'hands-free' shell removal device at a cost of £8000 (Fig. 21.3). Initial trials were successful, and a further two machines were installed in an acoustic booth to eliminate the associated dust and noise exposure. Apart from a small amount of chipping hammer removal on certain workpieces, the knock-out process was effectively automated.

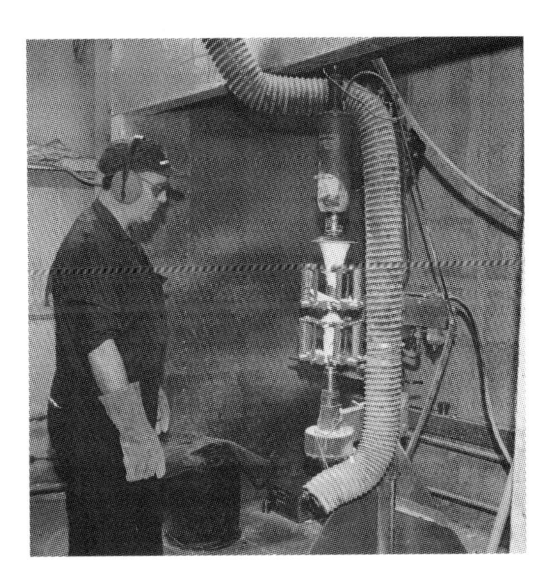

Figure 21.3 Trials using Herschal equipment to give 'hands-free' shell removal have proved to be successful.

The next stage was to look at the cut-off. A number of fixtures and jigs were designed to hold the cast clusters. A vibration isolating handle was used to present the grind wheel to the workpiece (Fig. 21.4). The $a_{h,w}$ value was reduced to below $2\,m\,s^{-2}$, amounting to a significant reduction in the magnitude of risk. However, the amount of fixtures and jigs that could be adapted for this type of machine was limited to a small number of parts. Further discussions with tool suppliers and employees' requirements led to the trial of a totally enclosed system. This equipment operated by fixing the workpiece and then feeding the grind wheel by an externally operated wheel. The whole cutting operation was viewed via a suitably placed mirror (Fig. 21.5).

The original cost of the machine was £21 000; after 6 months of use,

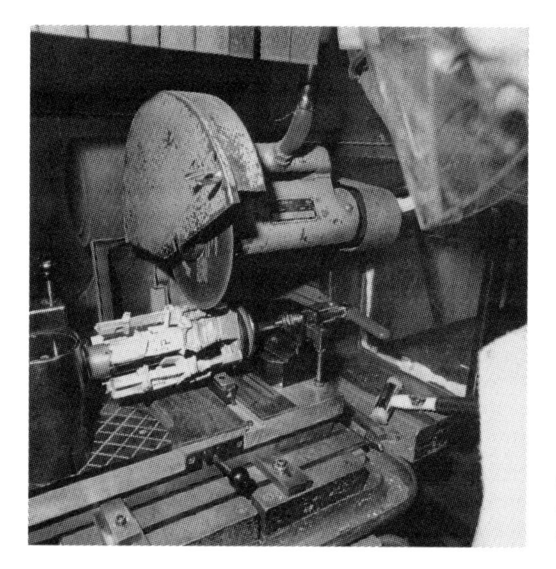

Figure 21.4 Cut-off process—intermediate solution removing the hazard of vibration and hand–wheel contact.

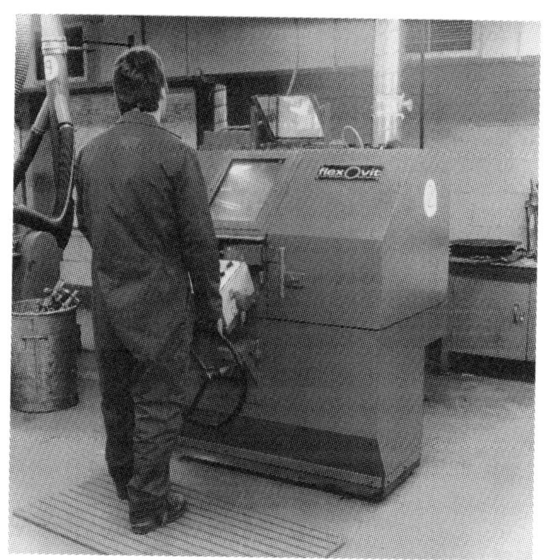

Figure 21.5 Totally enclosed cut-off machine eliminating all hazards.

it was realized that softer grind wheels could be employed, giving a 10-fold increase in usage time with the potential for £14 000 saving per year.

The mathematical relationship between the vibration magnitude and the exposure time, as shown by the equation given above, requires a large reduction in exposure time before any significant effect is seen on the vibration magnitude. There was little opportunity to rotate the tasks to those not involving HTV, and this was not seen by management as a practical option.

Information, instruction and training

The provision of information to employees on the hazard and associated risk of HTV was an integral part of the company policy. Information on the recognition of symptoms was given to all employees and supported by an advice leaflet. Employee leaflets have been produced by the HSE (HSE 1994b), and a modified version used at Rolls-Royce is shown in Table 21.4.

Following health surveillance, employees were advised of the stage that their condition had reached, and whether or not they needed to consider alternative employment. This advice was in accordance with guidance produced by the Faculty of Occupational Medicine of the

Table 21.4 Information leaflet. (From Lawson 1996.)

IMPORTANT ADVICE TO THOSE USING VIBRATING TOOLS AND EQUIPMENT

If you use vibrating tools or equipment, it is possible that you could develop a condition known as the 'hand–arm vibration syndrome' (HAVS) or 'vibration white finger' (VWF). If symptoms do develop they are usually mild, e.g. tingling, numbness or occasional whiteness of the fingertips; however, in some people, these symptoms may be more severe. The symptoms are normally triggered by cold weather.

Before you undertake work with vibrating tools or equipment, you should be aware of this risk and that, in exceptional cases, symptoms of HAVS could become apparent within a short time of taking on such work.

What can you do to reduce the possibility of this happening?

- Please report to the occupational health staff immediately any episodes of numbness or blanching in the fingers occur, or if there has been a deterioration in symptoms.
- Attend routine health surveillance when required to do so by the occupational health department.
- Try and keep yourself and your hands warm at all times.
- Tell your supervisor immediately if your machine or hand-held tool is vibrating abnormally.
- When using grinding wheels, ensure that the wheel is true, and always use the tool provided to dress the wheel.
- If the occupational health department gives you advice, take it.

Royal College of Physicians (1993). In a larger workforce, where there are opportunities for redeployment, this is considered to be a reasonable approach to take in the short term, whilst waiting for the effects of control measures in the longer term. Where there are limitations in terms of redeployment options, greater emphasis should be placed on the early control and reduction of an individual's exposure. It is also important to instruct and train the employee on good working practices, and to give guidance on how to grip tools appropriately without the need for excessive force. Although tool maintenance was implemented by management as part of a planned programme, advice was given to employees on the importance of reporting machines or tools that vibrated abnormally and were not running true. General advice was given on keeping the body and hands warm at work and during leisure activities.

Review

The incidence of new cases and the progression of established cases have significantly improved since the implementation of the company policy in the precision casting facility process. Management has seen the benefit in terms of the health of employees, their performance and the cost–benefit ratios of some of the control measures introduced. Since the original risk assessment, suppliers, manufacturers, designers, etc. have a responsibility under the Supply of Machinery Safety Regulations 1992 to provide information on vibration levels if hand-held or hand-guided machinery is likely to subject workers to vibration ($a_{h,w}$) exceeding $2.5\ \mathrm{m\,s^{-2}}$. Coupled with programmes to maintain the control measures, there should eventually be an elimination of HAVS from the precision casting facility.

References

Aw, T.C., Fox, J.E., Griffin, M.J., *et al.* (1993) *Hand-transmitted Vibration: Clinical Effects and Pathophysiology. Report of a Working Party.* Royal College of Physicians, London.

Brammer, A.J., Taylor, W. & Lundborg, G. (1987) Sensorineural stages of the hand arm vibration syndrome. *Scandinavian Journal of Work and Environmental Health* 13, 279–283.

BSI (1987) BS 6842. *Guide to Measurements and Evaluation of Human Exposure to Vibration Transmitted to the Hand.* BSI, London.

Griffin, M.J. (1990) *Handbook of Human Vibration.* Academic Press, London.

Hamilton, A. (1918) *A Study of Spastic Anaemia in the Hands of Stonecutters.* United States Bureau of Labor Statistics (part 19), Bulletin 236, pp. 53–66. United States Bureau of Labor, Washington DC.

HSE (1992) *Management of Health and Safety at Work Regulations 1992. Approved Code of Practice.* HMSO, London.

HSE (1994a) *Hand–arm Vibration.* HS(G)88. HSE Books, Sudbury, Suffolk.

HSE (1994b) *Hand–arm Vibration: Advice on Vibration White Finger for Employees and the Self-employed.* IND(G)126(L).
Lawson, I.J. (1996) Vibration. In: *Croner's Management of Health Risks* (ed. L. Falconer), Chapter 3-175–3-229, Fig. 7, p. 3-204. Croner Publications, Kingston-upon-Thames, Surrey.
Lawson, I.J. & Nevell, D.A. (1997) Review of objective tests for the hand arm vibration syndrome. *Occupational Medicine* **47**, 15–20.
Loriga, G. (1911) Il lavoro con i martelli pneumatici. *Boll Inspett Lavoro* **2**, 35–60.
Pelmear, P. (1995) Noise and vibration. In: *Epidemiology of Work Related Diseases* (ed. J. Corbett McDonald), pp. 185–205. BMJ Publishing Group, London.

Chapter 22 Risk management and manual handling

Philip Wynn and Keith Pilling

Introduction

Musculoskeletal problems are the single largest group of disorders seen by occupational health physicians working in industry. This includes overuse syndromes, such as tenosynovitis, but back pain forms the largest subgroup and is experienced by 80% of the working population during their working lives. Sickness absence from back pain alone has been estimated to result in £2000 million per year (1987–1988) in lost output in the UK and, in the USA, costs $18 000 in medical expenses for each back care patient and $22 000 in terms of loss of income and related benefits (Ratti & Pilling 1997). The case study in this chapter focuses primarily on back pain due to its importance as a cause of morbidity and economic cost.

Some low back pain (LBP) has a serious underlying cause, such as cancer, abscess or ankylosing spondylitis (less than 1% of total) or prolapsed intervertebral disc (15% of total). The majority, however, is classified as simple or 'mechanical' LBP, although only a small proportion of cases have an identifiable mechanical abnormality.

Manual handling carries a significant risk of back injury. In addition, the frequent bending and twisting movements involved in manual handling in many manufacturing jobs increases the likelihood of low back disability, doubling that of lighter occupations (Garg & Moore 1992).

However, the pathogenesis of back pain is not clearly understood; some estimates attribute only 20% of the incidence to manual handling in the general population. Low back pain is experienced in all professions—from heavy industrial to light office work—and despite a decline in numbers employed in heavy manufacturing in Western countries over recent years an exponential increase in sickness absence from back pain has been seen. The greatest risk factors for the development of back pain are previous history of the condition, smoking, psychological stresses at work (including job dissatisfaction, high workload and monotony), the operation of vibrating machinery and even the length of commuting (Niedhammer *et al.* 1994; Clinical Standards Advisory Group 1994). In those who develop mechanical LBP, those who keep active and exercise within the limits of the pain experience a faster recovery and an earlier return to work (Malmivaara *et al.* 1995).

Options for the prevention of back pain in industry

Medical screening

1 *Radiological screening.* The use of pre-employment low back X-rays to identify various structural abnormalities has been shown to have a high false negative and false positive rate when compared with symptoms, and the radiation exposure delivered by the investigation is an unacceptable health risk in radiological terms (Garg & Moore 1992).
2 *Medical history.* The strongest predictor for future back pain is a previous history, and this question is frequently included on pre-employment questionnaires. The sensitivity has been found to be limited to 25% by a lack of veracity in questionnaire responses. In addition, this approach can discriminate against older workers who are more likely to have had an episode of LBP, and it also has no predictive value in young workers who have yet to develop an episode (Garg & Moore 1992). However, the clinical examination and review of specialist reports (where available) by industrial occupational health physicians of potential employees with more severe back problems allow recommendations to be made regarding suitability or the need for job adaptation. This is of particular concern in meeting the requirements of legislation, e.g. the Disability Discrimination Act 1995 in the UK, which requires that those with disability should not be excluded from work that functionally they may be able to perform with or without reasonable adaptation.
3 *Anthropometry.* An overhead operation that can only be safely performed by a 6-ft employee should not be given to a 5-ft employee. However, more general attempts to predict the development of LBP based on age, sex, height, reach, etc. have been disappointing and can be discriminatory.
4 *Pre-employment strength testing.* The instinctive belief that those in jobs which require a lifting strength in excess of their own will experience more LBP has been borne out by research evidence. The use of isometric strength testing in the pre-employment examination has been shown to reduce the incidence of LBP, when such testing is based on the specific strength requirements of each individual job (Garg & Moore 1992). Although this approach has been adopted by some organizations, the logistical difficulties of assessing each job have resulted in single limits being set for relatively broad ranges of jobs which are of unproven value.

Training

The teaching of lifting and handling techniques has not been clearly shown to reduce the incidence of LBP when used alone. It may, however, have a role to play in combination with other interventions (Garg & Moore 1992).

Ergonomic job design

The use of ergonomic principles, intended to reduce workplace hazards by the better matching of the workplace to the employee, aims to minimize the risks inherent in manual handling tasks. Design changes to the workplace aim to reduce or eliminate load handling and bring all jobs within the capability of every employee. The strong evidence for the deleterious effect of manual handling on the incidence of LBP has made this approach the cornerstone of the primary prevention of LBP in many industrial companies.

Legislative requirements

To identify the possibility of manual handling injury, the UK Management of Health and Safety at Work Regulations 1992 (Health and Safety Executive (HSE) 1992a) state that employers should make a 'suitable and sufficient assessment of the risks to health and safety of their employees while at work. Where this general assessment indicates the possibility of risks to employees from the manual handling of loads, the requirements of the Manual Handling Operations Regulations (MHOR) 1992 should be considered' (HSE 1992b).

The MHOR apply to all employment in the UK requiring the manipulation of loads, involving repetitive movements, substantial forces, gross bodily movements or awkward postures, and are derived from European Union (EU) legislation. Their intention is to control these and related factors which may contribute to work-related musculoskeletal injury, i.e. back pain or related to any other part of the body.

Employers have the ultimate responsibility for assessments, but any competent individual (including health and safety personnel) may carry them out. In practice, they are usually performed by the line manager who has an understanding of the tasks to be performed. Those involved in the risk assessment of manual tasks require familiarization with the MHOR and guidance on work-related upper limb disorders to ensure competence. In combination with tuition in the ergonomic evaluation of the workplace, this background enables the identification of potential risks in the specific organizational environment, rather than simply seeking out well-recognized general risk factors, and should ensure a 'suitable and sufficient' assessment. If such training is not available, an independent, suitably qualified assessor is preferable.

Assessment of manual handling risks

Many processes identified as being a risk cannot be eliminated entirely for technological or economic reasons. Such processes require a more quantitative level of risk in order to identify and measure tasks that need to be adapted to within accepted limits. Two examples are given below.

1 *Handling capability under standardized conditions (e.g. Appendix 1 MHOR, National Institute for Occupational Safety and Health (NIOSH) guidelines)*. These data offer numerical guidelines for a range of basic manual handling procedures, such as lifting and lowering, twisting and pushing and pulling. They are based on research involving these simple processes performed under standardized conditions. The intention is for the assessor to estimate the actual risk in the more complex tasks performed from these basic 'building blocks'. Although there is no threshold below which manual handling operations may be regarded as 'safe', this guidance seeks to act as a filter, creating a boundary above which the need for a more detailed assessment and remedial action is likely. The figures quoted are not limits.

In the industrial environment, even mildly adverse ergonomic factors may lead to major problems due to the repetitive nature of the tasks performed. Consequently, *exposure* to potentially hazardous tasks requires assessment, in addition to the *biomechanical* factors outlined above. This aspect of assessment has been less clearly evaluated, but recommendations in UK legislation for biomechanical factors apply to those not exceeding around 30 operations per hour, where the pace is not forced, adequate pauses for rest or recovery are possible, and the load is not supported for any length of time. These quantitative targets are necessarily vague due to the difficulties of characterizing all possible handling tasks with reference to exposure times.

In general, these recommendations are too complex for use by non-ergonomically trained personnel. In a large organization with many manual handling problems, the assessment of all potentially hazardous operations poses logistical difficulties to a small health and safety department, making the use of assessment protocols requiring detailed ergonomic knowledge unfeasible.

2 *Ergonomic rating scales*. These scales have been formulated to quantify common risks within specific industries, and can be applied by trained health and safety professionals or line managers. The aim is to allow tasks to be adjusted to fall within safer levels set by the legislation using simple semiquantitative descriptions of common manoeuvres. Few, if any, have been validated.

Both approaches, whilst offering good general guidance, do not claim to offer protection to all workers and, in some instances, it may be acceptable to exceed the limits on the basis of a more detailed assessment. The guidance values given in Appendix 1 of MHOR aim to protect 95% of male workers and, for women, a reduction in loads by one-third is required to achieve the same level of protection. The approaches make little or no allowance for build, strength or age, necessitating a subjective estimate of capability in terms of these factors in the individual worker. As general guidelines, their application can be difficult, and they are of limited applicability to the complex manoeuvres required in manufacturing industry.

These approaches do, however, provide a goal which can be aimed

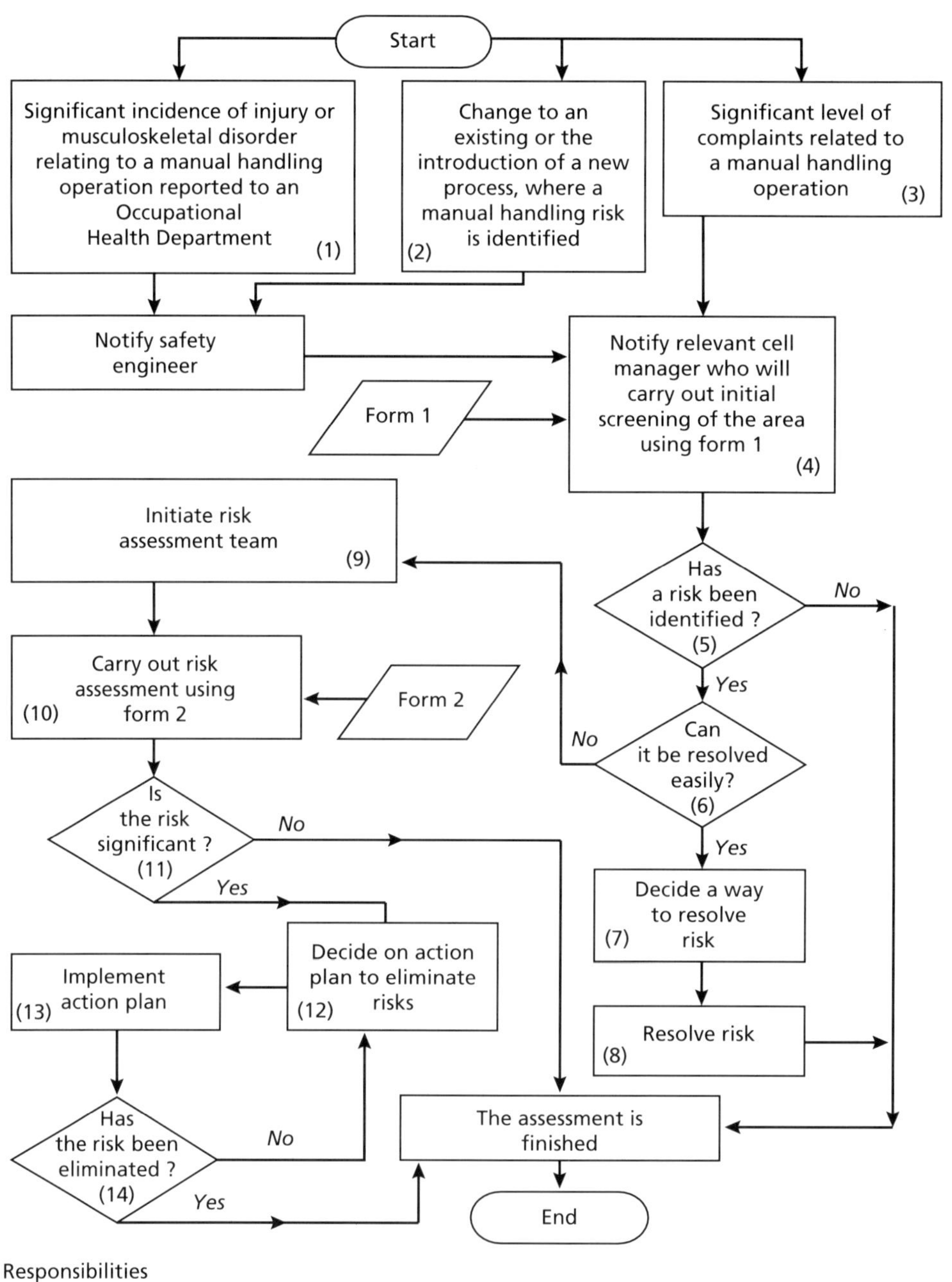

Responsibilities

1. Occupational Health Nursing staff
2. Process/Project Engineer
3. Supervisor/Team Leader
4. Safety Engineer
5. Cell Manager
6. Cell Manager
7. Cell Manager
8. Cell Manager
9. Cell Manager
10. Risk Assessment Team
11. Risk Assessment Team
12. Risk Assessment Team
13. Cell Manager
14. Cell Manager

Figure 22.1 Manual handling risk assessment procedure (note that form 1 is Fig. 22.3 and form 2 is Fig. 22.4).

for and exceeded, but do not replace the need to ensure that the task matches the individual employee.

Case study

Introduction

This case study relates to a large motor vehicle assembly plant employing 14 000, mostly male, workers. Each production line employee performs a restricted number of manual tasks, the cycle time (speed of repetition) of which is governed by the speed of the continuous track along which the vehicles travel, which is set within agreed limits.

Similar to other industrial sites, musculoskeletal problems are common. In 1993, back pain and other musculoskeletal disorders, both doctor and self-certified, resulted in 66 000 lost days at a cost of £3.3 million. This represented 3.7 days per person per year or 35% of all sickness absence. Consequently, the assessment and management of potentially high-risk procedures are seen by the company as an important part of employee care, with the byproducts of improved efficiency and quality of the final product.

The company policy for the primary prevention of ergonomic musculoskeletal problems has, where possible, been based on ergonomic research evidence as well as legislative requirements.

Hazard identification

Figure 22.1 outlines the routes by which concern regarding a manual handling task may arise and the subsequent management. In addition, each line manager applies a general risk assessment form (Fig. 22.2) to his/her area, which requires the consideration of all possible hazards covered by legislation, and this may highlight problems independently.

Line managers are responsible for the health and safety problems in their areas, as they are most aware of the tasks involved, and have a vested interest in minimizing lost time through injury and illness in order to meet production targets. This approach has been questioned due to a possible lack of training leading to the non-recognition of hazards (Graves 1993). To avoid this situation, line managers receive instruction in general risk assessment and basic ergonomics.

As a result of the assessment and the additional data outlined below, particular concern regarding the prevalence of low back problems on a section of the track involved in the fitting of car wheels was raised.

1 Sickness absence data—where the cause may be related to tasks performed at work.

2 Self-reported injury—of musculoskeletal problems to the local occupational health department.

3 Employee comments—to line managers and nursing staff.

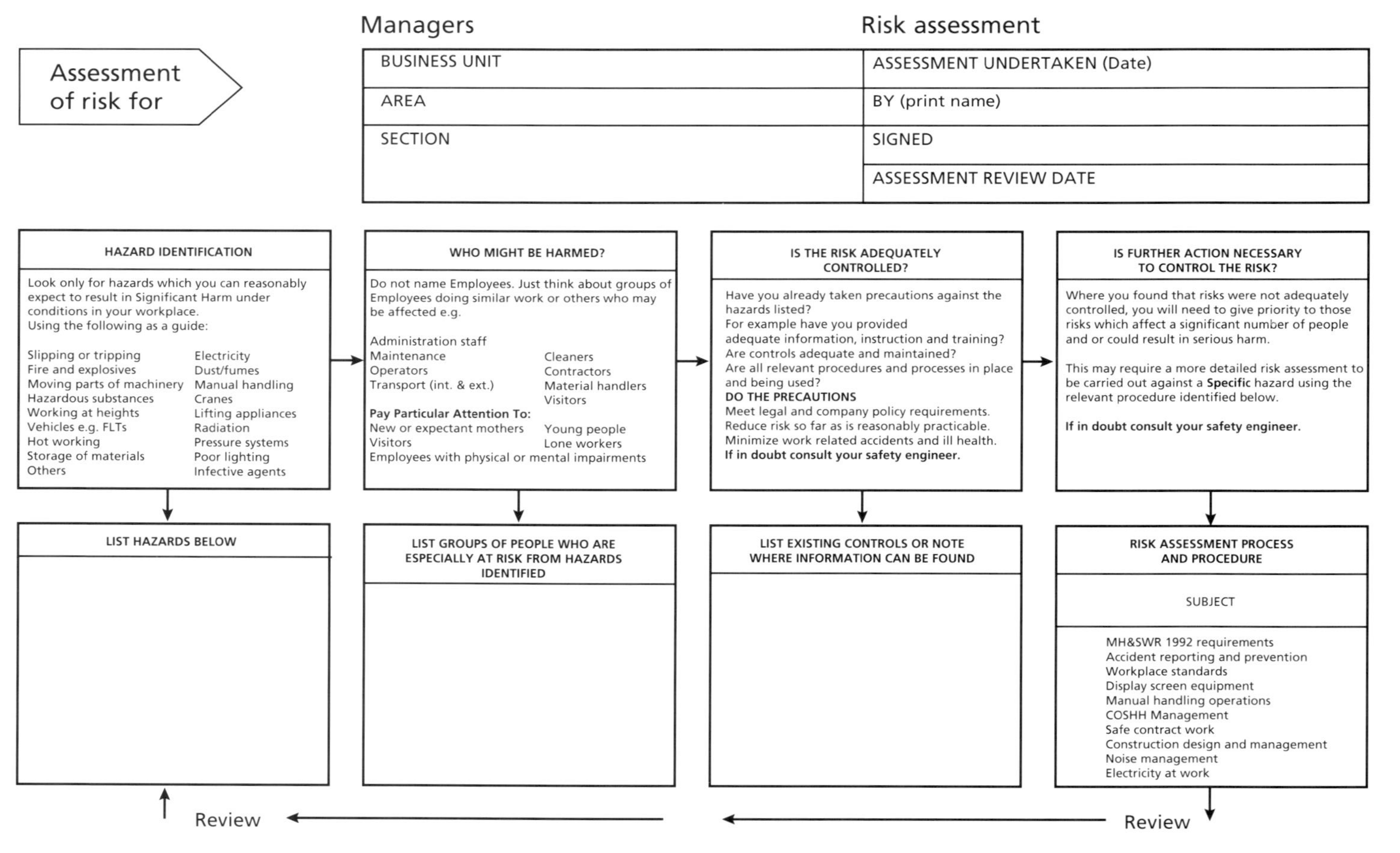

Assessment of risk for

Managers | Risk assessment

BUSINESS UNIT	ASSESSMENT UNDERTAKEN (Date)
AREA	BY (print name)
SECTION	SIGNED
	ASSESSMENT REVIEW DATE

HAZARD IDENTIFICATION

Look only for hazards which you can reasonably expect to result in Significant Harm under conditions in your workplace.
Using the following as a guide:

Slipping or tripping	Electricity
Fire and explosives	Dust/fumes
Moving parts of machinery	Manual handling
Hazardous substances	Cranes
Working at heights	Lifting appliances
Vehicles e.g. FLTs	Radiation
Hot working	Pressure systems
Storage of materials	Poor lighting
Others	Infective agents

WHO MIGHT BE HARMED?

Do not name Employees. Just think about groups of Employees doing similar work or others who may be affected e.g.

Administration staff	
Maintenance	Cleaners
Operators	Contractors
Transport (int. & ext.)	Material handlers
	Visitors

Pay Particular Attention To:

New or expectant mothers	Young people
Visitors	Lone workers

Employees with physical or mental impairments

IS THE RISK ADEQUATELY CONTROLLED?

Have you already taken precautions against the hazards listed?
For example have you provided adequate information, instruction and training?
Are controls adequate and maintained?
Are all relevant procedures and processes in place and being used?
DO THE PRECAUTIONS
Meet legal and company policy requirements.
Reduce risk so far as is reasonably practicable.
Minimize work related accidents and ill health.
If in doubt consult your safety engineer.

IS FURTHER ACTION NECESSARY TO CONTROL THE RISK?

Where you found that risks were not adequately controlled, you will need to give priority to those risks which affect a significant number of people and or could result in serious harm.

This may require a more detailed risk assessment to be carried out against a **Specific** hazard using the relevant procedure identified below.

If in doubt consult your safety engineer.

LIST HAZARDS BELOW

LIST GROUPS OF PEOPLE WHO ARE ESPECIALLY AT RISK FROM HAZARDS IDENTIFIED

LIST EXISTING CONTROLS OR NOTE WHERE INFORMATION CAN BE FOUND

RISK ASSESSMENT PROCESS AND PROCEDURE

SUBJECT

MH&SWR 1992 requirements
Accident reporting and prevention
Workplace standards
Display screen equipment
Manual handling operations
COSHH Management
Safe contract work
Construction design and management
Noise management
Electricity at work

Review ← ← Review

Figure 22.2 General workplace risk assessment form.

Risk assessment

Once a hazard has been identified, the line manager applies an initial screening tool (Fig. 22.3) and a risk assessment form (Fig. 22.4). This further assesses *biomechanical* risk factors in manual handling tasks. These are subdivided into the *task*, the *load*, the *working environment* and *individual capacity*, not all of which will be relevant in every case. The consideration of these factors, in tandem with a good understanding of the specific tasks required, enables the line manager to decide whether a more detailed assessment is required to establish a need to reduce such hazards.

The tasks performed in the suspect areas involved the transfer of the wheel and inflated tyre from a pallet across 1.5 m of level floor to the side of the track. There the wheel, weighing 20.2 kg (45 lb), was lifted 1.4 m from floor level to the axles, and fitted with nuts using a counter-

Name: Job/title:

Location:

Description of area/process(es):

Tick Yes or No to the following questions:

	Question	Yes	No
1.	**Do the Manual Handling Operations present a risk to injury?** Yes = Proceed No = Assessment finished		
2.	**Is there a significant manual handling risk?** Yes = Proceed No = Assessment finished		
3.	**Can the operations be avoided/mechanized/or automated, at a reasonable cost and without initiating Risk Assessment Team?** Yes = Do so and check the result is satisfactory No = Initiate Risk Assessment Team, assess the risk using form 2, decide upon and implement action plan to eliminate risk.		

Figure 22.3 Initial screening form.

Details of assessment (Operation(s) covered by this assessment)			
Process identification number: [ ] Location: [ ]			
Cell number: [ ] Team no.: [ ] Manager: [ ]			
Assessor(s) name(s):			No. of persons involved: [ ]
(A) Assessing the task: Does the Associate....	Yes	No	Comments
1. Hold or manipulate the load at a distance from the body?			
2. Twist their upper body when picking up or putting down the load?			
3. Reach upwards to lift or deposit the load?			
4. Move the load from a high to low point?			
5. Move the load from a low to high point?			
6. Carry the load across distances of approximately 10 m or more?			
7. Use a lot of effort to push or pull the object?			
8. Have to cope with unpredictable movement of the object?			
9. Handle the object repeatedly?			
10. Have sufficient time to rest and recover from the effort of the handling task?			
11. Have little or no control over their pace or rate of work?			
(B) Assessing the load: Is the load....			
1. Heavy? (use guidelines over page for reference)			
2. Of a shape or size which makes it difficult to pick up?			
3. Difficult to take a firm hold of?			
4. Likely to move unpredictably when picked up or, is it unstable?			
5. Likely to injure the Associate due to its sharp edges, rough surface, temperature, etc.?			
(C) Assessing the environment: Does the working environment have....			
1. Little space for the Associate to work comfortably and maintain good postures?			
2. Uneven, broken or slippy floor surfaces?			
3. Different floor levels or work surfaces on which the Associate works?			
4. Extreme temperature or climatic conditions such as being hot, cold or humid?			
5. Strong draughts, or poor ventilation?			
6. Poor lighting conditions?			
(D) Individual capability: Does the job....			
1. Require the Associate to have unusual strength, height, etc.?			
2. Place Associates with health problems in a problem situation?			
3. Place pregnant women at risk?			
4. Require special training to carry it out safely?			
(E) Assessing other factors			
1. Is the job made more difficult by clothing or the use of PPE?			
2.			
3.			

Figure 22.4 Manual handling operations risk assessment procedure form.

balanced air tool. Two employees divided the tasks thus: employee 1 performed the above tasks on the near side of the vehicle; employee 2 performed the same tasks on the far side of the vehicle, plus carrying a

Guidelines for acceptable weights

Forward lift		45 degree twist		90 degree twist	
10 kg	5 kg	9 kg	4 kg	8 kg	4 kg
20 kg	10 kg	18 kg	9 kg	16 kg	8 kg
25 kg	15 kg	22 kg	13 kg	20 kg	12 kg
20 kg	10 kg	18 kg	9 kg	16 kg	8 kg
10 kg	5 kg	9 kg	4 kg	8 kg	4 kg

The figures left, should only be used as a guide to acceptable weights. If other factors are acceptable themselves, the above weights may be exceeded. If other factors are unacceptable the weights may prove too high.

Notes of actions taken

Assessment undertaken by the following team:

Manager Signature Date	Others:

Figure 22.4 *Continued.*

spare tyre up four steps from the right side of the vehicle for placement in the boot.

The two operations described were shared full time between the employees. Each operation was alternated at 2-h intervals for an 8-h shift. The cycle time for each operation was approximately 2 min. This was interpreted as a high exposure as 30 cycles were performed per hour—involving at least 60 episodes of load (wheel) handling.

Other features of concern raised by the assessment were as follows.

1 The tasks:
- placement of the tyre on the axle required manipulation of the load at a distance from the trunk;
- removal of the tyre from the pallet and placement on the axle required stooping and reaching upwards;
- excessive lifting distances at axle and during placement of spare in the boot;
- excessive pulling forces to dislodge tyres from the pallet;
- frequent and prolonged physical effort;
- insufficient rest/recovery periods;
- a rate of handling imposed by the process.

2 The loads: in excess of range suggested by the MHOR.

3 The working environment: variations in levels of work due to steps up which the tyre needed to be carried for placement in the boot of the vehicle.

4 Individual capacity:
- the weight of the load and the carrying heights required a worker of greater than usual height and strength;
- the process would create a hazard to a pregnant worker.

5 Other factors: nil.

The company is piloting an ergonomic rating scale which rates manual handling activities (Fig. 22.5). Twenty parameters are measured, including the required height, mobility of arms, overhead work, lifting and carrying, noise, climate, lighting and shift work. This approach was chosen as the scale is industry specific, being used by other motor vehicle manufacturers, is straightforward to apply by the occupational health and safety team or line manager and allows a consistent company-wide approach. The activities are rated at one of three levels: g (green), design objective met; a (amber), action required; r (red), high priority action required. All r-rated processes are acted on immediately, whereas an a rating, if in isolation, will be addressed less urgently unless there is an exacerbating environmental factor, such as noise or lighting. In an attempt to gain an overall impression of the risk, the multiple processes performed by each employee with a- and r-rated activities are summed as a total ergonomic score. How this score equates with adverse clinical outcomes is currently being validated.

Risk control

Once the risk has been identified, the possibility of the elimination of handling is considered first, followed by the automation or mechanization of the process. Where these are not practical options, remedial

Analysis conducted: Date: .... by:	Short reference: ....

Workplace data: No.: ....

?: .... ?: ....

Plant: .... Brief ref: ....

Building: Floor:

Workplace designation:

....

Remarks:

....

Foreman	Present?
1st shift:	☐
2nd shift:	☐
Safety officer:	☐
Planner:	☐

Number of workers/shift involved: ......

010 Required height

Activity suitable for workers between 150 cm and 195 cm in height	g	011	
Activity suitable only for workers taller than 165 cm	g	012	
Activity suitable only for workers shorter than 185 cm	g	013	
Activity suitable only for workers with a height between 165 cm and 185 cm	a	014	

020 Mobility of arms (including shoulder joint)

Movements required for a reach up to 30 cm	g	021	
Movements required for a reach up to 60 cm	g	022	
Movements required for a reach up to 80 cm	a	023	

030 Frequent muscle load of arms and shoulders during activities when sitting

No handling or handling with expenditure of effort < 10 N	g	031	
Handling with expenditure of effort < 50 N	g	032	
Handling with expenditure of effort < 80 N	a	033	
Handling with expenditure of effort > 80 N	r	034	

Legend: *the abbreviations used in the second column mean:*
g = design objective met ***r = design work urgently required***
a = design work required

040 Frequent muscle load of arms and shoulders during activities when standing

No handling or handling with expenditure of effort < 25 N	g	041	
Handling with expenditure of effort < 120 N	g	042	
Handling with expenditure of effort < 180 N	a	043	
Handling with expenditure of effort > 180 N	r	044	

050 Load on lower arms/wrist caused by impact, pressure or turning movements

occasional load	g	051	
frequent load	a	052	
constant load	r	053	

060 Overhead work

No handling above shoulder height	g	061	
occasional handling without fundamental application of force < 10 N	g	062	
frequent handling without fundamental application of force < 10 N	a	063	
handling with brief application of force	a	064	
frequent handling with prolonged holding work	r	065	

070 Finger dexterity

No finger dexterity or operation only with closed fist	g	071	
full dexterity of fingers	g	072	
highest demands in difficult conditions	a	073	

080 Mobility of the trunk

slight turning and bending movements	g	081	
turning < 15 degrees, bending < 30 degrees	g	082	
full mobility: turning < 35 degrees bending < 90 degrees	a	083	
full mobility in difficult conditions	r	084	

090 Mobility of the hip joints

slight mobility, e.g. walking	g	091	
mobility (bending angle < 90 degrees)	g	092	
full mobility: bending angle > 90 degrees	a	093	
frequently more prolonged extension beyond 90 degrees	r	094	

100 Mobility of the knee joints

slight mobility, e.g. walking	g	101	
mobility (bending angle < 90 degrees) e.g. sitting	g	102	
full mobility: bending angle > 90 degrees	a	103	
frequently more prolonged extension beyond 90 degrees and/or twisting	r	104	

110 Mobility of the ankles

slight mobility, e.g. walking	g	111	
full mobility of ankles	g	112	
frequently more prolonged full extention	a	113	

Caution ! *the graduations used in the features have been defined as follows:*
occasional: *less than 5% of shift time*
frequent: *between 5% and 30% of shift time*
constant: *more than 30% of shift time*

Figure 22.5 Manual handling assessment form using ergonomic rating scales.

120 Lifting and carrying

no lifting/carrying or weight <1 kg	g	121	
frequent lifting/carrying <5 kg occasionally <10 kg	g	122	
frequent lifting/carrying <10 kg occasionally <18 kg	a	123	
lifting/carrying <18 kg occasionally <50 kg	a	124	
lifting/carrying >18 kg occasionally >50 kg	r	125	
constant lifting/carrying >10 kg	r	126	

130 Lifting and carrying: ergonomic preconditions

ergonomically favourable conditions	g	131	
occasional lifting and carrying in unfavourable conditions	a	132	
frequent lifting and carrying in unfavourable conditions	r	133	

140 Standing

standing, but possible to alternate with sitting/walking	g	141	
constant standing	a	142	
standing not possible or only occasionally	a	143	
constant standing in difficult conditions required	r	144	

150 Walking

walking, but possible to alternate with sitting/standing	g	151	
constant walking	g	152	
walking not possible or only occasionally	a	153	
constant walking in difficult conditions required	r	154	

160 Sitting

sitting, but possible to alternate with walking/standing	g	161	
constant sitting	a	162	
sitting not possible or only occasionally	a	163	
constant sitting in difficult conditions required	r	164	

170 Noise

Assessment level < ceiling value	g	171	
Assessment level < 90 dB(A) but > ceiling value	a	172	
Assessment level > 90 dB(A) or 85 dB(A) incl. pulsed noise	r	173	

Ceiling value: 55 dB(A) for predominantly mental activities
70 dB(A) for simple mental activities
85 dB(A) for other activities

180 Climate

Climatic conditions in comfort range	g	181	
climatic conditions outside comfort range, depending on season	a	182	
constant stress outside the comfort range	r	183	

Measured values:
illumination ______ *Lux*
noise: ______ *dB(A)*
max. weights: ______ *kg*

190 Visual power/illumination

Requirement of visual power under adequate lighting	g	191	
Requirement of visual power. Lighting does not correspond with the work task (lighting > 50% of the reference value)	a	192	
Requirement of visual power under poor lighting (<50% of the reference value)	r	193	

Reference values: simple visual tasks min. >250 Lux
higher visual tasks min. >500 Lux
fine visual tasks min. >750 Lux
very fine visual tasks min. >1000 Lux

200 Oscillations/vibrations

no particular load caused by oscillations	g	201	
increased load caused by oscillations	a	202	

210 Hazardous materials in the working area

not present	g	211	
present and tested < initiation threshold	g	212	
present and tested < initiation threshold, but annoying	a	213	
present and tested > initiation threshold	r	214	
present and not tested	r	215	

220 Wet

no load	g	221	
increased load	a	222	

230 Driving and steering activity

no driving and steering activity	g	231	
driving and steering activity	g	232	

240 Time-based workplace

no time and space connection to the work place	g	241	
time and space connection to the work place (relief required)	a	242	

250 (Performance) Pay

Hourly rate	g	251	
Group piece work	g	252	

260 Shift work

no shift work	g	261	
2 shift work	g	262	
3 shift work	a	263	

270 Permanent night shift

no permanent night shift	g	271	
permanent night shift	a	272	

280 Risk analysis

no special risk in the execution of the job	g	281	
risk possible in execution of job, but a risk analysis was done and precautions taken	g	282	
risk possible in execution of job, risk analysis was done but precautions were not taken	r	283	
risk possible in execution of job, a risk analysis was not done	r	284	

Figure 22.5 *Continued.*

action is considered under the same headings as the exposure assessment: the *task*, the *load*, the *working environment*, *individual capacity* and *exposure*.

In this case, the options for control fell into the following categories.

1 Engineering:
  - pallet less tightly packed—fewer wheels were loaded onto each pallet to reduce the friction between them;
  - introduction of a ramp with a gentle gradient from waist height at pallet to hip at track side; this reduced the distance required to carry the load;
  - pallets raised by 20 cm bringing the load closer to waist height;
  - pallets upright to reduce friction (to hang freely)—this resulted in rubber tyres no longer being in contact with the metal frame, reducing the pulling force required to remove each wheel from the pallet;
  - mechanical assister—to lift the wheel from the end of the ramp to the axle; this removed all lifting requirements at the side of the track.
2 Administration:
  - job rotation—the operations described were integrated into a job rotation schedule, such that no more than 2 h in any shift was spent performing either of the duties described;
  - lifting and handling tuition—a formal manual handling education programme, encouraging the reporting of problematic tasks and good handling techniques, was introduced for all employees.

The reapplication of the ergonomic rating scale revealed one remaining r-rated process: the continuing need to physically carry the spare wheel into the boot up the steps. The options for further manual assisters to help in this task, such as overhead delivery and drop or fitment of the spare tyre at a ground level area of track, are being evaluated.

Worker representative bodies, particularly safety committees, have an important role to play in raising the profile of manual handling issues with their members, and their involvement and support in the introduction of changes can have a large impact on their success.

Health surveillance

No formal health surveillance is performed, but health and safety personnel remain alert to reports of musculoskeletal problems through accident at work reporting, sickness absence and occupational health department attendance.

Record keeping

Any risk assessment requires a re-evaluation if the process changes significantly in terms of the nature of the task or cycle time. Assessment records are kept and maintained by line managers, as they are likely to be most aware of changes to their areas of responsibility possibly requiring a further manual handling evaluation.

Conclusions

Occupational health and safety teams in large organizations with significant and widespread manual handling hazards will be unable to identify and manage all risks. The multitudinous varieties of risk require a coherent, simple and effective approach which can be applied by suitably trained line managers or other delegated staff or contractor. Company policy should make health and safety issues a priority, and corporate culture which reinforces this should help to ensure that risk assessment is not neglected at the expense of other business priorities.

The role of the occupational health and safety team is to provide general ergonomic training to line managers with the goal of 'ergonomic independence'. In the early stages of this policy, more specific advice may be necessary in individual cases to ensure that appropriate conclusions and interventions are made.

Finally, although ergonomic factors for the development of LBP may be readily identified and controlled by ergonomically trained personnel, psychosocial factors remain of significant importance in the development and subsequent chronicity of LBP. Employee assistance schemes, workplace nurseries and other employee support should be considered as part of a wider preventative strategy.

References

Clinical Standards Advisory Group (1994) *Back Pain*. HMSO, London.
Garg, A. & Moore, J. (1992) Epidemiology of low-back pain in industry. *Occupational Medicine* 7 (4), 593–608.
Graves, R.J. (1993) Grasping the manual handling regulations—a burden for the safety practitioner? *The Safety and Health Practitioner* 11, 28–32.
HSE (1992a) *Approved Code of Practice. Management of Health and Safety at Work Regulations 1992*. No. L21. HSE Books, Sudbury, Suffolk.
HSE (1992b) *Approved Code of Practice. Manual Handling Operations Regulations 1992*. No. L23. HSE Books, Sudbury, Suffolk.
Malmivaara, A., Hakkinen, U., Aro, T., *et al.* (1995) The treatment of acute low back pain—bed rest, exercise, or ordinary activity? *New England Journal of Medicine* **332**, 351–355.
Niedhammer, I., Lert, F. & Marne, M. (1994) Back pain and associated factors in French nurses. *International Archives of Occupational and Environmental Health* **66**, 349–357.
Ratti, N. & Pilling, K. (1997) Back pain in the workplace. *British Journal of Rheumatology* **36**, 260–264.

Chapter 23 Risk management and display screen equipment

Rodney J. Graves and Janice E. Jones

Introduction

Risk management consists of three major components: risk identification, risk assessment and risk control (see Baker *et al.* 1996). This chapter describes some case studies and approaches illustrating examples of the practical application of risk management.

The Display Screen Equipment (DSE) Regulations 1992 (Health and Safety Executive (HSE) 1992) define a display screen equipment user as: 'an employee who habitually uses display screen equipment as a significant part of his normal work, where display screen equipment means any alphanumeric or graphic display screen, regardless of the display process involved'. The issues of work/workstation design which need to be dealt with are clearly identified by the DSE Regulations. Specific guidance relating to issues considered by the DSE Regulations can be found in British Standards BS 5940 (British Standards Institution (BSI) 1980) and BS 7179 (BSI 1990) and European Standard EN 29241 (European Committee for Standardization 1993). Although there is no requirement by law to comply with these standards, they provide a useful basis to highlight aspects of work design which could be improved in relation to the issues raised in the DSE Regulations.

The DSE Regulations are designed to deal with three main classes of hazard: discomfort and musculoskeletal problems; visual problems; and fatigue and stress. Typically, musculoskeletal problems will be related to the design of the equipment, workstation and tasks. Visual problems may occur in relation to the individual's visual system, including the task (e.g. size of detail) and environmental design (e.g. lighting and humidity). Stress can be a function of the nature of the task, e.g. its difficulty, as well as for how long it is being carried out.

Important sources of risk can be due to workstation design, and the guidance in the standards may not be comprehensive. It is therefore useful to examine the potential risk factors, and to identify the particular aspects of task and workstation design which relate to these. For example, some postural risk factors can be identified and related to aspects of workstation design by performing an analysis of how the design affects the reach requirements of a population of different sizes of operator. In addition, the postures being adopted, forces involved (hence the loads on the soft tissues) and exposure can be related to particular elements of tasks by observing a range of operators carrying out these tasks.

Musculoskeletal disorders

Musculoskeletal problems can affect the soft tissues of the body, such as the muscles, tendons, joints, nerves and circulatory system. Some types of musculoskeletal injury occur not as a result of accidents or sudden mishaps, but develop gradually as a result of mechanical stresses over time (Putz-Anderson 1988). Commonly affected areas include the hands, arms, shoulders, neck, lower back and legs. Conditions which affect the hands and arms are known as upper limb disorders, and are sometimes referred to as repetitive strain injuries. Those which are thought to be associated with work are described as work-related upper limb disorders (WRULDs).

From present knowledge, it is thought that there are four main ergonomic factors which need to be considered in relation to the risk of WRULDs. These are the posture being adopted, forces involved (and hence the loads on the soft tissues), repetition and exposure.

Any work situation which leads to awkward postures results in a degree of risk which is still being quantified. However, it is thought (HSE 1990) that, where there are awkward postures and static loads directly related to these postures, risk will increase. A combination of awkward postures, static loads and minimal recovery time from these (because of the nature of the exposure) can increase the risk further, particularly with continued overall exposure. It appears that as yet unclearly defined combinations of these factors increase the risk of ULDs.

Factors which are likely to cause awkward postures in keyboard work are the size of the individual concerned, working practices and the workplace layout. Fixed height work surfaces are often found in typing, and shorter people may be disadvantaged if adequate adjustment is not provided to allow them to adopt a comfortable posture in relation to the keyboard. For example, if the keyboard is not in the correct position, this can lead to awkward wrist postures. In addition, if the height at which they are working is too high, they may need to hold their arms and hands, and perhaps their shoulders, above a position where these would be relaxed and/or supported. This can result in their arms and wrists being held in a static posture. This is why it is important to have a range of adjustability available in workstation design.

Further musculoskeletal risk, especially in relation to the lower back and legs, can result from poor workstation design. Particular issues of importance include chair design and support for feet. Seat height should be adjustable to allow a range of operators to reach the work surface at an appropriate height. A chair whose seat height is positioned too high in relation to the work surface height, or whose backrest does not adequately support the lumbar region of the back, can lead to sustained poor back postures and hence the risk of back problems. An operator's feet should be supported at an appropriate height in relation to the seat height. This allows the legs to be supported by the seat without causing restriction to blood flow, which would increase risk. As a result, a footrest will be necessary to support the feet for small operators in particular, and where the work surface is relatively high.

Visual problems and stress

The DSE Regulations provide for users to have eye tests to take account of the risk of visual difficulties due to individual eye problems. Medical evidence shows that the use of display screen equipment does not lead to eye damage. Other aspects of display screens, such as temporary visual effects, can lead to impaired visual performance, red and sore eyes, headaches or the adoption of awkward postures. These can result from remaining in the same position and concentrating for a long time, poor positioning of the display screen equipment, poor legibility of the screen or document, poor lighting (e.g. glare and reflections) and unstable screen images.

Stresses which arise from display screen equipment tasks are likely to be caused by poor job design or work organization, particularly a lack of sufficient control of the work by the user, underutilization of skills, high-speed repetitive working or social isolation. The risks associated with physical fatigue and stress can be minimized by following the principles of careful design, selection and layout of display screen equipment, good design of the user's workplace, environment and task, and training, consultation and involvement of the user (HSE 1992). Any study needs to consider the implication of high-speed repetitive work.

Risk identification

In this section, a practical checklist approach is described for the identification of risk in office environments. Figure 23.1 shows an extract from an example of a practical DSE assessment worksheet made up of a number of sheets. This approach was used by one company to provide an overview of potential risk, i.e. to identify sources of risk. It was fairly comprehensive and depended upon a person with the appropriate level of skill to use it. The results provided a useful and practical overview of where the major problems were likely to occur. The data provided information on workstations which did not satisfy the requirements of the DSE Regulations. This enabled planning to be undertaken so that budgets could be agreed for purchasing equipment and training over a period of time. This type of approach enabled the objectives of the DSE Regulations to be achieved, i.e. to identify each user, carry out an assessment and record the observations, and put a plan into operation to control risk.

Risk assessment

This section describes a more detailed evaluation of risk in a non-office environment. Document reader encoder (DRE) operators are used in

Sheet 1
DISPLAY SCREEN EQUIPMENT
Record no.

Distribution:

LOCATION/SITE/COMPANY

DATE: WORKSTATION NUMBER & LOCATION:

PERSON BEING ASSESSED: PERSON CARRYING OUT ASSESSMENT:

WORKSTATION ASSESSMENTS

1. A 'NO' in any of the sections shall be considered for improvements during the Financial Years specified below.

(A) 1993/94 F.Y. (B) 1993/94/95 F.Y. (C) 1993/94/95/96 F.Y.

SOFTWARE CHECKS BEFORE CARRYING OUT SITE ASSESSMENT CATEGORY 'C' 1993–96

1. Have you checked the software with Management Services? YES/NO
2. Have you identified the software is to be satisfactory? YES/NO
3. Does the system provide feedback, enable the operator to monitor system performance? YES/NO
4. Is the system speed suitable YES/NO
5. Is information displayed at a pace intended to be comfortable to the operator? YES/NO
6. Is the format in which information is displayed suitable for the operator? YES/NO

Sheet 2
WORKSTATION ASSESSMENT
CATEGORY 'A' 1993/94

REFLECTIONS AND GLARE

1. Have you adjustable window blinds? YES/NO
2. Are wall surfaces low reflection? YES/NO
3. Are fixtures and fittings reflecting onto the workstation? YES/NO
4. Where the need cannot be avoided has an appropriate screen filter been fitted? YES/NO

LIGHTING

5. Is the lighting suitable? YES/NO

SPACE

6. Is there sufficient space to enable easy access to the workstation? YES/NO

TEMPERATURE

7. Is the temperature at the workstation satisfactory? YES/NO

CONDITION OF EQUIPMENT

8. Is the work equipment in good state of repair, thus ensuring the minimization of any risk? YES/NO

DISPLAY SCREEN EQUIPMENT

9. Does the display screen equipment have easily adjustable controls for brightness and contrast? YES/NO
10. Is it possible to easily tilt and swivel the screen? YES/NO
11. Does the screen stand upon a surface possible to achieve the correct height? YES/NO
12. Is the screen free from reflections or glare? YES/NO
13. Is the image on the screen stable and free from the flicker? YES/NO
14. Are the characters well defined? YES/NO

Figure 23.1 Example of two sheets from a checklist used by a company to identify DSE risk.

some bank environments to process a range of vouchers, including cheques, house credits/debits, bank giro credits and postal orders. This task involves the use of both a keyboard and a visual display terminal. The DSE Regulations apply to DRE work, and the employers in this case study wished to identify any potential risks.

An ergonomic study of a DRE workstation was carried out. The aims of this study were to identify potential ergonomic risk factors in DRE work, and to suggest ways of improving the nature of the work/workstation design to minimize the possible risks.

Video recordings were taken of two operators carrying out DRE work to provide examples of views of working postures. Photographs were taken to illustrate the actions performed. Measurements of workstation dimensions were recorded so that these could be examined in relation to reach criteria and guidance based upon the DSE Regulations. An informal description of the tasks was obtained from the processing centre manager. The analysis of the video was carried out off site by viewing the video to determine any possible risks due to awkward postures, forces, frequency and exposure.

The following findings were obtained.

1 For the present work surface height, the current chairs were inadequate, and the backrest of the chair did not provide adequate support in the lumbar region for a small operator.

2 The current work surface thickness was unacceptable and should be reduced substantially.

3 A footrest is recommended for workstations with fixed work surface heights, but none was provided.

4 There appeared to be potential musculoskeletal disorders risks in relation to the:

- back and neck from poor postures during writing as a result of a lack of work surface space and/or insufficient operator training in relation to risk factors and how to control them;
- left shoulder/arm as a result of poor posture from the use of an elbow/forearm rest which was non-adjustable;
- left elbow/forearm area as a result of localized pressure from the use of the elbow/forearm rest;
- right hand/palm area as a result of localized pressure from a lack of palm support due to the lack of free space in front of the keyboard;
- hands as a result of pinch gripping during the placement of vouchers, emptying of voucher pockets and removal of printer paper;
- right hand/wrist as a result of awkward wrist postures during the emptying of voucher pockets due to the orientation of voucher pockets;
- left hand/wrist as a result of strong flexion/extension movements of the wrist during voucher placement, because each voucher needed to be lifted over a bundle of vouchers;

- right hand/wrist during keying as a result of repetition and level of exposure;
- left hand/wrist during the placement of vouchers onto the track, exacerbated by the degree of repetition and level of exposure.

5 In relation to viewing issues, neither operator's line of sight angle was between 0° and 60° below the horizontal; the current document holder position did not allow eye, head and neck movement to be minimized.
6 The operators work under time pressure, which could place pressures on employees to work rapidly and take less breaks as a result, leading to less opportunity for the body to recover, and therefore increasing the risk.

Detailed recommendations were provided for changes to the workstation and organizational factors to reduce the potential risks.

Risk control

This section covers two methods of risk control. The first study describes a situation in which the workstation was redesigned to control the risk; the second study describes the control of risk in an administration department by user training.

Study 1: redesign of a workstation

On an offshore oil platform, a number of administration personnel had reported experiencing discomfort in their necks and shoulders while working in the helicopter administration area. They worked with a display screen and keyboard to check offshore personnel on and off the platform. Their work tasks involved mainly keyboard and screen work, communication with incoming and outgoing personnel and the weighing of baggage on the incoming flight (weigh-in).

An ergonomic assessment was undertaken, based on DSE criteria as described earlier, to establish whether the user discomfort could be linked to workstation risk, and to recommend a strategy for risk control.

During the assessment, the workstation layout was studied and photographed, key measurements were taken and the workstation layout and tasks were discussed with user personnel. It was concluded from the assessment that user discomfort was probably caused by the awkward postures adopted by personnel due to the lack of workspace and poor workstation design.

The following recommendations were made.

1 The workstation desk space must be increased as the area was too cramped to perform the necessary work tasks, e.g.:

- due to a lack of work space, the screen was positioned at right angles to the keyboard;
- there was no space in front of the keyboard to rest the hands and wrists;

- there was no available surface area for writing.

2 The area beneath the work desk should be free from obstructions. The space should allow adequate clearance for postural changes. This means adequate clearance for thighs, knees, legs and feet under the work surface and between furniture components. The current design did not allow for adequate clearance.

3 The baggage weigh-in point was at the opposite end of the workstation from the keyboard and screen. This was not practical or comfortable for the operator. The improved layout should include necessary modifications to streamline the check-in process.

4 The helicopter administration personnel must be provided with training on working with DSE, as prescribed by Regulation 6 of the DSE Regulations.

5 Detailed task analysis of the job function in helicopter administration should be carried out to confirm the impact of these recommendations.

6 The new workstation design and layout should be assessed after the recommended improvements have been implemented.

These recommendations were implemented by the company. Feedback from the users and the health and safety manager confirmed that the improvements had eradicated user discomfort.

Study 2: training users in a formal office environment

A number of DSE users had reported symptoms of upper limb discomfort to the organization's personnel manager. Interviews with DSE users suggested that the discomfort could be related to their limited knowledge of how to adjust their workstations. In addition, they did not have any knowledge of the health risks associated with display screen use, and thus were unaware of the necessary actions which could be adopted to reduce risks.

A training programme was set up to educate users on how to work with DSE safely and comfortably. The training programme covered the following topics.

1 Introduction to DSE and the user's health and safety.

2 The risks associated with working with DSE.

3 Actions to reduce the risk and prevent/reduce discomfort.

Follow-up discussions with the personnel manager indicated that the incidence of upper limb discomfort in the office had decreased. This shows the positive impact that training can have on risk reduction.

Conclusions

The risk management of DSE, as true of other work situations, involves many aspects. Firstly, the company must be in a position to identify the sources of risk (risk identification). This will involve the training of appropriate personnel in risk identification. Secondly, the priorities for risk reduction will be dependent upon risk assessment and a knowledge of the impact of risk on health and safety. Without the latter, it is difficult to establish budgets and obtain resources. Once these priorities have been established, it is possible to set up and implement a programme of work to reduce risk (risk control).

The latter will be successful only with the will and commitment of all those in the company, from senior management to shop floor worker.

References

Baker, M., Graves, R.J. & Kearney, M.K. (1996) A methodology for risk management in civil, mechanical and structural engineering. In: *Risk Management in Civil, Mechanical and Structural Engineering* (ed. M. James), pp. 67–86. The Institution of Civil Engineers, London.

BSI (1980) *BS 5940—Part 1. Office Furniture Specification for Design and Dimensions of Office Workstations, Desks, Tables and Chairs*. BSI, London.

BSI (1990) *BS 7179. Ergonomics of Design and Use of Visual Display Terminals (VDTs) in Offices*. BSI, London.

European Committee for Standardization (1993) *EN 29241—Part 3. Ergonomic Requirements for Office Work with Visual Display Terminals (VDTs). Visual Display Requirements*. European Standards Committee, Brussels.

HSE (1990) *Work Related Upper Limb Disorders. A Guide to Prevention*. HMSO, London.

HSE (1992) *Display Screen Equipment Work. Guidance on Regulations. Health and Safety (Display Screen Equipment) Regulations 1992*. HMSO, London.

Putz-Anderson, V. (1988) *Cumulative Trauma Disorders: A Manual for Musculoskeletal Diseases of the Upper Limbs*. Taylor and Francis, London.

Chapter 24 Biological agents

Jeremy R. Beach and Naveen Ratti

Introduction

For many people, the term biological agents conjures up images of rare infectious diseases, such as anthrax, restricted to relatively small occupational groups, and now encountered only as curiosities. However, the reality is that work-related diseases caused by microorganisms continue to occur, albeit attracting less attention than problems such as occupational asthma or upper limb disorders. A wide range of occupational diseases are attributable to microorganisms, from self-limiting and usually non-fatal conditions, such as orf in sheep farmers, to potentially life threatening infections, such as hepatitis in health care workers. Microorganisms may be encountered through specific work processes or through the work environment in general, as with Legionnaire's disease. Thus, biological agents remain an important cause of work-related illness in many of today's workplaces.

Biological agents, which for the purpose of this chapter are considered to be principally microorganisms and their products, occur ubiquitously in our environment and are an everyday feature of life. They occur in such variety that they can live in enormous numbers in almost any environment inhabitable by humans, and in many that are uninhabitable by humans. Although only a minority cause disease in humans, this is sufficient to have the potential to cause a great variety of disease. Risk assessment may be complicated, as the nature of their interaction with humans may depend on many factors in addition to the species and number of microorganisms encountered. The route through which microorganisms are encountered affects their potential to cause disease, as does the state of the immune system of their potential hosts, and a knowledge of both of these may be important in assessing the risk. To add further to this complexity, the pace of reproduction and hence evolution among microorganisms may be sufficiently fast that the risks arising are inherently unpredictable to a greater or lesser degree. Thus, risk assessment for biological agents remains an inexact science, with judgement and caution needing to be exercised.

Case 1

Defining the problem

Tuberculosis has been a recognized risk for health care workers for many years. However, as the disease decreased in prevalence in the second half of this century, and with the introduction of effective prophylaxis and treatment, it ceased to be an issue for many involved in occupational health. By the mid-1980s, there were relatively few cases of tuberculosis occurring due to exposure in the workplace: only six compensated cases in the UK in 1983/1984, seven in 1984/1985 and three in 1985/1986. With the emergence of acquired immunodeficiency syndrome (AIDS) in the 1980s, a range of diseases which were previously unusual became more frequently encountered, including tuberculosis. Although the risk to staff treating these and other patients remains small, there is still a potential risk of cross-infection from these patients.

This case was noted when a 35-year-old nurse presented to the clinic with a history of fatigue, night sweats, a worsening of her asthma, which had been ascribed to an ongoing 'viral' infection, and pleuritic chest pain which had progressively worsened over several months. A Heaf test gave a grade III reaction, and chest X-ray showed a pleural effusion; when this was drained, no mycobacteria were seen on direct microscopy and none grew on culture. The chest X-ray had previously been normal and she had received Bacillus Calmette–Guérin (BCG) vaccination. Nonetheless, she was treated for tuberculosis and initially improved, although her subsequent course was far from uneventful. She went on to have a pleural biopsy approximately 9 months after her treatment had been started, and live *Mycobacterium tuberculosis* were identified from this. She eventually completed 9 months of antituberculous treatment.

Hazard identification

Tuberculosis in humans is usually due to infection with *Mycobacterium tuberculosis*. Occasionally, infection may occur with *Mycobacterium bovis* or other 'atypical' mycobacteria, such as those of the *Mycobacterium avium/intracellulare* series, particularly in individuals who are immunocompromised. These microorganisms are commonly resistant to some of the agents used in their treatment, often necessitating treatment regimes incorporating a combination of three or more drugs. Worryingly, some of the strains seen in patients with AIDS have been resistant to almost all antituberculous drugs, causing great concern about how they may be effectively treated. Tuberculosis is usually spread from infected to uninfected individuals by droplet aerosols produced during coughing and sneezing. Although generally fairly close contact is required, there is some evidence that the tuberculosis of patients with AIDS can spread to others more easily than tuberculosis in patients without AIDS. The most infectious patients are those who have mycobacteria visible on direct microscopic examination of sputum (smear positive).

Exposure assessment

Estimating the exposure to biological agents is notoriously difficult, particularly the quantitative assessment of exposure to microorganisms which may be fastidious and difficult to culture. However, it seems likely that meaningful exposure probably occurred within the clinic where the nurse constituting the index case worked. She was employed as a nurse in charge of a chest clinic and, as part of her job, routinely interviewed patients with known or suspected tuberculosis to help with their investigation and treatment, and also to help with contact tracing. Following a site visit, it was clear that the room used for these interviews was small and poorly ventilated, and that no specific precautions were taken to try to prevent cross-infection from patients to staff. Staff, including the individual in this case, would almost certainly have had contact with a number of highly infectious smear positive patients. It is also probably relevant that several months before she presented, the nurse who became ill had interviewed a patient who, in hindsight, had been infected with a particularly virulent strain of *Mycobacterium tuberculosis*.

Risk characterization

For infectious diseases, the exact relationship between exposure and disease is complex, and consequently the risk of infection is difficult to estimate. The risk of becoming infected and developing disease may depend not only on the nature of the exposure (e.g. number of organisms encountered at a given site and their pathogenicity), but also on the characteristics of the potential host (e.g. current nutritional state and immune status). We identified some periods and activities which, in our evaluation, were likely to involve additional risk. We felt that coughing was likely to produce a droplet aerosol with a relatively high risk of transmitting disease, and sneezing was likely to act similarly. The poor ventilation in the interview room and the proximity of contact between the nurse and the patient were also likely to have played a role in determining the risk of infection (see Fig. 24.1).

Prevention and control

The first approach involved practical steps to try to reduce the exposure of the nurses interviewing patients to potentially highly infectious droplet aerosols. Patients were asked not to sneeze or cough towards the staff and, by sitting the nurse adjacent to the patient rather than directly opposite, droplet aerosols were directed away from the staff. The ventilation in the room was also improved, ensuring that the normal flow of air was away from the interviewer towards the patient and then to the outside rather than being recirculated. The communication of results from microbiology was also improved, so that staff could

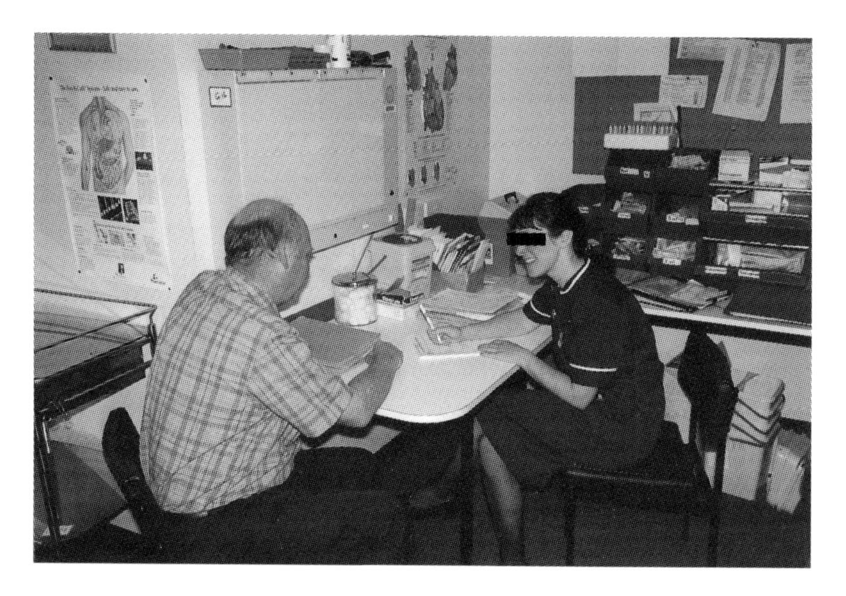

Figure 24.1 Contact with patients may entail exposure to biological agents sufficient for transmission to occur.

more quickly be made aware of those patients with smear positive tuberculosis who represented the greatest potential hazard, and could take appropriate extra precautions. The second approach for reducing risk centred around manipulating the immune status of staff. By ensuring that all staff were tuberculin tested, and by giving BCG to those without pre-existing immunity, the risk of tuberculous infection could be reduced, although staff needed to remain aware that no vaccine could provide 100% protection, and BCG would of course provide no protection against non-tuberculous infection.

Risk communication, training and information

It was felt to be important to ensure that some specific training for staff was provided, including information about the early signs of infection, even though the majority of staff were clinically experienced and so had a high pre-existing level of knowledge. Once adequately informed, staff could seek advice early if they were concerned about their health.

Health surveillance

In view of the fact that some residual risk almost certainly remained despite all precautions, health surveillance was felt to be appropriate. This constituted regular enquiry about respiratory and other non-specific symptoms, with further investigation where appropriate, and emphasizing to the staff the importance of reporting any suspicious symptoms early.

Review

A review of the processes used in the interview area was felt to be essential because of the rapid advancement of the knowledge of the disease and the accompanying evolution of new drugs and vaccines.

Case 2

Defining the problem

Individuals who work closely with animals have long been recognized as being at risk of developing a number of infectious diseases. Typical groups of workers affected include farmers, veterinary surgeons, butchers, abattoir workers and research workers. A wide range of diseases can be contracted from animals, and these are usually known as zoonoses. Humans are usually end hosts, i.e. infection is not usually transmitted from human to human, but must be caught from an animal host directly.

This case came to light when a patient was referred having had an acute illness over approximately 24 h, with nausea, headache, loss of appetite and fever. He was a 26-year-old offal porter who worked at a local abattoir. His own doctor prescribed oxytetracycline, and had arranged for a variety of further investigations. These showed a mild hepatitis and serological changes diagnostic of Q fever. By the time these results were available, he had made a good recovery.

Hazard identification

Q fever is a disease caused by infection with a rickettsial organism, *Rickettsia* or *Coxiella burnetii*. It is usually spread to humans from domestic goats, sheep or cattle by aerosol produced during parturition, when there may be contact with products of conception which contain a high concentration of the organism. It may also be transmitted by drinking infected unpasteurized milk, or by direct contact with infected animals or carcasses. The organism responsible is relatively resistant to heat and many disinfectants, and so can be difficult to eradicate. Q fever may develop in some individuals as an acute severe pneumonia or systemic illness with debilitating symptoms, while others may have only mild transient symptoms.

Exposure assessment

A site visit was arranged. The abattoir was fairly typical and dealt with a variety of animals, which were slaughtered and then separated into hide, meat and organs. Animals arriving at the abattoir were inspected by a vet, and any thought unfit were removed. Meat inspectors were also employed to try and ensure that no meat which appeared unfit for consumption was sold as food. Given the volume of work, we felt that this process of inspection would not be likely to identify all infected animals.

The patient was employed on a line processing internal organs. Animal intestines and liver would arrive by conveyer and he would separate intestines, fat and any other excess tissue from around the liver. The liver of each animal would then be placed in a tray for chilling and packing, the remaining tissue being passed to another section for further processing as offal. During a typical 10-h working day, as many as 3000–4000 lambs' livers might be processed.

Risk characterization

Although the process of inspection would allow the identification and removal of any obviously infected animals or meat, microscopic infection would not be identified. The patient wore some protective equipment, including overalls, an apron and a chain mail glove on his left hand. He was right handed and used his knife in this hand. He wore no glove whatsoever on his right hand, and consequently had obvious and frequent contact with animal products. Although the chain mail glove on his left hand provided protection against his knife or other sharp objects, it was not providing complete protection against animal products. Aerosols were produced during animal product processing, particularly when powered saws were used, but these were not especially evident in the area where the patient usually worked. He could not remember specifically any cuts or abrasions being present on either hand at the time of his illness, although this would have been the obvious route of infection. Other workers were also seen working without gloves.

Prevention and control

Ideally, animals for slaughter should be healthy and not infected with the causative organism of Q fever or any other disease. However, infection may, on occasions, cause little illness in the animal, and so may be impossible to identify through inspection, but may be more than adequate to cause an illness in somebody handling the animal. Thus, at present, there remains a need to consider that all animals may be a source of infection, and to act accordingly. Recommendations were made about the use of lined rubber gloves on both hands, thereby giving protection against direct skin contact with meat. Good general hygiene also needed to be enforced, so that protective clothing did not become unduly soiled. A requirement was also introduced stating that all employees with cuts and abrasions on their hands or other areas of potentially exposed skin should report these to the occupational health department. These could then be covered with a simple waterproof dressing. Dealing with aerosols produced by power tools proved to be more difficult, but careful shielding was used to direct any aerosol produced away from the workers, and good general ventilation ensured that any particles remaining airborne were removed as rapidly as possible. Vaccination is available for Q fever, but is not widely used as it is not always effective. It is not clear from a single case that the risk in this particular abattoir would justify vaccination. We also took into account that it may provide some false reassurance, when in fact it would give no protection whatsoever against other infections, and may have the undesirable consequence of allowing employees to be less careful about simple hygiene measures.

Risk communication, training and information

Again, this played an important role in preventing any further occurrences of problems. By educating employees about the nature of the risks they encountered, they were able to understand the measures introduced to reduce these risks and so were more willing to comply. In particular, the care needed for cuts and abrasions had to be emphasized to ensure that all employees realized the importance of covering these. Information about early symptoms of Q fever and other infections that could occur was also important as, although in this case the patient's doctor gave the appropriate treatment, such infections are relatively rare and it would have been foreseeable that treatment might have been delayed in other circumstances. By making all employees aware of the risks they face, they would be able to pass on this information to their doctors should they need attention.

Health surveillance

Although there is no simple, rapid and widely available technique to monitor infection with *C. burnetii*, some form of health surveillance is important in these circumstances. Many employees may not have been aware of the importance of reporting episodes of ill health such as this to their employer, and this could result in the employer underestimating the risk of disease. An active health surveillance programme, albeit largely reactive in nature, is therefore important.

Review

We emphasized that some regular reconsideration of the risks encountered in the work was important. If other cases of illness were to arise, this would certainly require a re-examination of the risk assessment.

Conclusions

These cases demonstrate some of the difficulties encountered when dealing with infectious agents in the workplace. Risk assessment may be very difficult as exposure assessment is often crude and at best semi-quantitative, while the development of disease depends not only on exposure but also critically on the potential host response. The prevention of such infections relies on the minimization of exposure and manipulation of the host so as to make the disease as unlikely as possible even if exposure occurs. Information and training are often central to this, as some of the most effective measures are the most simple, yet easy to forget.

Chapter 25 Risk assessment and management of asbestos in Malaysian industry

Lim Heng Huat

Introduction

Asbestos is a generic term which refers collectively to a group of naturally occurring fibrous mineral silicates. This includes the serpentines (chrysotile) and the amphiboles (actinolite, anthophyllite, tremolite, crocidolite and amosite). The basic chemical composition of asbestos consists of silicates of magnesium or other minerals, e.g. chrysotile—$(OH)_6Mg_6Si_4O_{11}.H_2O$.

Health effects from asbestos exposure are mainly due to inhalation, while the risks from ingestion appear to be negligible. The principal asbestos-related conditions in humans are bronchial carcinoma, mesothelioma, asbestosis and pleural plaques (World Health Organization (WHO) 1986).

International guidelines on occupational health and safety practices are given in the International Labour Office (ILO) Convention and Recommendations on Safety in the Use of Asbestos (ILO 1986), which have been ratified by various member countries. Many nations have also promulgated and gazetted specific regulations, such as the Factories and Machinery (Asbestos Process) Regulations 1986 in Malaysia, and the UK Control of Asbestos at Work Regulations 1987 and Control of Asbestos at Work (Amendment) Regulations 1992. These regulations stipulate the national safety standards and operational requirements for controlling the safe use of asbestos in industry. In addition, companies engaged in the mining, milling and manufacturing of asbestos products, particularly the larger multinational corporations, have also adopted their own corporate health and safety policies and programmes in their management structure, which enable them to comply with national regulations.

Defining the problem

The assessment of the health risks from asbestos is more complex than for many other substances due to its natural and physicochemical properties. The biological effect is influenced by many factors, including the type of asbestos, the diameter and length of the fibres, the durability and period of retention in the lung, the sources of the fibres and the method of manipulation in the industrial processes. It is thus difficult to derive a simple risk assessment or dose–response curve for asbestos.

Moreover, many cases of bronchial carcinoma may be attributed to cigarette smoking, which is a common habit in many male industrial workers. Currently, it is not possible to distinguish such cases from those due to asbestos exposure. In addition, combined exposure to asbestos and cigarette smoke appears to produce a more than additive effect. Thus, the risk of lung cancer from asbestos exposure may partly be contributed by cigarette smoking.

However, the majority of mesotheliomas are linked to asbestos exposure, not to smoking, although a small proportion have no demonstrable association with asbestos exposure. Asbestosis (interstitial fibrosis of the lungs) occurs within 5–20 years from initial exposure, depending on the dust exposure levels. The incidence of asbestosis seems to be declining with improved health and safety conditions in some countries. In addition, asbestosis does not appear to occur from exposure in the general environment.

The risk of cancer has thus become the major concern in asbestos exposure, especially in view of the 'no threshold' hypothesis for many carcinogens, although this has not been proven in the case of asbestos.

Characterization and estimation of risk

There are two broad approaches in estimating health risks from asbestos.

Qualitative approach

This approach uses various empirical observations from past experiences. In occupational groups, several studies have suggested that it may be possible to use asbestos under controlled situations with no detectable excess of lung cancer (Rossiter & Coles 1980; Thomas *et al.* 1982; Berry & Newhouse 1983; Ohlson & Hogstedt 1985). For mesotheliomas, the latency period is frequently longer than for lung cancer, and it occurs more often with exposure to amphiboles (particularly crocidolite). In para-occupational groups, the mesothelioma incidence was also found to be very high in crocidolite mining areas, but apparently undetectable in chrysotile areas in Zimbabwe and Swaziland (Wagner *et al.* 1960; Webster 1977). However, it is not possible to estimate the risks quantitatively due to extremely variable exposure data. For lung cancer, studies in chrysotile areas with high environmental pollution have not reported any significant excess risk (Siemiatycki 1983; Neuberger *et al.* 1984).

In the general population, the risk of mesothelioma and lung cancer attributable to asbestos exposure is undetectably low. For asbestosis, the risk is practically zero.

Quantitative approach

This approach takes into consideration the physicochemical properties of the fibre types, exposure measurement and biological response.

The fibre type appears to influence the incidence of asbestos-related diseases in occupational groups. Amphiboles have been linked with asbestosis, mesothelioma and lung cancer, while chrysotile has been associated with asbestosis and, less clearly, with mesothelioma. Variations in fibre size also appear to influence the variations in lung cancer ratio in different industries. Long fibres (> 5 μm) appear to be more biologically active than short fibres (< 5 μm). As the methods of counting are not strictly comparable, the database is insufficiently large or appropriate to estimate reliable dose–response relationships. The durability and period of residence in lung tissue are also variable for different fibre types. Chrysotile tends to split and degrade after inhalation, thus having a shorter residence time.

Lung cancer

The estimation of the cancer risk at low levels of asbestos exposure may be extrapolated from the observed incidence at high occupational exposure levels using a linear model, assuming that the relative risk increases approximately proportionally to the concentration and duration of exposure (WHO 1986):

$$I_A(d,f,a,s) = I_U(a,s) \times (1 + K_L df) \qquad (25.1)$$

where $I_A(d,f,a,s)$ represents the lung cancer incidence among asbestos workers aged '*a*', smoking '*s*' cigarettes per day and exposed to an average dose of '*f*' fibres per millilitre for '*d*' years. I_U represents the lung cancer incidence at age '*a*' in the unexposed population with comparable smoking habits. K_L is a constant derived from the asbestos mineral type and fibre dimensions.

However, the results derived from this formula may not be reliable due to the wide variations in the values of the different component variables. It can be used epidemiologically for very broad estimations of the lung cancer relative risk, although the results vary widely (US National Research Council/National Academy of Science 1984).

Mesothelioma

The estimation of the mesothelioma risk may also be carried out using the formula (WHO 1986):

$$I(t,f,d) = K_M f[t^4 - (t-d)^4] \qquad (25.2)$$

where I is the incidence of mesothelioma, t represents the number of years since first exposure, f is the exposure level in fibres per millilitre, d represents the number of years of exposure and K_M is a constant depending on the asbestos fibre type and dimensions (but cannot be used for chrysotile).

Basically, this model predicts that each exposure day contributes to the overall incidence, and its effect is proportional to the exposure level on that particular day.

The risks are considered to be independent of age or cigarette smoking. Again, the use of this prediction model is plagued with uncertainties and wide variations in results. Its main application is for very broad epidemiological estimations of mesothelioma risks (US NRC/NAS 1984).

The asbestos industry in Malaysia

There are no asbestos mining or milling operations in Malaysia, the main commercial activities being confined to the manufacture of asbestos products, such as building materials, pipes, friction materials and gaskets. About 2000 workers are employed in six large factories, with a number of smaller operations. The earliest factory was started more than 25 years ago. In 1984, the South Pacific Asbestos Association of Malaysia (SPAAM) was formed to group all companies engaged in asbestos product manufacturing together, with the objective of obtaining an organized approach towards the promotion of the safe use of asbestos in Malaysia. The SPAAM now has about 10 full and associate member companies.

Hazard identification

The type of asbestos product and the process of industrial manipulation contribute to the level of respirable fibre emission.

Asbestos cement products, such as sheets and pipes, form the largest group, containing 10–15% of asbestos, mainly chrysotile. The manufacture of such products is largely carried out in wet processes, although possible emission sources include the feeding of the asbestos fibres into the mix, blending, cutting or machining of the finished products and improper handling or transportation of the raw materials. Modern technology and control methods have greatly reduced the amount of dust emission in such processes, although appropriate working practices are also important in reducing personal exposure levels.

Friction materials, such as brake linings and clutch facings, are also important products in Malaysia. Asbestos fibres and other constituents are mixed with resin, and undergo various processes, such as thermosetting, curing, baking and grinding. Again, modern technology and dust control methods have significantly reduced the level of fibre emissions.

In the end products, asbestos fibres are physically and chemically bonded in a solid matrix. Thus, under normal circumstances, the amount of fibre released is small or negligible, although fibre emissions may occur during the manipulation of these products, such as sawing or cutting.

Exposure measurement

The standard method of exposure measurement is the membrane filter method, used by both government and industry. Personal monitoring of workers by representative sampling is carried out at intervals not longer than 3 months. Phase contrast microscopy is used for counting: only fibres greater than 5 μm in length, less than 3 μm in diameter and with an aspect ratio of greater than 3 : 1 are counted, because these are believed to be biologically active. The permissible exposure limit (PEL) set by the Malaysian government is 1 fibre ml^{-1} averaged over an 8-h period. Available data from industry show that the dust exposure levels are below the PEL in factories conducting exposure monitoring. In the UK, the 'control limits' for chrysotile are 0.5 fibre ml^{-1} averaged over any continuous period of 4 h, and 1.5 fibre ml^{-1} averaged over any continuous period of 10 min. The corresponding levels for other forms of asbestos, either alone or in mixtures, are 0.2 fibre ml^{-1} and 0.6 fibre ml^{-1}, respectively.

Prevention and control

The measures adopted for the prevention and control of asbestos dust exposures in factories are discussed below.

Work processes and practices

The use of crocidolite in any manufacturing process in any factory in Malaysia has been prohibited since the Asbestos Regulations were gazetted in 1986. In factories, wet manufacturing processes are also used where practicable. Appropriate working practices and the observance of good personal hygiene habits by workers are encouraged and enforced by supervisory personnel. Good housekeeping and cleanliness of machinery work areas, premises, furniture and fittings should be maintained at all times, although some small factories might be lax in these areas. Safe handling and disposal of asbestos materials, with storage in properly labelled receptacles, are also practised by employees and contractors. Smoking is also prohibited in work areas.

Engineering control

The installation, operation and maintenance of proper and adequate exhaust equipment are major factors in the reduction of dust exposure levels. Such equipment is inspected and tested regularly by competent persons.

Personal protective equipment

Workers exposed to asbestos dust are provided with proper protective clothing and respiratory protection equipment. These should be kept clean and properly maintained in good working order.

Health surveillance

Medical examinations for Malaysian asbestos workers are statutory, at intervals not exceeding 2 years. These are conducted by registered medical practitioners, and include:

- history (medical, occupational, smoking);
- physical examination;
- chest X-ray (posterior–anterior, 350 mm×430 mm);
- pulmonary function test (forced vital capacity and forced expiratory volume in 1 s).

Radiographs are read using the ILO International Classification of Radiographs of Pneumoconiosis. Medical reports must be provided to the employee if requested or his/her employer. In the UK, statutory medical examinations are performed at not more than 2 years before the beginning of exposure, and periodically at intervals of not more than 2 years. These must be conducted by an employment medical adviser or appointed doctor.

Health records must be kept for at least 20 years after the cessation of employment in Malaysia, and for at least 40 years from the date of the last entry in the UK.

Risk communication

Training programmes are also mandatory to communicate the health risks and preventive measures to workers. These programmes include information on the Asbestos Regulations, specific operations resulting in dust exposure, personal protective equipment, health effects, engineering controls and working procedures.

Regular seminars and workshops are organized by the SPAAM to communicate the safe use of asbestos to clients, contractors and the public. Speakers include local and foreign experts and scientists. At all times, close rapport and communication with relevant government departments are also maintained.

Conclusions

In summary, the health risks from asbestos are mainly in occupational groups where exposure may result in asbestosis, lung cancer and mesothelioma. Factors influencing these risks include the fibre type, fibre size, fibre dose and industrial processing. The risk of mesothelioma and lung cancer is generally much lower in the para-occupational groups (including household contacts and neighbourhood exposures), while the risk of asbestosis is very low. In the general population, the risks of mesothelioma and lung cancer cannot be reliably quantified and are probably undetectably low, while the risk of asbestosis is virtually zero.

Currently, there are few data available to quantify the health risks from asbestos in Malaysia. The problem is compounded by the relatively low autopsy rate and mortality certification by medical practitioners, and the lack of a National Cancer Registry. Hence, proactive research, in the form of health surveys, is being conducted to increase the database. In the meantime, it would seem prudent to adopt all necessary preventive and control measures in order to continue the safe use of asbestos in Malaysia.

References

Berry, G. & Newhouse, M.L. (1983) Mortality of workers manufacturing friction materials using asbestos. *British Journal of Industrial Medicine* 40, 1–7.

ILO (1986) *ILO Convention and Recommendations on Safety in the Use of Asbestos*. International Labour Office, Geneva.

Neuberger, M., Kundi, M. & Friedl, H.P. (1984) Environmental asbestos exposure and cancer mortality. *Archives of Environmental Health* 39, 261–265.

Ohlson, C.G. & Hogstedt, C. (1985) Lung cancer among asbestos cement workers. A Swedish cohort study and a review. *British Journal of Industrial Medicine* **42**, 397–402.

Rossiter, C.E. & Coles, R.M. (1980) H.M. Dockyard, Devonport: 1947 mortality study. In: *Biological Effects of Mineral Fibres. Proceedings of a Symposium held at Lyons, 25–27 September, 1979* (ed. J.C. Wagner), Vol. 2, pp. 713–721. International Agency for Research on Cancer (IARC) Scientific Publications No. 30. IARC, Lyons.

Siemiatycki, J. (1983) Health effects on the general population (mortality in the general population in asbestos mining areas). In: *Proceedings of the World Symposium on Asbestos*. Montreal, Canada, 25–27 May 1982. Canadian Asbestos Information Centre, Montreal.

Thomas, H.F., Benjamin, I.T., Elwood, P.C. & Sweetnam, P.M. (1982) Further follow up study of workers from an asbestos cement factory. *British Journal of Industrial Medicine* 39, 273–276.

US NRC/NAS (1984) Asbestiform fibres: non-occupational health risks. *US National Research Council, Committee on Non-occupational Health Risks of Asbestiform Fibers*, pp. 177–180. US NRC/NAS, Washington DC.

Wagner, J.C. (1963) Asbestos dust and malignancy. In: *Proceedings of the XIV International Congress of Occupational Health, Madrid, 1963*, pp. 3, 1066–1067.

Wagner, J.C., Sleggs, C.A. & Marchand, P. (1960) Diffuse pleural mesothelioma and asbestos exposure in the Northwestern Cape Province. *British Journal of Industrial Medicine* 17, 260–271.

Webster, I. (1977) Methods by which mesothelioma may be diagnosed. In: *Proceedings of Asbestos Symposium, Johannesburg, South Africa, 1977* (ed. H.W. Glen), pp. 3–8. National Institute for Metallurgy, Randburg.

WHO (1986) *Asbestos and Other Natural Mineral Fibres, Environmental Health Criteria 53*. World Health Organization, Geneva.

Chapter 26 Risk assessment for workers exposed to ionizing radiation

John Hipkin, Eric Spence and Alexander Sutherland

Introduction

Ionizing radiation is encountered in many different forms. It may consist of emissions from radioactive materials in the form of α- or β-particles or γ-rays, or as X-rays generated by machines. These radiations have one thing in common; they can damage humans by inducing changes in biologically important molecules. The consequences range from a small increase in the risk of cancer at low doses, to death in the short term at much larger doses.

At doses between these extremes, physical damage to individual organs and tissues, such as erythema (including skin burns) and depilation (loss of hair), can occur. These effects are referred to as deterministic effects, where the severity of the injury depends directly on the magnitude of the radiation dose. They also have a threshold, i.e. a level of radiation exposure below which they would not occur. In the case studies described in this chapter, there is the potential for such effects.

An increased risk of deleterious effects (cancer and hereditary defects) is assumed to be a consequence of even small exposures. These effects are referred to as stochastic effects. It is assumed that there is no dose threshold below which there is no risk of stochastic effects, and the risk to the individual is proportional to the dose.

In order to evaluate the health risk to an individual, the potential dose of radiation that the individual might receive must be determined. The absorbed dose is the mean energy imparted by ionizing radiation to the mass of matter in a volume element. It is expressed in a unit called the gray (Gy). The effective dose is the name given to a quantity intended to measure the detriment from stochastic effects; it is derived from the absorbed dose, and takes into account the risk and the seriousness of these effects. It is expressed in a unit called the sievert (Sv). Annual dose limits are normally expressed in units of millisieverts (mSv). Dose rates are expressed in units of microsieverts or millisieverts per hour ($\mu Sv\,h^{-1}$, $mSv\,h^{-1}$). High, acute exposures are normally expressed as the absorbed dose in grays.

Activity is the term used to indicate the amount of radioactive material. It defines the rate at which the material spontaneously decays, and is expressed in becquerels (Bq).

Evidence for health effects

Evidence for the deterministic effects of ionizing radiation has been gathered from a variety of sources. Such effects are known from accident situations and from the radiotherapy treatment of cancer. Examples of effects and the doses that cause them are given in Table 26.1.

The principal sources of information concerning stochastic effects are the epidemiological studies carried out on the survivors of the two atomic bombs dropped on the Japanese cities of Hiroshima and Nagasaki, studies of cancer induction in miners exposed to radon and studies of patients undergoing radiation treatment. Estimates of risk are kept under review, and a recent publication by the International Commission on Radiological Protection (ICRP) summarizes the current position (ICRP 1991). The recommendations of this publication are intended to prevent the occurrence of deterministic effects and limit the probability of stochastic effects, both to individuals and their immediate and second generation offspring, to an acceptable level. Table 26.2 summarizes the dose limits recommended by ICRP (1991). Among the ICRP recommendations is a risk coefficient for workers. This is mainly based on the risk of death, but also takes into account morbidity and the risk to future generations from hereditary effects. The numerical risk coefficient recommended for fatal cancer in workers is $4 \times 10^{-2}\,Sv^{-1}$. The ICRP's recommendations have been endorsed by the National Radiological Protection Board (NRPB) for use within the UK (NRPB 1993).

Table 26.1 Doses and effects.

Effect	Threshold dose (Gy)
Whole body exposure	
Detectable chromosome change	0.1
Detectable blood count changes	1
Radiation sickness	1
Possible death	3
Probable death	10
Localized exposure	
Erythema	5
Depilation	4

Table 26.2 Summary of ICRP 60 dose limits. (From ICRP 1991.)

Radiation workers	50 mSv in any 1-year period, but not more than 100 mSv in any 5-year period (implied average dose of 20 mSv per year)
General public	1 mSv per year; in special circumstances, a higher effective dose could be allowed in a single year, but the average dose must not exceed 1 mSv per year during the person's lifetime

There is no change to the dose limits for individual organs or for the eye lens.

In the UK, the principal pieces of legislation are the Ionizing Radiation Regulations 1985 (SI 1985 No. 1333) made under the Health and Safety at Work, etc. Act 1974 and the Radioactive Substances Act 1993. The former is administered by the Health and Safety Executive (HSE) and the latter by the Environment Agency (EA). The Ionizing Radiation Regulations 1985 and their accompanying Approved Code of Practice (ACOP) formed the first comprehensive set of regulations which covered all users of ionizing radiation. Table 26.3 summarizes the legally permitted dose limits of the Ionizing Radiation Regulations 1985. It should be noted that the new ICRP recommendations cannot be embodied in the present Ionizing Radiation Regulations 1985 without parliamentary approval. To take note of the ICRP recommendations, the HSE issued a Part 4 ACOP which advises on stricter constraints on radiation exposures, requiring investigations and subsequent reports to the HSE if the dose exceeds 75 mSv in any 5-year period (HSE 1985).

The work described in the case studies is subject to the above regulatory controls in the UK, and many of the precautions taken are necessary to comply with these requirements. The precautions form part of an overall radiation protection programme whose aims are as follows.
1 To prevent deterministic effects.
2 To minimize the stochastic risks so that they are as low as reasonably practicable.
3 To limit the risk of stochastic effects in any individual so that they are within acceptable bounds.

Site radiography, the subject of case study 1, is also governed by guidance from the Engineering Construction Industry Association.

Case studies

Two case studies are outlined below; both involve industrial radiography, but are quite different. In the first, a source containing a radionuclide is taken to the site where radiography takes place. On completion of the work, the source is removed. A particular characteristic of this type of work is that complete control of the exposure of workers to the source is not possible, because the source has to be exposed in

Table 26.3 Summary of UK permitted annual dose limits (mSv). (From Ionizing Radiation Regulations 1985.)

	Whole body	Individual organs	Lens of eye
Radiation workers	50	500	150
Trainees under the age of 18	15	150	50
Non-radiation workers and members of the public*	5	50	15

*The dose limit to the abdomen of a woman of reproductive capacity is 13 mSv in any 13-week period. The dose limit to the abdomen of a woman who is pregnant is limited to 10 mSv during the period of pregnancy.

places not specifically designed for radiography. The second case deals with a fixed installation with an X-ray source, where engineered solutions can operate to control the exposure very effectively.

In this chapter, the annual dose limit of 20 mSv (Table 26.2) is used for comparative purposes. The annual whole body dose limit that applies in the UK is 50 mSv (Table 26.3). Whilst dose limits are important elements of radiation protection, the most important principle is that of optimization of protection. The assumption that all doses of radiation are associated with some risk inevitably leads to the requirement to keep all doses as low as reasonably practicable.

Case 1

Hazard identification

In this case study, two industrial radiographers are given the job of testing a series of welds in pipes. They are equipped with a projection-type container that contains a radioactive source with an activity of 120 GBq of iridium-192. Rope barriers, signs and signals are provided to delineate a controlled area and to warn persons who may approach the area during radiography. The radiographers also have personal dosimeters and dose rate monitors.

During radiography, a cable is used to initiate the exposure by remotely winding the source out from the shielded container along an external guide tube to the exposure position. The duration of each exposure is less than 1 min. At the end of each exposure, the source is retracted into the shielded container. Figure 26.1 illustrates the arrangement.

Exposure assessment

A 120-GBq iridium-192 source will produce a dose rate of 15.6 mSv h^{-1} at 1 m from the source. Thus, a person exposed at 1 m from the source for a period of 1.3 h would receive a dose equal to 20 mSv. The dose rates at various distances from the source vary with the inverse square of the distance. The dose rate close to the source is therefore considerably greater. For instance, the dose rate at 1 cm from the source is 156 Sv h^{-1}, and 2 min of exposure would be sufficient to produce erythema, although the effects may not be apparent immediately. A person exposed in close proximity to the source for a period of several tens of hours could die within a matter of weeks.

Because the dose rate varies with the inverse square of the distance from the source, distance is used very effectively to limit the exposure of both the radiographer and his/her assistant, who should retire from the vicinity of the source for the duration of the exposure sequence. Similarly, other workers are restricted from entering the controlled area by the rope barriers put in place by the radiographers. It is a current

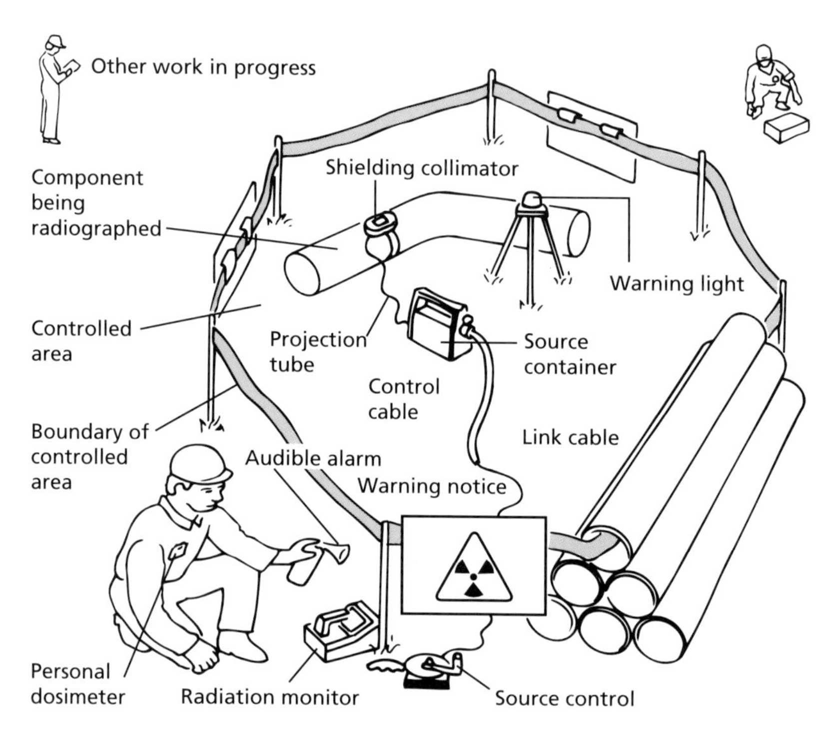

Figure 26.1 Typical arrangement for site radiography using a γ-source. (Reproduced from an NRPB Radiation at Work Leaflet on Industrial Radiography.)

requirement in the UK that barriers are placed at positions at which the dose rate is no greater than $7.5\ \mu Sv\ h^{-1}$.

During routine radiography, using good practices, radiographers should not receive a dose that is excessive, but experience has shown that, for high workloads in adverse environmental conditions, it is possible for doses to be significant fractions of the dose limits. There are a number of contributions to the exposure that cannot easily be avoided. These are outlined below.

1 Exposure to the dose rate from the source container while transporting and carrying it to the site.

2 Exposure to relatively high dose rates for short periods of time while winding out the source at the start of a radiograph and retracting it at the end.

3 Exposure during radiography.

The combination of these factors could lead to an annual dose to a busy radiographer of about 5 mSv.

Radiography does not, however, always run smoothly. The most frequently encountered mishap is when a source cannot be retracted into its shielded container at the end of the planned exposure. The dose that can result from this event depends critically upon its early detection by the proper use of dose rate monitoring procedures. As long as the occurrence is recognized immediately and safe recovery procedures are implemented, exposures are likely to be small. If the event is not immediately recognized, the consequences can be serious, and there is a high potential for dose limits to be exceeded. In a worst case scenario, where the source becomes detached from the exposure equipment, is left behind on the site and is picked up by an unsuspecting other party, there is the potential for major injury. The deaths of a number of individuals in several countries have resulted from such a series of events.

Risk management

Prevention and control

A number of factors require attention if the aims of the radiation protection programme are to be achieved. Prior to the work being undertaken, the company will need to ensure the following.

1 The exposure container should have been chosen so that it provides sufficient protection whilst the source is in the shielded position, and should be designed to ensure that the transfer of the source in and out of the container operates smoothly and efficiently during exposure procedures.

2 When newly acquired, the equipment should have been subjected to a prior radiological assessment to ensure that it operates in a satisfactory manner, particularly with respect to shielding and source movement.

3 The exposure equipment should be properly maintained to ensure that its efficacy does not deteriorate.

4 Radiation dose rate monitors should be provided and properly maintained and tested so that barriers can be monitored and the retraction of the source after radiography can be confirmed.

5 Emergency recovery equipment should be provided to deal with a source becoming stuck or detached during radiography.

6 Back-up assistance should be available and should be able to be obtained swiftly if needed.

7 Written procedures, referred to as Local Rules in the Ionizing Radiation Regulations 1985, should have been provided so that there is no ambiguity about what is required; this also means that written material is readily available for reference.

8 Suitable training should have been provided for the radiographers.

9 Suitable arrangements should have been made for the supervision of the radiographers whilst on site, and for the routine auditing of all safe working procedures.

The team of radiographers must include a radiation protection supervisor whose function is to supervise the work and ensure that the Local Rules are followed. The following actions should be observed where radiographers are working to a high standard of radiation safety.

1 A barrier should be set at an appropriate distance from the source exposure position, taking into account local shielding; access to the

radiography area should also be restricted from areas above and below.
2 Local shielding close to the source, e.g. a collimator, should be used to provide a radiation shadow into which the radiographer can retire during the exposure.
3 The radiographers should use the portable radiation dose rate monitor provided to check after every exposure that the source has fully retracted.
4 The action in 3 is the most crucial to prevent accidental exposure and, as a separate back-up to this, the radiographers should wear personal alarm monitors; these must not be employed instead of the proper use of a portable dose rate monitor.

Routine inspections of this work are the responsibility of senior management, and should be performed randomly, but at intervals of no more than 3 months, by the safety officer. The audits are also the responsibility of senior management, but should also be carried out at 3-year intervals by an external consultant.

Emergency planning
The most frequently encountered mishap, the failure of the source to retract, has been described above. It is important that procedures to deal with this are well developed, rehearsed and therefore familiar to at least one of the radiographers on a site. In the case described here, a contingency plan would have formed a part of the 'Local Rules', and the radiographers would have had appropriate emergency recovery equipment, including shielding materials and a bolt cutter.

Risk communication
It is vitally important that radiographers and their managers have a basic grasp of the hazards of ionizing radiation, and, in particular, they must understand the importance of the safety procedures and the plans to deal with emergencies. Appropriate instruction and training are therefore essential elements in risk management. In order to deal with emergencies, this must include rehearsals of emergency procedures using simulated accident situations. The importance of dose rate monitoring after each use of the radiography equipment must be stressed. Monitoring must be practised until it becomes second nature. The managers must have a good grounding in radiation safety principles, and a sound understanding of the importance of providing and ensuring adherence to written procedures.

Health surveillance
Radiographers involved in site radiography are amongst the most exposed workers in the UK and in many other countries. Their potential exposures could exceed nationally set annual dose limits and, as they are designated as 'classified radiation workers', the monitoring of their exposure and of their health is mandatory. The radiographers involved in the case study described here should wear personal dosimeters. An

audit would confirm that they were subject to annual medical reviews and that appropriate dose records were being kept.

Case 2

Hazard identification

This involves the use of an X-ray cabinet to assess the integrity of small castings. The item to be assessed is placed inside the cabinet with radiographic film, the cabinet is closed and radiography is undertaken with the X-ray set typically used at a rating of 150 kV, 5 mA. A typical exposure period of 2 min is set using an automatic timer that is part of the control system of the cabinet.

Exposure assessment

The output from an X-ray set operating at a rating of 150 kV, 5 mA would typically be about 15 Sv h^{-1} at 1 m from the anode. This is enough to deliver a dose of 20 mSv in a period of about 4 s at this distance. At the exit window of the X-ray tube head, the dose rate could be as high as 5000 Sv h^{-1}, sufficient to deliver in a few seconds a dose that would cause erythema. In practice, the possibility of such eventualities is prevented by engineered safety features.

The X-ray set is enclosed inside a substantial cabinet that provides sufficient shielding to ensure that dose rates outside the cabinet do not exceed 7.5 μSv h^{-1}. Typically, dose rates are a few microsieverts per hour. Access to the inside of the cabinet is through a door that has to be opened to place the items to be radiographed inside the cabinet. The door is interlocked so that X-rays cannot be generated when the door is open and, during an exposure, the generation of X-rays will stop if the door is opened.

Exposures may be substantial if an operator deliberately overrides the door interlock system, or if the interlock system fails and a door is opened during an exposure. Under these circumstances, exposure of the hands and arms may occur, with doses approaching those that could cause erythema. Whole body doses from scattered radiation may also be substantial.

Risk management

Prevention and control

Again, a number of factors require attention. The following actions must be taken.

1 The equipment should be chosen for the shielding provided and the effectiveness of the interlock and warning systems; these systems should be designed, as far as practicable, to fail-to-safety.

2 Before it is brought into routine use, the equipment should be sub-

jected to a prior radiological assessment to ensure that the shielding and interlocks operate in a satisfactory manner.

3 The cabinet should be properly maintained.

4 Arrangements should be made for routine tests to confirm that the interlocks and warning systems operate correctly.

5 Radiation dose rate monitors should be provided and properly maintained and tested, so that the shielding can be routinely assessed and any deterioration noted and remedied in good time.

6 Procedures should exist to inform management of any malfunction of the safety features of the equipment, so that prompt action can be taken to avoid exposure and to remedy the faults.

7 Written procedures (Local Rules) should be provided so that there is no ambiguity about what is required, and written material should be readily available for reference.

8 Suitable training should be provided for the radiographers.

9 Suitable arrangements should be made for the supervision of the radiographers and for routine auditing of the safe working procedures.

In addition to the routine tests of the operation of the interlocks and warning systems carried out by the operators, the radiation protection supervisor should carry out similar inspections and radiation surveys of the cabinet at intervals of 3 months. Again, audits should be carried out at 3-year intervals by an external consultant.

Emergency planning

Contingency plans that include the actions needed to remedy faults which may develop in the safety features of the equipment must be prepared. These plans should also include the need to summon medical assistance in the event that an individual is exposed because of failure or overriding of the door interlocks. Appropriate contingency plans should be part of the Local Rules.

Risk communication

Operators and managers need to be made aware of the nature of the hazard, and the way in which the cabinet has been engineered to overcome it. They need to be told that the risks are small in routine use, but that any deterioration in the safety features must be attended to as soon as possible. A safety audit should assess whether appropriate training has been provided.

Health surveillance

The routine exposures should be so low that there is no need for the assessment of individual doses or for routine medical surveillance. In the unlikely event of an accident situation, medical advice may be needed.

References

HSE (1985) *The Ionizing Radiations Regulations 1985. Statutory Instrument No. 1333 and Associated Approved Code of Practice.* HMSO, London.
ICRP (1991) *Annals of the International Commission on Radiological Protection* **21** (1–3). ICRP Publication 60. *Recommendation of the ICRP on Radiological Protection.* Pergamon Press, Oxford.
NRPB (1993) *Documents of the NRPB* **4** (2). HMSO, London.

Chapter 27 Stress

Wilfred Howe

Introduction

The assessment and management of health problems related to stress in the workplace are complicated by two factors which do not usually apply when managing chemical, physical or biological risks. Firstly, many causes of stress originate outside of work and are less open to influence by normal risk management techniques. Thus, although occupational causes of stress may have been identified and controlled, employees may still be affected and underperform because of stress from out-of-work sources. Secondly, there is significant variation in the amount of stress with which each individual can cope. This depends on a person's inherent coping skills, their response to those factors causing pressure, which may be cumulative, and the timeframe in which the stressors operate. Each person has a limit beyond which any further pressure will cause adverse effects. Thus, there is an interaction between work and non-work pressures and the ability of the individual to cope with these pressures at any period in time.

This case study reviews the author's experience of the introduction of strategies for the management of stress in the workplace. In this context, occupational stress is defined as: 'the adverse mental or emotional reactions to environmental factors occurring in the workplace which result in lowered efficiency, job satisfaction, performance and mental well-being'. Every job has its own set of demands which put pressure on the individual and, indeed, some pressure is essential to promote optimum performance and motivation. Excessive pressure, whether from the workplace alone or in combination with outside sources, can lead to an inability of people to cope, resulting in harmful effects to the individual, group or organization.

Risk assessment and management process

The objectives of the risk assessment and management process are to identify the risks to health, control them so as to eliminate or minimize any risk to health and monitor the process to ensure compliance with the objective. The process for managing chemical, physical or biological risks is well established and has been described elsewhere in Section 3. However, the process for managing psychosocial risks is less well developed in terms of hazard identification, exposure assessment, risk characterization or primary prevention. In examining occupational hazards likely to cause stress, such as inappropriate culture or poor management policies, it is difficult to state with any certainty that the stress experienced by an individual or group is caused by workplace factors, or to put a numerical value on the degree of exposure to such a hazard. In searching for a measurement for psychosocial hazards, the effect on the individual or group becomes an important exposure estimate. Data on adverse health effects can target work groups or processes, and health surveillance becomes an important tool for the identification of the risk from stress. This is a significantly different approach to that of risk management for chemical exposure, where a key objective of health surveillance is to ensure that all measures have been taken to control the hazard, and the absence of any adverse effects demonstrates successful control.

In searching for a systematic approach for the prevention of psychosocial risks, the medical model of primary, secondary and tertiary prevention is used to describe the development of stress management priorities (Bell & Bishop 1995).

Medical model for prevention

In this model, primary prevention aims to identify and eliminate the health risks at source. Secondary prevention involves the early detection of adverse health effects, preferably before clinical disease is evident, and intervention to halt, reverse or retard the progress of the effect. Tertiary prevention aims to minimize the effect of clinical disease by interventions to cure or prevent further deterioration. Each of these strategies can be applied at the individual or group level, and Table 27.1 lists the possible approaches which can be taken.

Primary preventive measures can be applied to the assessment and management of workplace stressors. Secondary and tertiary prevention can be used to deal with both work and non-work stress.

In the author's experience, it is relatively easy to introduce secondary and tertiary strategies, but more difficult to produce assessment data

Table 27.1 Prevention of stress-related effects.

Prevention	Individual	Group
Primary	Preplacement assessment, e.g. psychometric tests Education and training in stress management	Assess work cause of stress Opinion surveys Stress management workshops
Secondary	Routine health assessment Support to those identified	Stress surveys to target hazards
Tertiary	Disease identification and management Counselling, EAP	Epidemiology to target hazards

EAP, employee assistance programme.

that will allow management to target appropriate primary preventive measures. This problem is complicated by stress being perceived by some managers and employees as a weakness, rather than an outcome where people are at the limit of or beyond their ability to cope. Management may be reluctant to accept evidence that its company's policies or style of management may be a major factor in causing occupational stress, but may be more open to dealing with problems that are perceived to be of a non-work-related causality. The result of these perceptions is that there may be little commitment to introduce measures to tackle the root of the problem, but more acceptance of the introduction of strategies to support troubled employees. An awareness of these sensitivities allows a more flexible approach to risk assessment and management, in which tertiary and secondary preventive measures may be established in parallel with initiatives to tackle the root of the problem. This is how several companies have established stress management policies, and the following account describes their implementation using examples over the past 10 years, commencing with tertiary and moving to primary prevention at both individual and group levels.

Tertiary prevention

At an individual level, tertiary prevention seeks to help people who are finding it difficult to cope with the pressures they are experiencing, whether from work or non-work sources. It has traditionally been the role of personnel advisers in human resources departments, health professionals in occupational health departments or industrial chaplains to support troubled employees. In recent times, it is rare for there to be a dedicated welfare officer, and industrial chaplaincy was never extensive.

A strategy which has been successfully implemented has been to encourage occupational physicians and nurses to become proficient at giving first-line help to individuals who present with stress-related symptoms. The skills required are to be able to recognize the physical, behavioural and emotional signs of stress and the likely causes, and to be able to provide support, counselling and advice on coping skills to the individual. Many employees are reluctant to disclose to others that they are not coping—they may see it as a sign of weakness or feel that their supervisors will perceive it that way—and access to a trained health professional provides a 'safe haven' for them to share their concerns. This may be the only support required to help an employee regain optimum well-being. Health professionals are encouraged to undergo training in stress management and counselling skills to enable them to understand the basis for helping stressed employees and to recognize when to refer to expert services outside the workplace. Basic courses, lasting from 3 to 5 days, can be organized using appropriate specialists. As addictive disease is often an outcome in individuals with poor coping skills, health professionals are also encouraged to attend training courses in substance abuse.

Some employees may be reluctant to attend the occupational health department, but may approach their human resource adviser or supervisor. Alternatively, supervisors themselves may have concerns about an employee's behaviour or performance, but may not know how to approach the issue. An additional strategy has been to train human resource staff and key supervisors in basic stress management and counselling skills, so that individuals with problems can be identified, helped and referred either to occupational health professionals or outside support.

A further strategy which has been used for tertiary prevention has been the introduction of an employee assistance programme (EAP); EAPs have been available in the UK over the past 10 years. They offer employees and their immediate families an independent and confidential counselling and information service available, by telephone, on a 24-h basis. Assistance is provided immediately and, if more in-depth counselling is felt to be appropriate, this can be arranged with a 'face-to-face' counsellor. Services can be organized 'in house' or by using outside contract organizations, usually on a 'per capita' payment basis.

Individuals are using EAP services for stress-related problems and, although no individual data are provided back to the company, regular statistics are supplied. In one company, contact was made to the EAP by 20% of employees per year; 15% of these calls were from family members or 'significant others'; 25% of the calls were for emotional or relationship problems, and 10% of the calls resulted in face-to-face counselling for a significant problem; only 5% of problems were reported as being work related, suggesting that most of an employee's stress was experienced outside of the workplace.

The final strategy for tertiary prevention has been to give more support to those individuals who absent themselves from work because of stress or other psychological disease. For these individuals, a policy has been promoted for their managers to make contact with them to offer support, followed up, where appropriate, by contact with an occupational health professional to continue support and, with the family practitioner's agreement, referral to the EAP programme.

These strategies for tertiary prevention have been well supported by management and employees. Their success has been demonstrated by the anecdotal feedback from individuals who have used the services, and from managers who now have a high regard for these services during a period when all costs are being critically appraised.

On a group level, tertiary prevention can be focused on the collection and analysis of epidemiological data on psychosocial illness. The data can be used to demonstrate to management the presence of a significant risk to health.

Mortality data are not usually useful, although death by suicide due to stress-related problems is often sufficient to catalyse management into some sort of action.

Morbidity data are often difficult to collect. The Health and Safety

Executive's *Labour Force Study* (HSE 1994) showed that stress-related illness was the second most prevalent illness perceived as being work related.

In the occupational setting, data on the causes of sickness absence can be useful. For example, an analysis in 1995 of the causes of sickness absence in one business showed that 12% of days lost were reported as mental illness. Although this was the third most frequent cause of sickness absence, it probably represents a significant underreporting of psychological illness.

Data such as these, particularly if they can be quantified into monetary costs to the business, have been useful in demonstrating that action taken to minimize the effects of stress makes good business sense.

Secondary prevention

Secondary prevention for individuals involves the detection of adverse effects, preferably before there is clinical evidence, and intervention to halt, reverse or retard the progress of these effects.

As stated above, employees may be reluctant to seek help until the pressure they are experiencing is adversely affecting their lives. In order to help people who would benefit from an understanding of the causes and effects of stress, and to improve their coping skills, two strategies have been used.

The first is based on the premise that, at some time in their lives, everyone may experience stress-related effects. Training and education in stress management techniques for all employees would help them to recognize the effects and causes of stress and to improve their coping skills.

An interactive workshop has been established which uses written material, questionnaires, visual aids and audio video support.

Using this core material, the workshop is tailored to suit the needs of supervisory and production employees, and can last from 2 to 6 h. The workshop is designed to be led by health professionals who have been trained as facilitators. The workshop explores the nature of stress, its causes and effects and the variety of coping skills which can be used. A maximum of 15 participants are guided through the workshop, as far as possible using their own experience of stress and coping skills, to impart knowledge to the group. Coping skills cover physical measures, such as exercise and relaxation, emotional skills, such as being able to relate their feelings to others, behavioural skills, such as defining goals and making choices, and cognitive skills, such as challenging outdated or irrational belief and value systems.

Included in the workshop is an analysis of the factors which participants themselves experience as being major causes of stress in their own lives. A picture of work- and non-work-related causes of stress has been built up over the past 3 years, and is presented in Table 27.2.

The workshops have been well received, and feedback questionnaires

Table 27.2 Causes of stress.

Too much work
More work than can be handled
Time pressure/tight deadlines
Conflicting objectives
Overambitious and unachievable goals
Inadequate communication, training and development
Lack of information on what is happening
Lack of knowledge of new jobs
Unclear or ambiguous roles
Unclear objectives
Change
Speed of change in the environment
Lack of control
Feeling of 'no choice'
Changing goals
Threat of redundancy
Job insecurity
Fear for the future
Uncertainty
Values/beliefs/behaviours
Lack of trust
Lack of recognition
Feeling of not being valued
Fear of revealing an inability to cope
Lack of care, concern or value for the individual
Relationship problems
Personality clashes
Sexual harassment
Conflict with colleagues
Individual and lifestyle factors
Balancing work and family needs
Financial worries
Health concerns
New baby/crying/lack of sleep/toilet problems
Marriage/divorce
Moving house
Difficult parents, children, partners or in-laws
Lack of self-confidence
Lack of self-esteem
Psychiatric problems—anxiety, depression

give overwhelming support for the workshop to be given to all employees. At present, the workshops are voluntary, and so there may be an element of self-selection.

In order to cascade the workshop to all employees as soon as possible, a pilot scheme is in operation to train non-health professionals to act as facilitators.

The second strategy has been to introduce a three yearly occupational health nurse-based health assessment programme for all employees. This personal health assessment (PHA) process includes a confidential computerized stress questionnaire which takes 10–15 min to complete. The results of the questionnaire are provided to the individual as scores on three factors: the propensity for having Type 'A' behaviour, the degree of stressful changes (work and non-work related) in their lives and an indication of their physical and emotional stress levels.

As part of the PHA programme, those scoring significant stress are given immediate advice on stress management by the nurse, and are recommended to attend one of the stress management workshops. Those reporting considerable stress are additionally recommended to seek further help from the EAP or appropriate specialists through their family practitioners. Although voluntary, the PHA programme has been well accepted by employees with up to 95% take up in some locations.

Action that can be taken at the group level has been to collect and analyse data on early indicators of stress. This has been possible using the PHA system which allows for data analysis. For example, the data which have been collated over the past 3 years are presented in Table 27.3.

The data show that about 20% of employees have a Type 'A' personality, almost 40% have experienced moderate to major stressful events over the past 12 months, 25% report significant symptoms of stress and 9% report considerable symptoms of stress.

The questionnaire has been validated 'in-house' against the general health questionnaire (version with 30 questions) (Goldberg & Williams 1988), and showed good correlation.

It is felt to be a pragmatic tool for the collation of information on the level of stress prevalent in the workplace, and feedback of the information to managers and employees has raised the awareness of stress as an issue which requires positive management.

The stress questionnaire should be able to identify the prevalence of work-related stresses. Unfortunately, this has not been possible with the

Table 27.3 Analysis of stress questionnaires, 1993–1995.

Total numbers	2066
Type 'A' personality	437 (21%)
Causes of stress—moderate/major	778 (38%)
Number with significant stress	515 (25%)
Number with considerable stress	185 (9%)

tool used, and there is a pressing need to develop a simple questionnaire which will identify workplace causes. The data could be used to demonstrate to managers the likely primary source of work-related stress, so that changes and improvements could be made.

Qualitative data on the source of workplace stress have also been made available through the factor analysis in Table 27.2. However, the data are subjective and relate to the perceived stresses of groups of employees. To date, this method has lacked the specificity or credibility for managers to be concerned that action needs to be taken to tackle fundamentally the primary source of stress.

Primary prevention

Primary prevention aims to identify and eliminate the health risks at source, and is the preferred first-line approach to the management of occupational risks.

As discussed earlier, it is relatively easy to assess and manage chemical, physical and biological risks in the workplace. Health surveillance, in these circumstances, is likely to reveal little ill health, as the risk management process is designed to prevent illness from occurring.

The assessment and management of psychosocial hazards in the workplace are more complicated, because it is difficult to identify and quantify the stressors inherent in management policies or organizational culture. As discussed in the sections on 'Secondary prevention' and 'Tertiary prevention', health surveillance takes on a more important role in the quantification of stress-related problems. However, the analysis of the prevalence of stress effects from sickness absence data, stress questionnaires or EAP data provides little quantitative information on the nature or extent of occupational psychosocial risks.

Other data may act as a surrogate for the identification of such risks, such as a reduction in output, decrease in quality, judgemental errors, increased industrial relations' problems, decreased sales, increased overtime or poor timekeeping. However, these measurements can be affected by many different factors and, although they may indicate that an organization is under stress, they contribute little to the targeting of the source of stress.

At the group level, formal studies to identify specific stress hazards are possible using tools such as the Occupational Stress Indicator (Cooper *et al.* 1988) or employee opinion surveys. Experience suggests that these tools are best implemented by specialists in organization and development, who should use them as part of an overall assessment of an organization's effectiveness.

These studies usually reveal factors which need to be changed or improved, and an illustrative list produced from the author's experience is provided in Table 27.4.

Experience has shown that the conclusions from this type of study may not be welcomed by management who may see them as a direct

Table 27.4 Significant factors, the absence of which may be associated with stress at work.

Management and culture	Clear vision, goals and objectives Good two-way communications Well-trained managers Good training and development of staff Humanistic values Open and honest culture
Relationships at work	Fair and consistently implemented personnel and management policies Fair systems for dealing with interpersonal conflict or grievance
Job design	Proper training and resources Role and responsibilities well defined Workload matches skills, knowledge and ability
Employee contribution	Design of job Involvement in change processes Consultation
Physical factors	Appropriate environment with absence of excessive noise, heat and cold

criticism of its policies and style. It is imperative for such studies to receive commitment from both management and staff representatives before implementation. The aims and objectives of the study, methods of analysis and interpretation of the results need to be agreed before commencement. It is particularly important that the likely outcome and actions are also considered.

Unless all of these factors are considered, management may be presented with data which it finds difficult to agree with, and no action will be taken.

At a more practical level, much good has been accomplished by ensuring that senior management and employee representatives are aware of the primary causes of workplace stress, and how organizational factors can adversely affect individual and group psychological health. A 1-day stress management workshop targeted specifically at these issues has been found to be helpful in raising awareness of the issue of stress at work. The outcome should be for management to accept that stress is a business issue which requires positive management similar to any other business need. Training in stress management should, in the future, be incorporated as a standard module in management training courses.

Primary prevention at the individual level is problematical. Psychometric testing is a technique which has been used as a preplacement tool to match an individual's psychological profile with the job. Similar techniques have been used for employees and their families who are to be placed on assignments overseas.

The usefulness of this type of technique to the individual has been to identify any gaps in his/her psychological make-up which could be improved with further education, training or counselling. However, to achieve this same end-point, individual education and training for all employees by the attendance of stress management workshops, as described in the section on 'Tertiary prevention', has been encouraged.

Policy on stress management

The management of stress should be incorporated into company health and safety policies, with an agreed strategy for implementation.

There is no specific legislation on the control of stress at work in the UK. However, implicit in the Health and Safety at Work, etc. Act 1974 and the Management of Health and Safety Regulations 1993 is the requirement for employers to ensure that their workplaces are safe and healthy, and that risks to health are assessed and control measures instituted. Ill health from stress at work should be treated in the same way as ill health due to other physical causes present in the workplace, and should be explicit in a company's health and safety policy.

It is hoped that this case study provides sufficient practical information for companies to adopt such a policy, and to implement programmes to assess and manage stress at work.

References

Bell, J.G. & Bishop, C. (1995) A systematic approach to health surveillance in the workplace. *Occupational Medicine* 45, 305–310.

Cooper, C., Sloan, S. & Williams, S. (1988) *Occupational Stress Indicator*. NFER-Nelson Publicity Company Limited, London.

Goldberg, C. & Williams, S. (1988) *A User's Guide to the General Health Questionnaire*. NFER-Nelson Publicity Company Limited, London.

HSE (1994) *Labour Force Study*. HMSO, London.

Chapter 28 Violence at work

Stuart C. Whitaker

Introduction

Violence at work is causing increasing concern to government bodies, health and safety professionals, employers and employees in many industrialized countries. The risk of violence at work seems to have spread from what were traditionally considered to be high-risk jobs, such as police, prison or security officers (Haapaniemi & Kinnunen 1997), to a large number of what were previously considered to be relatively safe jobs in the service and retail sectors (Aromaa 1997). Employees in diverse environments, such as transport, entertainment, health care, social services and retail sales, are reporting a growing number of incidents. Fortunately, severe injuries and fatalities still remain rare but, where they do occur, they attract wide public attention. Whilst media attention can help to heighten public awareness and encourage organizations to review their arrangements to deal with violence at work, news reports can also serve to increase employees' anxieties about the risk of violence at work without necessarily offering accurate information on the actual degree of risk which they might face or solutions to the problem.

Employers have a responsibility and a legal duty to address the risk of violence at work in the same way as they are required to address other occupational risks. Employees also have duties to co-operate and comply with health and safety arrangements. There are also sound economic reasons why an employer should address the risk of violence at work. Violence can lead to impaired performance at work, high rates of sickness absence, high levels of staff turnover and difficulties for the organization in recruiting or retaining staff (Braithwaite 1992). Increased insurance premiums and the costs of compensation and litigation are all factors to consider in a cost–benefit analysis. Many employers, trade unions and individual employees recognize that violence at work is a legitimate concern, and are working together to seek effective solutions to the problem.

Whilst the risk of violence at work should be assessed and managed in exactly the same way as other occupational risks, violence does have a number of unique characteristics which need to be considered. The clear definition of violence (the hazard), the quantification of the risk and the assessment of the potential severity of incidents can be problematical. This is largely because of the individual perceptions, experiences and expectations of people in relation to violence at work. Strong emotions are often aroused by violence, and some employees may have difficulties in reporting incidents or expressing their concerns due to the fear of appearing inadequate amongst their peers. The potential involvement of the police, criminal prosecution and the prospect of facing the perpetrator in court are additional factors which may influence the willingness of employees to report incidents.

Hazard identification

A clear definition of the hazard is central to any effort to discuss, assess and control the risk of violence at work. Efforts to measure, monitor and report incidents of violence at work are largely dependent upon being able to define clearly what incidents should be reported, recorded and analysed. However, the perception of violence by individual employees is a very personal and subjective issue, often dependent upon the person's culture, values and previous experience. It cannot be assumed that customers and clients, managers, employees and health and safety professionals share a common definition of what constitutes violence at work.

Violence is often defined as much by the context of the actions as by the actions themselves. A push from a patient with senile dementia may not be perceived as a violent attack by a nurse caring for that patient, but the same action from a drunk patient may well be regarded as such. Verbal abuse and swearing may be tolerated to a greater degree in some situations, such as customer complaints' departments, simply because it occurs more often, rather than because it is more acceptable.

In many respects, what an individual perceives as a violent incident is subjectively defined by the experience of the recipient. Regardless of the real intention of the aggressor, if the individual feels threatened, they will define the actions or behaviour as potentially violent. Within groups, there may be clear agreement that extremes of behaviour, such as pushing, punching or kicking, are acts of violence, but perhaps less consensus agreement on whether to include swearing or rude behaviour in a definition of violence. Fortunately, bodies such as the Health and Safety Executive (HSE), the enforcement agency for health and safety in the UK, and the Association of Directors of Social Services have explicit definitions of what they consider violence at work to be. The HSE have defined work related violence as:

> Any incident in which a person is abused, threatened or assaulted in circumstances relating to their work. (HSE 1997a)

The Association of Directors of Social Services (1987) define violence as:

> Violence is behaviour which produces damaging or hurtful effects physically or emotionally on other people. This definition is not limited simply to physical assault but permits the inclusion of equally distressing and intimidating verbal aggression.

These definitions can be useful in helping staff to recognize and define violence in their own workplaces. The definitions can also be used to make explicit statements to customers or clients about what the organization considers to be violence. The important points from these definitions are that violent behaviour is not limited only to physical acts, but also includes intimidation and verbal abuse. Even where there is no direct physical assault, an attempt to abuse, hurt or intimidate employees in the course of their duties is considered to be an act of violence.

Exposure assessment—exposure modelling

Defining violence and recognizing that its effect can be both physical and psychological are important when attempting to assess the probability and the severity of the risk. Whilst exposure to some types of violent behaviour at work may be shrugged off by some employees, others experience long-term damaging effects which can appear to be out of all proportion to the incident. It is well recognized that much of the harm which employees suffer from intimidation or verbal abuse is emotional trauma which may occur some time after the event, and that repeated exposure can be debilitating. The effects of abuse can be cumulative over time, and may impair performance not only at work, but also in an individual's personal life.

An additional problem to consider when assessing potential exposure to violence is that some employees may have difficulty in admitting to feeling fearful in situations which are common, because they feel that they should be able to cope with such circumstances. Employees may feel that, if it were known that they found these situations difficult to cope with, it may affect their career opportunities. Such concerns can affect the employees' willingness to discuss openly or define clearly violence at work for fear of appearing inadequate and unable to cope with situations which others accept.

Despite the growing fear of violence at work, it would appear from published reports that only a minority of employees report such incidents each year, but that there has been a dramatic increase in the number of reported incidents across a wide range of occupational groups (Beale & Cox 1996). Fortunately, despite the relatively few, high-profile cases where employees have suffered major injuries or have been killed, the majority of employees who report being involved in a violent incident do not require inpatient hospital treatment and are usually allowed to go home (More & Maguire 1995). Little is known of the long-term impact of violence at work based upon studies of groups, or of the incidence and prevalence of violence at work based upon the HSE definition. The failure to report, record and investigate incidents or fund research into this important area means that there is limited information on the immediate and long-term effects of what is considered to be the most common form of violence: abuse, intimidation and threat without physical assault.

Within one workplace, an assessment of the potentially high-risk situations can be undertaken either by an investigation performed by a competent person or by the involvement of staff in the identification and evaluation of high-risk situations. The results from this assessment can then be discussed between managers, trade unions and employees. These discussions should focus upon an attempt to identify all of the situations which have resulted in some form of violence in the past and all other situations in which employees consider themselves to be at risk.

A typical list for office workers may include the following.

1 Working alone or on other peoples' premises.
2 Telling people things that they do not want to hear.
3 Withdrawing services.
4 Travelling or staying away from home overnight.
5 Dealing with the public where drugs or alcohol may be encountered.
6 Dealing with people with a mental illness.
7 Leaving the office at night.
8 Using public transport, car parks or 'seedy' hotels.
9 Being late for appointments, overworked and subject to time pressures.

When balancing the probability and severity of an incident, staff can be encouraged to use this information to prioritize risks. Objective data from accident or incident reports, sickness absence records and insurance assessments can help with these discussions. Where objective data are not available, the results of staff surveys, questionnaire studies or the views of focus groups can be used to try to quantify the incidence and severity of incidents. Using their experience of these situations, staff can be encouraged to discuss the possibility of changing working practices, the environment or the range of services being provided in order to reduce the risks.

One model which identifies many of the potential contributory factors which may lead to a violent incident in the health services is described in Fig. 28.1. This model can be used with staff groups to help them identify those factors in their own working environments which may put them at increased risk from violence.

For example, in one case, district nurses had experienced a number of attacks and had felt intimidated when visiting one particularly rough area of a city at night. The accident reports showed that a small number of incidents had been reported, and that none of these had resulted in severe injury. However, when staff where surveyed by questionnaire, the results showed that many of them had experienced unpleasant incidents, mainly of verbal abuse, which had not been reported on accident or incident forms. Staff felt that they were at risk and wanted to take action before a serious incident occurred. They felt unable to work safely in this area even in pairs, and were unable to secure a police escort for all visits. The group proposed that routine visits should be scheduled only during daylight hours, and visiting services should be withdrawn during the night. A central clinic was staffed during the night, which

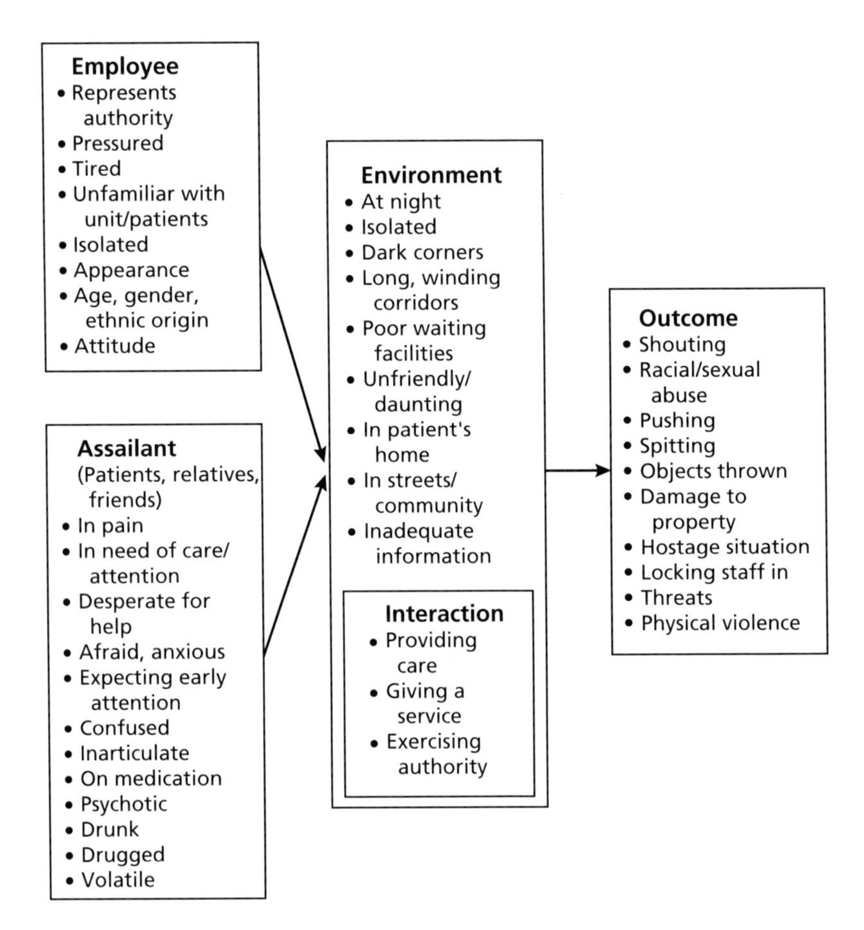

Figure 28.1 Model of a violent incident (HSE 1997b).

enabled patients and relatives to contact the nurses for advice and help in dealing with situations as they arose. This solution helped to eliminate a particular risk, but reduced the level of service which the district nurses would have liked to deliver in this area.

Where the risk cannot be eliminated through changing working practices, efforts to reduce the risk as far as reasonably practicable should be considered. For example, where employees are concerned about staying away from home in 'seedy' hotels, efforts should be made to bring several colleagues together at one hotel in the evening or to find acceptable hotels, which may include only those with *en suite* facilities, a telephone in the room and with staff on duty to respond in the event of an emergency (Faupel 1993). Some hotels now offer a women only floor, and do not place unaccompanied women in ground floor rooms. In an effort to remain attractive to the growing number of business women who may be travelling alone, some hotels advertise that they are happy to serve full evening meals in the privacy of the customer's room.

Risk characteristics—quantitative risk assessment

Where possible, exposure assessment should be based on the quantification of risk based upon objective information. Where records of incidents are available, these can be used to help to quantify the risk. For example, where social workers are required to remove children from their parents against the will of the parents, the records may show that, in nine out of 10 cases, the parents will be angry and try to physically stop the removal of their children. In these circumstances, an incident of some kind can reasonably be expected to happen and a clear strategy is called for.

In high-risk jobs, generally where the public are being dealt with under difficult circumstances or where there may be a risk of robbery, the probability of a violent incident occurring at some point can reasonably be foreseen. Therefore, the need for assessment and control is clear (Standing & Nicolini 1997). However, the quantification of risk can be useful in deciding upon the nature, scale and scope of arrangements. The quantification of risk can be a useful component of a cost–benefit analysis and, in some cases, can help to identify where unacceptable risks are occurring.

For low-risk jobs, the likelihood or probability that a violent incident will occur within a specific timeframe can often be difficult to predict. Rare events, particularly when they do not follow a pattern, offer little information on which to base preventive action. This is particularly so when considering the risk of violence for new organizations or new ventures, where there is little or no information available on incidents from previous records. In these circumstances, the assessment of risk is often based on individual views, the balance of probabilities from a knowledge of other sources and, ultimately, a management decision based upon the available information.

The most difficult incidents to predict are those for which there is no previous information on which to base decisions (Isotalue & Saarela 1997). Many workers are faced with dealing with the public in situations in which they have little information on or knowledge of the behaviour of the people they serve. In order to gather accurate data on which to base decisions, accurate recording and reporting of incidents are essential. Where several organizations are willing to combine together, perhaps through shop owners' associations, local groups or trade unions, data on the type and nature of incidents can be combined to give more information. Examples of how different situations are addressed can be shared and, through co-operation with the police, the perpetrators of violence can be pursued.

Prevention and control

The risk of violence at work can be eliminated or controlled in the majority of cases by the planning, training and maintenance of safe systems of work. As with all risk management strategies, prevention is the key to success, and efforts should be concentrated primarily on this aspect. When all that can reasonably be done to eliminate the risk of violence at work has been performed, strategies to reduce the risk and mitigate the consequences should be considered.

In the same way that many inexperienced managers will inappropriately purchase personal protective equipment (PPE) to protect their employees from exposure to chemicals as the first step in a risk management strategy, many managers will automatically think of self-defence training as the first response to violence at work. Self-defence training should be considered as a last resort only when all other efforts to eliminate or control the risk have failed. Self-defence training, in the form of teaching employees to block punches, stop kicks or effectively break free from strangle holds, requires many years of training to develop a high level of skill, a good standard of physical fitness and the ability to react instinctively under combat situations. If employees are frequently faced with being punched, kicked or strangled at work, the risk management strategy has failed. This is also true for high-risk jobs, such as police or prison officers and psychiatric nurses, where the prospect of having to deal with physical violence is relatively common. Good planning, manpower, training, equipment and teamwork in these situations can effectively reduce the risk of injury and in many situations prevent an incident from occurring in the first place.

Efforts to prevent violence at work should start by considering the causes of violence. If customers become aggressive because of the way in which they are being treated, methods to improve the way in which they are handled should be examined. In accident and emergency departments, one of the most common complaints from aggressive clients was that they were not told anything and did not know how long they might be kept waiting. Now it is common to see the waiting time displayed in most departments; efforts have also been made to provide reading material, televisions and other diversions, such as children's toys, to help clients cope with the often long delays (Carter & Kenkre 1997).

If the environment is thought to contribute to the level of aggression, perhaps through inadequate seating, shabby facilities or inadequate privacy, attempts should be focused upon the provision of an environment which is suitable for its purpose. Some organizations have introduced pastel colour schemes, soft furnishings and reading materials into their waiting areas. Other changes to the environment, such as video cameras, screens separating potentially aggressive customers from staff, alarm systems, security doors and the fixing of movable objects which could be used as weapons, can also be considered. All changes proposed must be thought through in detail; cameras do not prevent violence of themselves, but simply record information. Making customers aware that they are being recorded on camera and that any incident will be followed up vigorously are just as important. Security doors are of no value if they are propped open.

Staff should be involved in the identification and evaluation of violence at work and should contribute to plans to control this violence. Personal training is essential in order to educate employees to recognize the early warning signs when a situation is escalating, to be clear about their role in the operational policies for dealing with potentially aggressive clients and to provide the personal skills necessary to help diffuse aggressive situations, disengage themselves from arguments and seek help from others without feeling inadequate.

Senior management needs to ensure that the decisions reached on how to reduce the risk of violence at work are actually being implemented in practice. By setting targets for implementation, managers can monitor progress towards agreed goals and, through a regular review of performance, can evaluate the effectiveness of their arrangements for managing this risk.

The health and safety policy can address the risk of violence, and may include specific sections on the organization's commitment to the management of the risk of violence at work. The policy may contain the following sections.

1 *Statement of intent*: states that the organization is totally committed to maintaining the health and safety of its staff, including in relation to violence.

2 *Definitions of violence*: includes acts of aggression, verbal abuse and hostility. The clarity of what is included in the definition of violence is important.

3 *Prevention of violence*: details the procedures to be used to reduce the risk of all types of violence at work, including risk assessment, audit and review procedures. Also includes a commitment to training and the provision of suitable premises, equipment and safe working practices.

4 *Procedures to be followed in all cases of violence*: includes the immediate action to be taken to prevent further abuse or harm, procedures for reporting, recording and analysing data from incidents and future management. Also includes the company policy on the legal representation for staff subjected to violence at work.

Audit and review

Finally, every incident should be treated as an opportunity to review and refine the risk management strategy, near-miss incidents should be learned from and regular reviews should be held to share examples of good practice. Information and objective data on violence at work should be published in order to ensure that discussions are based on objective information and to allay unnecessary fears. A lead person in the organization should be chosen who has the responsibility to monitor, co-ordinate and advise managers (Simonowitz & Rigdon 1997).

The following steps should be taken after any incident.

1 The employee must be supported at the time and on his/her return to work. This can be through informal peer support, by the line manager or

through formal arrangements with a counselling service. Employees may need time off from work or may be allowed to move to another job until their confidence is restored. Reassurance and support from senior management are often valued by the individual and other members of staff.

2 The incident must be recorded in sufficient detail to be useful, and must be brought to the attention of senior management. Detailed investigation can lead to recommendations being made which can help in the future.

3 The incident may have to be reported to the police. This can be useful not only to pursue a conviction, but also to enable the police to gather information and to help to address the problem. This may help to reduce the risk in future for the affected and other sites.

4 The impact on others should be considered, e.g. customers who witnessed the incident, other staff who may be afraid and relatives of the employee who may need to be reassured that all that can be done is being done.

5 Experiences and best practices should be shared with others who may be similarly exposed, through trade associations, trade unions, professional meetings and training days.

References

Aromaa, K. (1997) The EC is focusing attention on work related violence. *Tyoe ja Ihminen* 11 (1), 47–52.

Association of Directors of Social Services (1987) *Guidelines and Recommendations to Employers on Violence Against Employees*. Internal Document. Directors of Social Services, London.

Beale, D. & Cox, T. (1996) Work related violence—is national reporting good enough. *Work and Stress* 10 (2), 99–103.

Braithwaite, R. (1992) *Violence. Understanding, Intervention and Prevention*. Radcliffe Professional Press, Oxford.

Carter, Y.H. & Kenkre, J.E. (1997) The development of a training pack on the management of aggression and violence in primary care. *Safety Science* 25 (1–3), 223–230.

Faupel, P. (1993) The lone worker. *Safety and Health Practitioner* 11 (8), 34–36.

Haapaniemi, M. & Kinnunen, A. (1997) Changed violence at work 1980–1993. *Tyoe ja Ihminen* 11 (1), 14–23.

HSE (1997a) *Violence at Work: A Guide for Employers*. HSE Books, Sudbury, Suffolk.

HSE (1997b) *Violence and Aggression to Staff in Health Services. Guidance on Assessment and Management*. p.31. HSE Books, Sudbury, Suffolk.

Isotalue, N. & Saarela, K.L. (1997) Preventing violent injuries and threatening situations in the retail trade. *Tyoe ja Ihminen* 11 (10), 24–34.

More, W. & Maguire, J. (1995) *Handling Aggression and Violence in Health Services. A Training Programme*. PEPAR Publications, Birmingham.

Simonowitz, J.A. & Rigdon, J.E. (1997) Workplace violence: prevention efforts by the occupational health nurse. *American Association of Occupational Health Nurses Journal* 45 (6), 305–316.

Standing, H. & Nicolini, D. (1997) *Review of Workplace Related Violence*. HSE Contract Research Report No. 143/1997. HSE Books, London.

Appendices

Appendix 1 Examples of UK legislation for different occupational hazard types

General requirements including reporting and pre-employment

Health and Safety at Work, etc. Act 1974
Management of Health and Safety at Work Regulations 1992
Health and Safety (First-Aid) Regulations 1981
Workplace (Health, Safety and Welfare) Regulations 1992
Personal Protective Equipment at Work Regulations 1992

Social Security (Industrial Injuries) (Prescribed Disease) Regulations 1985
Reporting of Injuries, Diseases and Dangerous Occurrences Regulations 1995

Diving Operations at Work Regulations 1992
Road Transport Act 1988

Chemical hazards

Control of Substances Hazardous to Health Regulations 1994
Chemical (Hazard Information and Packaging for Supply) (CHIP 2) Regulations 1994
Control of Asbestos at Work Regulations (CAWR) 1987, amended by CAWR 1992
Asbestos (Licensing) Regulations 1983
Asbestos (Prohibition) Regulations 1985
Control of Asbestos (Amendment) Regulations 1992
Control of Lead at Work Regulations 1980
Notification of New Substances Regulations 1988

Physical hazards

Noise at Work Regulations 1989

Legal reference to *vibration* is contained in various regulations including:
Provision and Use of Work Equipment Regulations (PUWER) 1992
Pressure Systems and Transportable Gas Containers Regulations 1989
Use of Explosive in Mines Regulations 1988

Supply of Machinery (Safety) Regulations 1992
Ionizing Radiation Regulations 1985
Ionizing Radiations (Outside Workers) Regulations 1993
Supply of Machinery (Safety) Regulations 1992—particular duties for protection against lasers
Radioactive Materials (Road Transport) Act 1991

Biological hazards

Control of Substances Hazardous to Health Regulations 1994
Notification of Cooling Towers and Evaporative Condensers Regulations 1992
Genetically Modified Organisms (Contained Use) Regulations 1992
Genetically Modified Organisms (Deliberate Release) Regulations 1992

Machinery hazards including pressure systems

Provision and Use of Work Equipment Regulations 1992
Supply of Machinery (Safety) Regulations 1992
Construction (Design and Management) (CDM) Regulations 1994
Pressure Systems and Transportable Gas Containers Regulations 1989
Simple Pressure Vessel (Safety) Regulations 1992

Ergonomics (posture and repetitive movement)

Manual Handling Operations Regulations 1992
Health and Safety (Display Screen Equipment) Regulations 1992

Electricity, flammable liquids and fire safety

Electricity at Work Regulations 1989
Fire Precautions Act 1971
Fire Precautions (Places of Work) Regulations (proposed)
Fire Precautions (Factories, Shops and Railway Premises) Order 1976
Highly Flammable Liquids and Liquefied Petroleum Gases Regulations 1972
Fire Certificate (Special Premises) Regulations 1976
Petroleum (Consolidation) Act 1928

Stress

European Union (EU) Directive on Display Screen Equipment (90/270/EEC) stipulates that the analysis of the workstation should evaluate the problem of mental stress, and the Supply of Machinery (Safety) Regulations 1992 require a designer to consider psychological stress together with comfort and fatigue.

Safety cases

Regulations which require safety cases or safety reports include:
Control of Industrial Major Hazard Regulations 1984, amended by the Control of Industrial Major Hazard (Amendment) Regulations 1990
Offshore Installations (Safety Case) Regulations 1992
Railway (Safety Case) Regulations 1994

Appendix 2 Schedule 3 to RIDDOR 1995

Schedule 3 to RIDDOR 1995 is reproduced below to show the range of diseases required to be reported in the UK. The information presented also provides a useful guide of work activities and associated diseases which is an important element of risk assessment.

Conditions due to physical agents and the physical demands of work.

Column 1 Diseases	Column 2 Activities
1 Inflammation, ulceration or malignant disease of the skin due to ionizing radiation.	Work with ionizing radiation.
2 Malignant disease of the bones due to ionizing radiation.	
3 Blood dyscrasia due to ionizing radiation.	
4 Cataract due to electromagnetic radiation	Work involving exposure to electromagnetic radiation (including radiant heat).
5 Decompression illness.	Work involving breathing gases at increased pressure (including diving).
6 Barotrauma resulting in lung or other organ damage.	
7 Dysbaric osteonecrosis.	
8 Cramp of the hand or forearm due to repetitive movements.	Work involving prolonged periods of handwriting, typing or other repetitive movements of the fingers, hand or arm.
9 Subcutaneous cellulitis of the hand (beat hand).	Physically demanding work causing severe or prolonged friction or pressure on the hand.
10 Bursitis or subcutaneous cellulitis arising at or about the knee due to severe or prolonged external friction or pressure at or about the knee (beat knee).	Physically demanding work causing severe or prolonged friction or pressure at or about the knee.
11 Bursitis or subcutaneous cellulitis arising at or about the elbow due to severe or prolonged external friction or pressure at or about the elbow (beat elbow).	Physically demanding work causing severe or prolonged friction or pressure at or about the elbow.

Continued p.462

Conditions due to physical agents and the physical demands of work.

Column 1 Diseases	Column 2 Activities
12 Traumatic inflammation of the tendons of the hand or forearm or of the associated tendon sheaths.	Physically demanding work, frequent or repeated movements, constrained postures or extremes of extension or flexion of the hand or wrist.
13 Carpal tunnel syndrome.	Work involving the use of hand-held vibrating tools.
14 Hand-arm vibration syndrome.	(a) The use of chain saws, brush cutters or hand-held or hand-fed circular saws in forestry or woodworking; (b) the use of hand-held rotary tools in grinding material or in sanding or polishing metal; (c) the holding of material being ground or metal being sanded or polished by rotary tools; (d) the use of hand-held percussive metal-working tools or the holding of metal being worked upon by percussive tools in connection with riveting, caulking, chipping, hammering, fettling or swaging; (e) the use of hand-held powered percussive drills or hand-held powered percussive hammers in mining, quarrying or demolition, or on roads or footpaths (including road construction); or (f) the holding of material being worked upon by pounding machines in shoe manufacture.

Infections due to biological agents.

Column 1 Diseases	Column 2 Activities
15 Anthrax.	(a) Work involving handling infected animals, their products or packaging containing infected material; or (b) work on infected sites.
16 Brucellosis.	Work involving contact with: (a) animals or their carcasses (including any parts thereof) infected by brucella or the untreated products of same; or (b) laboratory specimens or vaccines of or containing brucella.

Continued

Infections due to biological agents.

Column 1 Diseases	Column 2 Activities
17 (a) Avian chlamydiosis.	Work involving contact with birds infected with *Chlamydia psittaci*, or the remains or untreated products of such birds.
(b) Ovine chlamydiosis.	Work involving contact with sheep infected with *Chlamydia psittaci* or the remains or untreated products of such sheep.
18 Hepatitis.	Work involving contact with: (a) human blood or human blood products; or (b) any source of viral hepatitis.
19 Legionellosis.	Work on or near cooling systems which are located in the workplace and use water; or work on hot water service systems located in the workplace which are likely to be a source of contamination.
20 Leptospirosis.	(a) Work in places which are or are liable to be infested by rats, fieldmice, voles or other small mammals; (b) work at dog kennels or involving the care or handling of dogs; or (c) work involving contact with bovine animals or their meat products or pigs or their meat products.
21 Lyme disease.	Work involving exposure to ticks (including in particular work by forestry workers, rangers, dairy farmers, game keepers and other persons engaged in countryside management).
22 Q fever.	Work involving contact with animals, their remains or their untreated products.
23 Rabies.	Work involving handling or contact with infected animals.
24 Streptococcus suds.	Work involving contact with pigs infected with streptococcus suds, or with the carcasses, products or residues of pigs so affected.
25 Tetanus.	Work involving contact with soil likely to be contaminated by animals.
26 Tuberculosis.	Work with persons, animals, human or animal remains or any other material which might be a source of infection.

Continued p.464

Infections due to biological agents.

Column 1 Diseases	Column 2 Activities
27 Any infection reliably attributable to the performance of the work specified in the entry opposite hereto.	Work with microorganisms; work with live or dead human beings in the course of providing any treatment or service or in conducting any investigation involving exposure to blood or body fluids; work with animals or any potentially infected material derived from any of the above.

Conditions due to substances.

Column 1 Diseases	Column 2 Activities
28 Poisonings by any of the following: (a) acrylamide monomer; (b) arsenic or one of its compounds; (c) benzene or a homologue of benzene; (d) beryllium or one of its compounds; (e) cadmium or one of its compounds; (f) carbon disulphide; (g) diethylene dioxide (dioxan); (h) ethylene oxide; (i) lead or one of its compounds; (j) manganese or one of its compounds; (k) mercury or one of its compounds; (l) methyl bromide; (m) nitrochlorobenzene, or a nitro- or amino- or chloro-derivative of benzene or of a homologue of benzene; (n) oxides of nitrogen; (o) phosphorus or one of its compounds.	Any activity.
29 Cancer of a bronchus or lung.	(a) Work in or about a building where nickel is produced by decomposition of a gaseous nickel compound or where any industrial process which is ancillary or incidental to that process is carried on; or (b) work involving exposure to bis(chloromethyl) ether or any electrolytic chromium processes (excluding passivation) which involve hexavalent chromium compounds, chromate production or zinc chromate pigment manufacture.
30 Primary carcinoma of the lung where there is accompanying evidence of silicosis.	Any occupation in: (a) glass manufacture; (b) sandstone tunnelling or quarrying; (c) the pottery industry;

Continued

Conditions due to substances.

Column 1 Diseases	Column 2 Activities
	(d) metal ore mining; (e) slate quarrying or slate production; (f) clay mining; (g) the use of siliceous materials as abrasives; (h) foundry work; (i) granite tunnelling or quarrying; or (j) stone cutting or masonry.
31 Cancer of the urinary tract.	1 Work involving exposure to any of the following substances: (a) beta-naphthylamine or methylene-bisorthochloroaniline; (b) diphenyl substituted by at least one nitro or primary amino group or by at least one nitro and primary amino group (including benzidine); (c) any of the substances mentioned in subparagraph (b) above if further ring substituted by halogeno, methyl or methoxy groups, but not by other groups; or (d) the salts of any of the substances mentioned in subparagraphs (a)–(c) above. 2 The manufacture of auramine or magenta.
32 Bladder cancer.	Work involving exposure to aluminium smelting using the Soderberg process.
33 Angiosarcoma of the liver.	(a) Work in or about machinery or apparatus used for the polymerization of vinyl chloride monomer, a process which, for the purposes of this subparagraph, comprises all operations up to and including the drying of the slurry produced by the polymerization and the packaging of the dried product; or (b) work in a building or structure in which any part of the process referred to in the foregoing subparagraph takes place.
34 Peripheral neuropathy.	Work involving the use or handling of or exposure to the fumes of or vapour containing *n*-hexane or methyl *n*-butyl ketone.

Continued p.466

Conditions due to substances.

Column 1 Diseases	Column 2 Activities
35 Chrome ulceration of: (a) the nose or throat; or (b) the skin of the hands or forearm.	Work involving exposure to chromic acid or to any other chromium compound.
36 Folliculitis. 37 Acne. 38 Skin cancer.	Work involving exposure to mineral oil, tar, pitch or arsenic.
39 Pneumoconiosis (excluding asbestosis).	1 (a) The mining, quarrying or working of silica rock or the working of dried quartzose sand, any dry deposit or residue of silica or any dry admixture containing such materials (including any activity in which any of the aforesaid operations are carried out incidentally to the mining or quarrying of other minerals or to the manufacture of articles containing crushed or ground silica rock); or (b) the handling of any of the materials specified in the foregoing subparagraph in or incidentally to any of the operations mentioned therein or substantial exposure to the dust arising from such operations. 2 The breaking, crushing or grinding of flint, the working or handling of broken, crushed or ground flint or materials containing such flint or substantial exposure to the dust arising from any of such operations. 3 Sand blasting by means of compressed air with the use of quartzose sand or crushed silica rock or flint or substantial exposure to the dust arising from such sand blasting. 4 Work in a foundry or the performance of, or substantial exposure to the dust arising from, any of the following operations: (a) the freeing of steel castings from adherent siliceous substances; or (b) the freeing of metal castings from adherent siliceous substances:

Continued

Conditions due to substances.

Column 1 Diseases	Column 2 Activities
	(i) by blasting with an abrasive propelled by compressed air, steam or a wheel; or (ii) by the use of power-driven tools.
	5 The manufacture of china or earthenware (including sanitary earthenware, electrical earthenware and earthenware tiles) and any activity involving substantial exposure to the dust arising therefrom.
	6 The grinding of mineral graphite or substantial exposure to the dust arising from such grinding.
	7 The dressing of granite or any igneous rock by masons, the crushing of such materials or substantial exposure to the dust arising from such operations.
	8 The use or preparation for use of an abrasive wheel or substantial exposure to the dust arising therefrom.
	9 (a) Work underground in any mine in which one of the objects of the mining operations is the getting of any material; (b) the working or handling above ground at any coal or tin mine of any materials extracted therefrom or any operation incidental thereto; (c) the trimming of coal in any ship, barge, lighter, dock or harbour or at any wharf or quay; or (d) the sawing, splitting or dressing of slate or any operation incidental thereto.
	10 The manufacture or work incidental to the manufacture of carbon electrodes by an industrial undertaking for use in the electrolytic extraction of aluminium from aluminium oxide and any activity involving substantial exposure to the dust therefrom.
	11 Boiler scaling or substantial exposure to the dust arising therefrom.

Continued p.468

Conditions due to substances.

Column 1 Diseases	Column 2 Activities
40 Byssinosis.	The spinning or manipulation of raw or waste cotton or flax or the weaving of cotton or flax, carried out in each case in a room in a factory, together with any other work carried out in such a room.
41 Mesothelioma. 42 Lung cancer. 43 Asbestosis.	(a) The working or handling of asbestos or any admixture of asbestos; (b) the manufacture or repair of asbestos textiles or other articles containing or composed of asbestos; (c) the cleaning of any machinery or plant used in any of the foregoing operations and of any chambers, fixtures and appliances for the collection of asbestos dust; or (d) substantial exposure to the dust arising from any of the foregoing operations.
44 Cancer of the nasal cavity or associated air sinuses.	1 (a) Work in or about a building where wooden furniture is manufactured; (b) work in a building used for the manufacture of footwear or components of footwear made wholly or partly of leather or fibre board; or (c) work at a place used wholly or mainly for the repair of footwear made wholly or partly of leather or fibre board. 2 Work in or about a factory building where nickel is produced by decomposition of a gaseous nickel compound or in any process which is ancillary or incidental thereto.
45 Occupational dermatitis.	Work involving exposure to any of the following agents: (a) epoxy resin systems; (b) formaldehyde and its resins; (c) metalworking fluids; (d) chromate (hexavalent and derived from trivalent chromium); (e) cement, plaster or concrete; (f) acrylates and methacrylates; (g) colophony (rosin) and its modified products; (h) glutaraldehyde;

Continued

Conditions due to substances.

Column 1 Diseases	Column 2 Activities
	(i) mercaptobenzothiazole, thiurams, substituted paraphenylene-diamines and related rubber processing chemicals; (j) biocides, antibacterials, preservatives or disinfectants; (k) organic solvents; (l) antibiotics and other pharmaceuticals and therapeutic agents; (m) strong acids, strong alkalis, strong solutions (e.g. brine) and oxidizing agents including domestic bleach or reducing agents; (n) hairdressing products including in particular dyes, shampoos, bleaches and permanent waving solutions; (o) soaps and detergents; (p) plants and plant-derived material including in particular the daffodil, tulip and chrysanthemum families, the parsley family (carrots, parsnips, parsley and celery), garlic and onion, hardwoods and the pine family; (q) fish, shellfish or meat; (r) sugar or flour; or (s) any other known irritant or sensitizing agent including in particular any chemical bearing the warning 'may cause sensitization by skin contact' or 'irritating to the skin'.
46 Extrinsic alveolitis (including farmer's lung).	Exposure to moulds, fungal spores or heterologous proteins during work in: (a) agriculture, horticulture, forestry, cultivation of edible fungi or malt-working; (b) loading, unloading or handling mouldy vegetable matter or edible fungi whilst same is being stored; (c) caring for or handling birds; or (d) handling bagasse.
47 Occupational asthma.	Work involving exposure to any of the following agents: (a) isocyanates; (b) platinum salts; (c) fumes or dust arising from the manufacture, transport or use of hardening agents (including epoxy resin curing agents) based on phthalic

Continued p.470

Conditions due to substances. (*Continued*)

Column 1 Diseases	Column 2 Activities
47 Occupational asthma.	anhydride, tetrachlorophthalic anhydride, trimellitic anhydride or triethylenetetramine; (d) fumes arising from the use of resin as a soldering flux; (e) proteolytic enzymes; (f) animals including insects and other arthropods used for the purposes of research or education or in laboratories; (g) dusts arising from the sowing, cultivation, harvesting, drying, handling, milling, transport or storage of barley, oats, rye, wheat or maize or the handling, milling, transport or storage of meal or flour made therefrom; (h) antibiotics; (i) cimetidine; (j) wood dust; (k) ispaghula; (l) castor bean dust; (m) ipecacuanha; (n) azodicarbonamide; (o) animals including insects and other arthropods (whether in their larval forms or not) used for the purposes of pest control or fruit cultivation or the larval forms of animals used for the purposes of research or education or in laboratories; (p) glutaraldehyde; (q) persulphate salts or henna; (r) crustaceans or fish or products arising from these in the food processing industry; (s) reactive dyes; (t) soya bean; (u) tea dust; (v) green coffee bean dust; (w) fumes from stainless steel welding; (x) any other sensitizing agent, including in particular any chemical bearing the warning 'may cause sensitization by inhalation'.

Appendix 3 Information sources for the assessment and management of occupational health hazards

Compiled by Sheila Pantry, Steven S. Sadhra and Christine McRoy

This section provides examples of CD-ROM databases, commercial software packages available in the UK and textbooks for further reading that may assist occupational health professionals when conducting workplace risk assessments.

CD-ROM databases

There are numerous databases available on occupational health and related disciplines. The databases are either bibliographic or full text: the former give citations and abstracts to books, reports and journals in various subject areas and the latter provide publications in full on the database. The following examples may provide useful infozrmation on the assessment and management of occupational health risks.

CHEMINFO

A database available from the Canadian Centre for Occupational Health and Safety (CCOHS), which provides details of the health effects of chemicals, personal protective equipment, trade names and regulatory requirements. Although the regulatory information relates to Canadian legislation, EU classification and labelling requirements have been introduced. The health hazard information is applicable in any country.

EuroOSH

A full text health and safety database produced by Chapman and Hall Electronic Publishing Division. It contains full text and summaries of European Union legislative and regulatory instruments and International Labour Conventions and Recommendations.

OSH-ROM

A bibliographic database produced by SilverPlatter Information Ltd. There are six databases on OSH-ROM (listed below), which together contain over 350 000 citations taken from 500 journals and 100 000 reports and publications.

CISDOC, produced by the International Labour Office Health and Safety Centre, Geneva, covers references from many countries which are linked into the Centre. These include legislation, research results, materials and chemical safety data sheets, conference proceedings and journal articles.

RILOSH, produced by the Ryerson Technical University, Toronto, covers a wide range of references from worldwide sources with an emphasis on American and Canadian information.

OEM, is a subset of the US National Library of Medicine information and covers references in occupational and environmental medicine.

HSELINE, produced by the Health and Safety Executive (HSE) Information Service, UK, contains worldwide information. This database cites publications produced by the HSE Information Service. In addition, references from international publications, UK legislation, European Commission Directives, UK Acts and Statutory Instruments, Codes of Practice and HSE translations are included.

NIOSHTIC, produced by the National Institute for Occupational Safety and Health, USA, contains references to NIOSH documents, such as Criteria Documents, Occupational Hazard Assessments, Special Hazard Reviews, Manual of Analytical Methods, Current Intelligence Bulletins and Joint Occupational Health Recommendations, and also references from international books, journals and reports.

MHIDAS, developed by AEA Technology Ltd., UK, provides summaries of major chemical accidents and incidents that have occurred worldwide.

OSH-CD

A full text database produced by the HSE Information Service and published by SilverPlatter Information Ltd and Stationery Office (formerly HMSO). It contains the full text of all HSE publications, including Approved Codes of Practice, Guidance Notes and Leaflets. There are also abstracts from over 1600 British Standards relating to health and safety.

OSH-OFFSHORE

This is produced by the HSE Information Service and published by the Stationery Office, and provides access to essential health and safety information specifically relevant to the offshore oil and gas industry. It contains the full text of all relevant legislation and guidance from the Health and Safety Commission (HSC) and HSE, and all Offshore Technology Reports—OTH and OTI series. In addition, the full text of journals, such as *Offshore Research Focus*, *HSC Newsletter* and *Toxic Substances Bulletin*, is also included.

RTECS (Registry of Toxic Effects of Chemical Substances)

This is the computerized version of the NIOSH compendium of toxicity data and is available from CCOHS, the Canadian Centre for Occupational Health and Safety. It gives information on the toxic effects of chemicals, health hazards and mutagenic and carcinogenic data. It is also available with four other chemical databases on CHEMBANK produced by SilverPlatter Information Ltd.

TOXLINE

This is produced by the USA National Library of Medicine and supplied by SilverPlatter and CCOHS. It is an international bibliographic database containing toxicological information published in journals, books and reports. The records date from 1966 to the present day.

Textbooks are available on CD-ROM, e.g. the new edition of the *ILO Encyclopaedia*, *SAX's Dangerous Properties of Industrial Materials* and *Hawley's Condensed Chemical Dictionary*.

Software packages

The following list illustrates examples of the software packages available in the UK which may assist occupational health professionals both in the conduct of workplace assessment and in the recording and analysis of the data collected. No assessment of the relative merits of the packages listed has been attempted, as this will depend on the user requirements. Furthermore, inclusion in this list does not indicate approval of the products. The supplier should be contacted for further information and demonstration disks. The software packages are listed in alphabetical order.

Name. AIMS—ACCIDENT INFORMATION MANAGEMENT SYSTEMS
Scope. Aids compliance with the Reporting of Injuries, Diseases and Dangerous Occurrences Regulations (RIDDOR) 1995 and the Social Security Act. Records accidents, diseases and dangerous occurrences. Analyses incidents to reveal patterns.
Supplier. Deltasoft Ltd., PO Box 107, Tasburgh, Norwich, Norfolk NR15 1QT. Tel.: 0707 1233 234. Fax: 0707 1250 910.

Name. ARRAN, AUDIT, RISK and COSHH
Scope. Four systems covering Accident Reporting and Analysis (ARRAN), Health and Safety Auditing (AUDIT), Quantified Risk Assessment (RISK) and Control of Substances Hazardous to Health (COSHH). Packages available for both DOS and Windows environments.
Supplier. Norton Waugh Computing Ltd., The Old School, Weston-under-Lizard, Shifnal, Shropshire TF11 8SZ. Tel.: 01952 850333. Fax: 01952 850649.

Name. BDH HAZARD DATA DISK
Scope. Contains around 5000 hazardous products and is fully compliant with the Chemical (Hazard Information and Packaging for Supply) (CHIP 2) Regulations 1994. It runs under Microsoft Windows™.
Supplier. Warehouse Merck Ltd., Hunter Boulevard, Magna Park, Lutterworth, Leicestershire LE17 4XN. Freephone: 0800 223344. Fax: 01455 558586.

Name. BRETHERICK'S REACTIVE CHEMICAL HAZARDS DATABASE
Scope. Bretherick's classic *Handbook of Reactive Chemical Hazards* has been updated and converted to a database for IBM and compatible PCs, giving electronic access to a collection of data concerning the reaction hazards associated with various elements, compounds, mixtures and reaction processes. With over 140 000 chemical products and 90 000 searchable chemical structures.

Supplier. Aldrich Chemical Co. Ltd., The Old Brickyard, New Road, Gillingham, Dorset SP8 4XT. Tel.: 01747 822211. For orders: Tel.: 0800 717181; Fax: 01747 823779; Telex: 417238 AldrchG.

Name. CAM HEALTH VERSION 5
Scope. Fully compliant with RIDDOR 1995, and can be used to print F2508 style reports. Includes causal tree analysis, costing, status, etc. For accidents/incidents and general risk assessment.
Supplier. CamAxys Ltd., 8 The Meadow, Meadow Lane, St Ives, Cambridgeshire PE17 4LG. Tel.: 01480 497739. Fax: 01480 497759.

Name. CDM Range™
Scope. A complete system for the Construction (Design and Management) (CDM) Regulations 1994. Contains the *Planning Supervisor*, which produces and manages all the necessary CDM documentation, *Safe Designer*, which guides designers through the processes required to produce relevant information for the *Planning Supervisor*, and *Principal Contractor*, which allows the user to develop the construction plan and file. Risk assessments and method statements can be produced. *Safe Contractor* provides comprehensive tools for the production of information that the *Principal Contractor* will want to receive.
Supplier. ErgoSystems wmb, 17 Dorset Square, London NW1 6QB. Tel.: 0171 7245200. Fax: 0171 7246055. E-mail: ergosystems@compuserve.com. www.ergosystems.co.uk.

Name. CHASE—Complete Health and Safety Evaluation
Scope. Available in both manual and software formats. Has a number of sections on a range of general workplace health and safety matters. There is *CHASE I* for small organizations (less than 100 employees) and *CHASE II* for larger employers; *CONSTRUCTION CHASE* is for the construction industry and there is also an *ENVIRONMENT CHASE*.
Supplier. Health and Safety Technology and Management Ltd. (HASTAM), Aston Science Park, Love Lane, Aston Triangle, Birmingham B7 4BJ. Tel.: 0121 3590981. Fax: 0121 3590734.

Name. CHEMDATA
Scope. Contains information on over 93 000 product names in the chemical product information database. Provides hazard information and emergency action advice for dealing with land- and sea-based incidents, including the International Maritime Organization (IMO) Dangerous Code, Emergency Schedules.
Supplier. AEA Technology, National Chemical Emergency Centre, F6 Culham, Abingdon, Oxfordshire OX14 3DB. Tel.: 01235 463060. Fax: 01235 463070.

Name. DATASHEET+
Scope. A multilanguage safety data sheet generator to help chemical manufacturers, traders and distributors to produce safety data sheets for any substance in the format required by the European Union Preparations Directive and its UK counterpart—the Chemicals (Hazard Information and Packaging for Supply) Amendment Regulations (CHIP 96, etc.).

Supplier. AEA Technology, National Chemical Emergency Centre, F6 Culham, Abingdon, Oxfordshire OX14 3DB. Tel.: 01235 463060. Fax: 01235 463070.

Name. DNV PRO.
Scope. Hazard study software for hazard and operability (HAZOP) studies, failure mode effect analysis (FMEA), 'what if?', checklists and audit, for operation under Windows™.
Supplier. DNV TECHNICA, DNV, Software Products and Development, Palace House, 3 Cathedral St., London SE1 9DE. Tel.: 0171 3576080. Fax: 0171 3577297. www.dnv.com/technica.

Name. ECOSCI
Scope. This is version 2 (1997) of the *COSHH Expert* software. Allows access to over 10 000 prepared materials safety data sheets (MSDSs) in the European format. Also allows modifications to existing MSDSs, creates new sheets and copies sections to a new record. Customer and MSDS Revision Control automatically informs which customers require updated sheets. Products in this range include: *COSHH Expert 1—Materials safety data sheets*, *COSHH Expert 2—Chemical labelling*, *COSHH Expert 3—TREM cards* and *COSHH Expert 4—Dangerous goods notes.*
Supplier. H & H Scientific Consultants Ltd., PO Box MT27, Leeds LS17 8QP. Tel.: 0113 2687189. Fax: 0113 2687191. E-mail: ecosci@dhscient.demon.co.uk. www.demon.co.uk/dhscientific/.

Name. ENVY
Scope. A plant management information system, developed with the Royal Sun Alliance, for the recording of information associated with the maintenance of engineering plant, particularly that covered under the Pressure Systems Regulations 1989. Windows based, ENVY has additional modules recording lifts, lifting and general plant inventories and inspection procedures. Examination schedulers provide management information for plant maintenance.
Supplier. Warwick I.C. Systems Ltd., Warwick House, Woodhouse Road, Horsley Woodhouse, Derbyshire DE7 6AY. Tel.: 01332 781882. Fax: 01332 781410.

Name. EQS-INFORMATION MANAGEMENT SOFTWARE
Scope. EQS is an integrated management system designed to facilitate and promote management systems compliant with today's regulations and standards relating to:
- environment: BS 7750, the ISO 14 000 series and Eco Management Audit Scheme;
- quality: BS 5750 and BS EN ISO 9000;
- health and safety: COSHH, CHIP and other legislation on health and safety at work.

EQS consists of these three core components, together with the management facility, which manages common information.
Supplier. Granherne Information Systems Limited, Chester House, 78–86 Chertsey Road, Woking, Surrey GU21 5BJ. Tel.: 01483 729661. Fax: 01483 750418. E-mail: ashar@granherne.co.uk.

Name. Fault EASE™ Windows™
Scope. Windows-based software for fault tree analysis.
Supplier. A.D. Little Inc., Process Safety and Risk Management Practice, Acorn Park, Cambridge, MA 02140-2390, USA. Tel.: +1617 4985476.

Name. HAZDATA
Scope. Contains information on over 2700 substances, providing the basis for good hazard assessment and storage records. The database can be searched via product names/synonyms, CAS, EC, RTECS and UN numbers.
Supplier. AEA Technology, National Chemical Emergency Centre, F6 Culham, Abingdon, Oxfordshire OX14 3DB. Tel.: 01235 463060. Fax: 01235 463070.

Name. HEALTH AND SAFETY MANAGER
Scope. A complete health and safety information system with full auditing system; includes CDM Regulations 1994, accident recording and near-misses, management of health and safety personnel and training, control of hazardous substances, security, fire safety, noise control, safe use of electricity, first aid, food safety and chemical hazard information and packing. The range covers: *HSM Health and Safety Assessor*, *HSM Health and Safety Advisor* and *HSM Health and Safety Co-ordinator*.
Supplier. Torq Computer Systems, Communications House, Mayors Road, Altrincham WA15 9RP. Tel.: 0161 9299110. Fax: 0161 9299440.

Name. PLANT
Scope. Monte Carlo simulation software for availability analysis of complex systems.
Supplier. W.S. Atkins, Woodcote Grove, Ashley Road, Epsom, Surrey KT18 5BW. Tel.: 01372 726140. Fax: 01372 740055.

Name. PSI—PERFORMANCE SUPPORT INTERNATIONAL
Scope. Risk management solutions covering: risk assessment, incident/event reporting and analysis and corporate stress management.
Supplier. PSI Ltd., 6–16 Huntsworth Mews, London NW1 6DD. Tel.: 0171 7248599. Fax: 0171 7248627.

Name. SHE^6—SAFETY, HEALTH AND ENVIRONMENT MANAGEMENT SOLUTIONS
Scope. Scaleable health and safety systems that meet the needs of all organizations in terms of functionality and price. Choose from 13 modules including COSHH, incident/accident reporting, risk assessments, audit and custom. Extensive database analysis with full management graphics.
Supplier. Lexware International Ltd., Brunel Building, Scottish Enterprise Technology Park, East Kilbride G75 0QD. Tel.: 01355 272444. Fax: 01355 272445. E-mail: mail@lexware.co.uk. www.lexware. co.uk.

Name. SAFETY ORGANIZER FOR WINDOWS
Scope. Computerized risk assessment programme which fully integrates with *COSHH Organizer*. Modules for all regulations including Manual Handling, Display Screen Equipment, Personal Protective Equipment, Workplace, Work Equipment, Fire and First Aid Directives.

Supplier. E.O. Associates, 18 Shepperton Close, Castlethorpe, Milton Keynes MK19 7BR. Tel.: 01908 510034. Fax: 01908 510901.

Name. VDUWorkstation
Scope. Consists of three main components. The User Module carries out an interactive ergonomic risk assessment of the workstation, identifies problems and offers training and more in-depth questions. The built-in VDU Timer gives a reminder to the user that the time spent in front of a visual display unit (VDU) should be broken up with other tasks. Office Manager collects data from each VDU user, including laptops and home workers, and creates specific, dated charts of each employee assessment and their findings.
Supplier. ErgoSystems wmb, 17 Dorset Square, London NW1 6QB. Tel.: 0171 7245200. Fax: 0171 7246055. E-mail: ergosystems@compuserve.com. www.ergosystems.co.uk.

Further reading

Andrews, J.D. & Moss, T.R. (1993) *Reliability and Risk Assessment.* Longman Scientific and Technical, Harlow.
Covello, V.T. & Merkhofer, M.W. (1993) *Risk Assessment Methods. Approaches for Assessing Health and Environmental Risks.* Plenum, New York.
Deshotels, R. & Zimmerman, R. (1995) *Cost Effective Risk Assessment for Process Design.* McGraw-Hill, New York.
European Centre for Ecotoxicology and Toxicology of Chemicals (ECETOC) (1995) *Assessment Factors in Human Health Risk Assessment.* ECETOC Technical Report No. 68. ECETOC, Brussels.
European Centre for Ecotoxicology and Toxicology of Chemicals (ECETOC) (1996) *Risk Assessment for Carcinogens.* ECETOC Monograph No. 24. ECETOC, Brussels.
European Commission Directorate General for Employment, Industrial Relations and Social Affairs (1996) *Guidance on Risk Assessment at Work.* OOPEC, Luxembourg.
Fan, A.F. & Chang, L.W. (eds.) (1996) *Toxicology and Risk Assessment. Principles, Methods and Applications.* Marcel Dekker, New York.
Hallenbeck, W.H. (1993) *Quantitative Risk Assessment for Environmental and Occupational Health*, 2nd edn. Lewis Publishers, Chelsea, MI.
Higson, N. (1996) *Risk Management. Health and Safety in Primary Care.* Butterworth–Heinemann, Oxford.
HSE (1993) *Risk Assessment: International Conference, October 5–9, 1992, Queen Elizabeth II Conference Centre, Westminster, London.* HSE Books, Sudbury, Suffolk.
HSE (1994) *Risk Assessment of Notified New Substances. Technical Guidance Note.* HSE Books, Sudbury, Suffolk.
HSE (1996) *Use of Risk Assessment Within Government Departments.* HSE Books, Sudbury, Suffolk.
Lu, F.C. (1996) *Basic Toxicology: Fundamentals, Target Organs and Risk Assessment*, 3rd edn. Taylor & Francis, Basingstoke.
National Research Council Committee on Risk Assessment of Hazardous Air Pollutants (1994) *Science and Judgement in Risk Assessment.* National Academy Press, Washington DC.

Roach, S. (1992) *Health Risks from Hazardous Substances at Work. Assessment, Evaluation and Control*. Pergamon, Oxford.
Royal Society (1992) *Risk: Analysis, Perception and Management*. Royal Society, London.
Smith, C.M. & Christiani, D.C. (1994) *Chemical Risk Assessment and Occupational Health: Current Applications, Limitations and Future Prospects*. Auburn House, Westport, CT.
Stranks, J. (1996) *The Law and Practice of Risk Assessment: A Practical Programme*. Royal Society for the Prevention of Accidents (Health and Safety in Practice). Pitman Publishing, London.
Turney, R. & Pitblado, R. (1996) *Risk Assessment in the Process Industries*, 2nd edn. UK Institution of Chemical Engineers, Rugby.
Wang, R.G.M. & Knaak, J.B. (1993) *Health Risk Assessment. Dermal and Inhalation Exposure and Absorption of Toxicants*. CRC Press, FL.
Wells, G. (1996) *Hazard Identification and Risk Assessment*. UK Institution of Chemical Engineers, Rugby.
World Health Organization (WHO) (1993) *Biomarkers and Risk Assessment: Concepts and Principles*. Environmental Health Criteria 155. WHO, Geneva.

Index

Note: page numbers in **bold** refer to tables, those in *italic* refer to figures

abattoir case study 417–19
absorbed dose 85, 428
absorption toxicokinetics 43
acceptable risk
  definition 9–11, **11**
  risk communication 279
  risk perception 269–72
accident rates 60–1
accident ratios (accident triangles) 222–3, *222*, *223*
accident statistics
  analysis 107, 221
  compensation claims 230–1
  costs 232–7, *233*, *235*
  hazards identification 105–7
  monetary value of injuries 242
  prevention 237, 238
    loss control 221–2, 223
  screening for workplace inspections 113
acquired immunodeficiency syndrome (AIDS) 290, 414
active sampling techniques 132
acute toxicants
  assessment tests 49
  exposure sampling duration 147
  risk perception 270
  standard setting for protection 121, **121**
acute toxicity test 42, 49–50
  eye irritation 50
  skin irritation 50
  substances classification/labelling 50
Advisory Committee on Toxic Substances (ACTS) 124
aerosols 79–81
  classification 80
  direct reading instruments 116
  Q fever case study 418–19
  tuberculosis case study 414, 415
age
  as confounding factor 71
  risk perception differences 273
age-adjusted death rates 62
air flow
  models 167, 168, 169
  ventilation system design 202–3
airborne contaminants *see* atmospheric exposure monitoring
ALARA (as low as reasonably achievable) 187
ALARP (as low as reasonably practicable) 6, 15, 186, 187
  tolerability of risk 10
alcohol intake and liver function tests 303
allergens
  health surveillance 304
  respiratory sensitizers 43, 48, 238, **291**
allergic reactions 147
analytical studies 63
annual health business plan 27
annual radiation dose limits 429, 430, 431
anthrax 94
anthropometry
  back pain pre-employment screening 391
  ergonomics 90
antibody levels determination 299
Apollo-13 264–5
asbestos 66, 72, 75, 122, 134, 220, 308
  cancer risk 422, 423
  case study 421–7
    characteristics of industry 424
  chest X-ray surveillance 296, 298
  chrysotile 81, 421, 422, 423, 424
  crocidolite 81, 421, 422, 423, 425
  damages awards 231
  dust suppression 201
  fibre types 81, 423
  health and safety enforcement actions 239
    international guidelines 421
  health surveillance 293, 304, 426
  latent period 309
  mineral species 81, 421
  qualitative risk assessment 422
  quantitative risk assessment 423–4
    lung cancer 423
    mesothelioma 423–4
  tobacco smoke synergism 298, 422
Asbestos (Licensing) Regulations (1983) 239, 348
asbestosis 226, 227, 422
  fibre type influences 423
asphyxiants 82
Assessment Team 34

assessment units 33
Associated Octel 350
asthma/occupational asthma 94, 226, 227
damages awards 231
isocyanates sensitization 369
lung function tests 294–5
respiratory symptom review 291
sensitizing agents **291**
see also respiratory sensitizers
atmospheric exposure monitoring 129–58
active sampling 132
analytic method selection 137–8, 139
bulk sampling 132–3
definition 129
exposure variation 139, *140*
instantaneous monitoring 130
integrated monitoring 130–1
interpretation of exposure data 153–8
comparisons with exposure standards 154, 156
probability plots 153–4, *154*, **155**
working hours variations 156
minimum sampling volumes 138
passive sampling 132
path of emission modelling 167
box models 168–9, *168*
diffusion models 169–70
personal sampling 131
prioritization 135–7, *136*
purpose 133–4
quality assurance (QA) 139, 141–2
record keeping 156, *157*, 158
sample contamination 138
sampling method selection 137, 139
sampling strategies 142–51
for compliance 151–3
static sampling 131
see also exposure assessment
attributable risk 62
audiometry 295–6, *296*
audit 315–42
benefits to organizations 316, 342
compliance *see* compliance auditing
components of programme *318*
occupational health programme 31
types 316–18
violence at work 454–5
workplace hazards identification 107–8
see also management systems assessment
audit report 332–3
distribution 333–4
structure 332–3
style of writing 333, **334**
Australia
legislation 5
standards setting 124, 125
autoignition temperature 83
avoidance of risk-associated operations 198, 220

Bacillus Calmette–Guérin (BCG) immunization 299, 416
back pain 91
display screen equipment hazards 407
manual handling 390
motor vehicle assembly plant case study 390, 395–404
ergonomic rating scales 400, *401–2*
preventive measures 391–2
ergonomic job design 392
medical screening 391
training 391
risk factors 390
back X-rays 391
background risk 10
bacteria 94, 96
barotrauma 90
bead blasting cabinets 203–4
benchmark guidance values (BGVs) 301
benzo[a]pyrene (BaP) 62, 75
benzene 57, 75, 220, 256
statutory medical surveillance 306
Bhopal 247
bias (systematic error) 70–1, 138
bioactivation 44, **44**
bioaerosols 81
biological effect monitoring 119, 302–3, 307
organophosphate pesticides 365, *366*
biological exposure indices (BEIs) 119, 185, 300–1
biological hazards 94–6, **94**, **95**
case studies 413–20
exposure assessment 415
exposure modelling 163–4
UK legislation 460
biological monitoring 119, 129, 300–2, 307, 308
benchmark guidance values (BGVs) 301
health guidance values (HGVs) 301
organophosphate pesticides 364–5
substances and metabolites **301**
biological monitoring guidance values (BMGVs) 119
biological tolerance values (BATs) 119
bladder cancer 227, 308
bladder carcinogens 306
bladder cytology 298
box models 168–9, *168*
receiver exposure modelling 171
brain cancer 68
breathing apparatus 261
breathing zone 144, *145*
sampling (personal sampling) 131
brucellosis 94
bulk bag delivery methods 199–200, *201*
bulk sampling 132–3
burden–damage relationship 147

'burn-down' philosophy 252
business environment 22–6
  health policy development 26–7
  line management responsibilities 22–3
  occupational health programme organization 22–6, *23*, 28, 30–1
  quality management aspects 23–4
business interruption control 225
byssinosis 64, 65, 227

cadmium 45, 75, 303
cancer 226
canopies 204–5
capture velocity 205, 210, 213
carbon monoxide 44, 82, 164
carbon tetrachloride 45, 306
carcinogenicity assessment 57
  epidemiological studies 57
  tests 49, 51–2
carcinogens 47, 48, 220, 268–9
  exposure levels 12, 43, 124
    reduction 127
    USA legislation 5
  health surveillance 296–7, 304, 309
    statutory requirements 306
  International Agency for Research on Cancer (IARC) classification 74–6
  latent periods 309
  standards setting 127–8
case control studies 65, *69*
case series 63
case studies 63
causal associations 72–3
causes of hazard 99, *100*
CD-ROM databases 471–2
Central Assessment Team 34
ceramic fibres 75
chance associations 70
checklist for hazard identification 108, *109*, *180–1*
  display screen equipment *408*
chemical fume cupboards 204, 213
chemical hazards 79–84
  aerosols 79–81, *80*
  classification 16
  complex mixtures 127
  consequence analysis 181
  exposure modelling 162, *162*, 164
  FMEA 104
  HAZOP 103
chemical mixtures 127
  atmospheric monitoring 132–3
  vapour pressure/evaporation models 165–6
Chemicals (Hazard Information and Packaging for Supply) Regulations (1994) (CHIP 2 Regulations) 79
Chernobyl 247
chest X-ray 296–8
  asbestos case study 426
cholinesterase serum levels 302
chromic acid 47, 134
  health surveillance procedures 292
chronic toxicants
  exposure sampling duration 146–7
  risk perception 270
  standard setting for protection 121, **121**
civil law 352–5
  general health and safety requirements 353
classification of hazardous substances 54–5
coal dust
  chest X-ray surveillance 297
  suppression 201
cohort studies 66, *69*
cold stress 89–90, 120
colophony 144
combustion characteristics 83
communications, emergency response 257, 258
  media involvement 262–3
compensation 225, 227, 228, 230–1, 344
  awards from criminal courts 347
  employers' liability insurance 347
  punitive damages 356
complex mixtures *see* chemical mixtures
compliance auditing 317, 318–34, *318*, *338*
  coverage 320
  key characteristics 322–3
  objectives 318–19
  on-site activities (audit steps) 326–32, **327**
    evidence evaluation 330–1
    gathering evidence 329–30
    internal controls assessment 328–9
    management systems familiarization 328
    reporting findings 331–2
    setting priorities 328, *328*
    site tour 328
  organization 320–1
  post-site activities 332–4
    audit report 332–3
    report distribution 333–4
  pre-audit activities 324–6
    information requirements 325, **326**
    pre-audit questionnaire 324–6
    protocol design 324, *325*
  procedure 323–34, *323*
  resources 321
  scope 319–20
compliance testing
  atmospheric monitoring sampling strategies 151–3
    NIOSH method 152
    zoning method 152–3
  exposure sampling duration 146
confidentiality 311
confounding factors 71–2

consequence analysis 181–2
Control of Asbestos at Work Regulations 5, 219, 239, 421
  punishment of breaches 348
control of exposure 35, 197–217
  asbestos case study 425–6
  assessment by exposure monitoring 134, 135
  costs 208–9
  hand-transmitted vibration case study 384–7, *385*, *386*
  handling/transfer-associated exposure 197
  hardware (engineering) solutions 197, 202–7
    canopies/hoods 204–5
    dilution/general ventilation 205–7
    displacement ventilation 207
    partial enclosure with extract ventilation 204
    total enclosure under negative pressure 203–4
    see also ventilation systems
  hierarchy of measures 207–8
  isocyanates case study 376–7
  management aspects 207–17
    selection of controls needed 207–8
  organophosphate pesticides 366
  software (organizational) solutions 197, 198–202
    elimination of process or substance 198
    form of raw materials 199
    production procedure changes 199
    substitution by less toxic substance 198–9
    suppression of substance 200–2
    worker awareness/training 202
  tuberculosis case study 415–16
Control of Industrial Major Accident and Hazard (CIMAH) Regulations (1984) 5, 9, 101, 247, 347
Control of Lead at Work Regulations (1980) 4, 219, 304, 308
control limits (CLs) 124
Control of Major Accident and Hazard (COMAH) Regulations 101
Control of Substances Hazardous to Health (COSHH) Regulations 5, 13, 79, 124, 219, 346, 367
  control methods (COSHH hierarchy) 197
  exposure monitoring 134
  health surveillance 305–6, 307
    records 312
  punishment of breaches 348
  risk assessment requirement 346
corporate damage 256
cost benefit analysis 15, 123, 185–6, 240–2
  health and safety law compliance 345
  standards setting 118–19
  value of human life/good health 242
cost benefit assessments (CBAs) 16–17
counselling skills 440
cross-sectional studies 64
Cullen Report 4, 252

damage control 223–4
Dangerous Substances Directive 49, 54
decompression sickness 90
delayed consequences, risk perception 270–1
dermal exposure modelling 171–2
descriptive studies 63
design stage
  exposure risk prevention 198
  hazard identification 101–5
diesel engine exhaust 75
  substitution of less toxic fuel 198
diffusion models 169–70
diisocyanates 369, *370*
  respiratory sensitization 369
  see also isocyanates
dilution ventilation 206
  isocyanates exposure case study 375
N,*N*-dimethylformamide (DMF) 45, 47
Disability Discrimination Act (1995) 344, 391
displacement ventilation 207
display screen equipment operators 120, 405–12
  document reader encoders (DRE) 409–10
  musculoskeletal problems 405, 406–7
  risk identification 407
    checklist *408*
  safety policies 346
  stress 405, 407
  visual problems 405, 407
  visual status screening 299, 407
  workstation adjustment training 411
  workstation design 405–6
    changes 410–11
Display Screen Equipment (DSE) Regulations (1992) 405
distribution toxicokinetics 43
disulphur dichloride 305–6
DNA adducts 303
document reader encoder (DRE) operators 409–10
dose–response relationship 17, 42–3, 120, 126, 147
  health surveillance 304
Dow Index 102, 103
drum filling methods 199, *200*
dust explosions 84
dusts 80
  chest X-ray surveillance 297
  particle size 80–1
  personal exposure sampling device location 144
  powdered raw material delivery methods 199–200, *201*

powdered vs. pelleted raw materials 199
suppression methods 200–1

ear plugs 172
effect modification (interaction) 72
ejection injuries 92
electricity, UK legislation 460
electromagnetic fields exposure 68, 268
emergencies 246–7
categories 246
follow-up investigations 265
ionizing radiation case studies 434–6
media response 262–4
recovery planning 265
relatives' response 264
risk assessment 246–7, 249, 252
emergency response 246–65
'burn-down' philosophy 252
callout and mobilization 256–7
communications 257, 258
contingency planning 264–5
emergency teams 251
back-up 256
corporate emergency management (crisis management) 255–6
leadership 252
local management 254–5
on-site response 252, 254
facilities 257–8, *258–9*
hazard information communication to emergency services 254
levels of response 250
non-legislative guidelines 248
organization 250–6, *251*, *252*
procedure manual 259–60
statutory requirements 247–9
training 260–2
exercises 261–2
initial familiarization 260
media interviews 264
specific roles 260–1
emission sources exposure modelling 162, 163–7, **163**
empirical rates 163–4
evaporation models 164–7
theoretical prediction of rates 164
employee assistance programme (EAP) 441
Employers' Liability (Compulsory Insurance) Act (1969) 225, 228
employers' liability insurance 221, 225 30, 234, 235, 347
alternative approaches 228–9
claim settlement costs 227, 228
claims for compensation 226–7, 230–1
liability limitation 228, 347
occupational diseases latency period 227
retrospective rating scheme 229
Environment Act (1995) 347
environmental contamination
emergency response 261
loss control in prevention 224
epidemiological studies 56–76
appraisal 73–4, **74**
causal associations 72–3
data sources 57–8
definitions 56–7
disease–exposure relationships 61–3
effect modification (interaction) 72
exposure assessment 57, 58, 134, 135
hazard identification 56–76
health surveillance records 310, 311, 312
limitations 73
measurements 58–61
age adjustments, direct/indirect 62–3
comparison of rates 61–2
meta analysis 68, 70
outcome measures 57, 58
sample size selection 150–1
spurious associations
bias 70–1
chance 70
confounding factors 71–2
types of study 63–70, *64*, **67**
ergonomic rating scales 393, 400, *401–2*
ergonomics 90–2
job design 392
work-related upper limb disorders (WRULDs) 406
European Health and Safety Directives 5
European Inventory of Existing Commercial Chemical Substances (EINECS) 48
European Union (EU) standards setting 123–6
evaporation models 164–7
outdoor conditions 166–7
SUBTEC model 167
evaporation suppression 201–2
excretion toxicokinetics 44–5
exhaust ventilation 135
asbestos case study 425
isocyanates exposure case study 377
experimental studies 63
expired air sample monitoring 300
explosion hazards 83, 84
costs 232
identification at planning/design stage 102
exposure assessment 17, 20
asbestos case study 425
biological hazard 415
epidemiological studies 57, 58, 134, 135
hand-transmitted vibration case study 382–3, **383**
ionizing radiation case studies
industrial site radiography 431–3
X-ray cabinet operation 435

isocyanates exposure case study 369, 373–6
legislation 134
pesticides 364–5, *366*
Q fever case study 417–18
tuberculosis case study 415
violence at work 450–2
see also atmospheric exposure monitoring, exposure modelling, health surveillance
exposure modelling 161–74
applications 161, **161**
dose and effect relationship 162, *162*
limitations 172–3
model components 162–3, *162*
Monte Carlo simulations 173, *173*
path of emission 162, 167–70
receiver 162, 170–2
sources of emission 162, 163–7, **163**
extent of risk 7
external inspections 317
extrinsic allergic alveolitis 94
Exxon Valdez oil spill 256
eye irritation test 50
eye tests 298–9, 407

Factories and Machinery (Asbestos Process) Regulations (1986) 421
failure mode and effect analysis (FMEA) 104–5, 181
fibres 81
asbestos-related diseases 81, 423
financial aspects 219–43
accidents 232–7, *233*, *235*
risk management 16–17
Fire and Explosion Index 102
fire point 83
fires
costs 232
health and safety offences 239
emergency response 248
training 261
hazard identification at design stage 102
prevention 224
UK safety legislation 460
first aid 248
training 261
flammable limits 83
flammable substances 83–4, **84**
direct reading instruments 116
HAZOP (hazard and operability) study example 182–4, **183**
UK legislation 460
flash points 83
Flixborough 247
FN curves 9
freezing injuries 90
frequency rates 60
fume 81
complex mixtures 127
exposure modelling 164
composition prediction 165
receiver exposure 171
personal exposure sampling device location 144, *145*
fume cupboards 204, 213
fungi 94, 96

gas chromatography-mass spectrometry (GC-MS) 132
gases 82–4
direct reading instruments 116
exposure modelling 164
instantaneous monitoring instruments 130
odour 84
toxicity in divers 90
gender differences in risk perception 273
general ventilation 206
genetic effects *see* mutagens
Germany
health surveillance 308
standards setting 125
glare 90, 407
glove boxes 203
gloves 172
Grangemouth refinery fire 232, 239

hand–arm vibration syndrome 88, 379
hand-transmitted vibration 91, 379
average frequency-weighted acceleration ($a_{h,w}$) measurement 382
health surveillance procedures 293
precision casting process case study 379–88
casting process 380–1
exposure measurement (BS 6842) 382
action levels 383
questionnaire 384
Stockholm classification 384
health surveillance 384, **384**
preventive measures 384–7, *385*, *386*
information leaflet **387**
hazard
assessment 126
causes 99, *100*
continuous/non-continuous 99, 114, 115
definition 6–7, 98
prevention/control 17
relative risk studies 61–2
types 78–96, **78**
hazard identification 17, 18–19, 33, 41, 105–8, 134, 179, 181
accident/ill health analytical investigations 107
accident/ill health statistics 105–7
asbestos case study 424
audits 107–8
back pain case study 395
checklists 108, *109*, *180–1*

definition 6–7, 98
epidemiological aspects 56–76
existing substances 48, 52
hand-transmitted vibration case study 381–2, *381*, *382*
ionizing radiation case studies
industrial site radiography 431, *432*
X-ray cabinet operation 435
isocyanates case study 372
new substances 48, 49–52
pesticides information 364
planning/design stage 101–5
Q fever case study 417
techniques 98 117, 181
workplace hazards 105–8
workplace inspections 108–17
tuberculosis case study 414
violence at work 449–50
hazard indices 102–3
hazard and operability (HAZOP)
method *102*, 103–4
guide words **104**
study 99, 181, 220
example 182–4, **183**
hazard rating 7
health guidance values (HGVs) 301
Health Management System 24
Health and Safety at Work etc. Act (1974) 4, 219, 345, 366, 447
'catch-all' requirements 348–50
control of premises 350–1
costs of enforcement actions 239
delegation of liability 352
emergency response duties 247–8
employees' duties 351
other people's premises 350–2, 354
personal liability of directors 351
persons on premises 350–2
self-employed contractors 350
subcontractors 350, 352
unforseeable events 352
wrongful use of premises 351
Health and Safety (Display Screen Equipment) Regulations (1992) 348
health and safety legislation
costs of enforcement actions 238–9
enforcement 237–8
general principles 345–7
Prohibition Notices 348
punishment of breaches 239, 240, 347–8, 349–50
risk assessment requirement 345–6
health surveillance 20, 288–312
asbestos case study 426
availability of effective treatment 308
back pain case study 391, 403
definition 288
detection of early effects 307–8
extent of provision 289
hand-transmitted vibration case study 384, **384**
indications 303–4
ionizing radiation case studies
industrial site radiography 434–5
X-ray cabinet operation 436
isocyanates exposure case study 373–4
legislative requirements 304–7
long-term following cessation of exposure 309–10
pesticides 366
procedures *see* health surveillance procedures
Q fever case study 419
records 310–12
risk management aspects 289
secondary prevention role 288–9
target populations 308
tuberculosis case study 416
health surveillance procedures 289–303
assessment by health care professional 292–3
biological effect monitoring 302–3
biological monitoring 300–2
immune status determination 299
medical examination 293
self-examination 292
special investigations 293–9
audiometry 295–6, *296*
bladder cytology 298
chest X-rays 296–8
lung function tests 293–5
periodic eye tests 298–9
symptom review 290–2
hearing protection 172
heat stress 88–9, 120
hepatitis B 94
immunization 299
hepatotoxicants 45
n-hexane 47–8, 290
hierarchy of control 35
high altitude effects 90
high velocity low volume (HVLV) extraction 205
human error 114
hydrocarbons 132, 133
exposure modelling 164, 165
hypothermia 90

ill health
analytical investigations 107
compensation claims 230–1
monetary value 242
prevention 238
workplace hazards identification from statistics 105–7
see also sickness absence
illuminance 90, **91**, 120
immune status determination 299
impact injuries 92
impact noise 87, 88
incidence rate 59
prevalence rate relationship 59–60

individual risk 8–9, 272–3
information bias 71
information sources 471–7
infrared photography 115
infrared radiation (IR) 86, 87
infrasound 88
instantaneous monitoring instruments 130
insurance 225
  costs of accidents 234, 235
  legal expenses 240, 347
  risk retention 220
  risk transfer 220–1
  sites distant from home site 353, 354
  see also employers' liability insurance
integrated monitoring 130–1
inter-risk comparisons 3
interaction (effect modification) 72
internal inspections 316–17
International Agency for Research on Cancer (IARC) carcinogens classification 74–6
interviewer bias 71
intolerable risk 186
involuntary risk 9, 268–9
ionizing radiation 84–5, 120
  absorbed dose 85, 428
  annual dose limits 429, 430, 431
  damages awards 231
  direct reading instruments 116
  effective dose 428
  exposure modelling 162, 163, 164
  health effects 428, 429–30
    dose relationships 429, **429**
  ICRP dose limit recommendations 429, **429**
  industrial radiography case study 431–5
    radiation protection programme 433–4
    risk management 433–5
  occupational exposure 86
  stochastic/non-stochastic biological effects 86, 428
  total enclosure under negative pressure (hot cells) 203
  UK legislation 430
  X-ray cabinet operation case study 435–6
Ionizing Radiation Regulations (1985) 5, 430
  permitted annual dose limits **430**
irritation thresholds 85
ISO 14001 *335*, 336
isocyanates 82, 369
  automotive industry case study 369–76
  polyurethane formation 369, *370*
  respiratory sensitization 369, 371
isothermal evaporation model 167

job rotation 202

labelling of hazardous substances 16, 50, 54–5, 284
lasers 86, 120
  hazard classification scheme 86
latent period 227
  health surveillance 309
  lung fibrosis 298
LD_{50} 49
lead 45, 63, 65, 75, 119, 134, 270
  biological effect monitoring 302
  health surveillance 304, 308
legal expenses
  insurance 240, 347
  occupational disease claims 227
Legionnaires' disease 96
legislation 4–6, 459–60
  civil law 352–5
  common law duties 347
  costs of compliance 346
  demonstrating compliance 344–56
  equal opportunities 344
  exposure monitoring 134
  health surveillance requirements 304–7
  product labelling requirements 284
  risk assessment requirements 345–6, 348, 349, 354–5
  risk communication requirements 283–4
  'six-pack' of regulations 5, 346, 347
  see also Health and Safety at Work etc. Act (1994); health and safey legislation
leptospirosis 94
lifestyle health assessment programmes 288
  see also health surveillance
lifting strength testing 391
lighting in workplace 90, **91**
  direct reading instruments 116
  display screen equipment 407
likelihood rating 7
liquids
  drum filling methods 199, *200*
  exposure limits 132–3
liver function tests 303
loss control 221–5
  accident ratios (accident triangles) 222–3, *222*, *223*
  business interruption 225
  damage control 223–4
  definition 221
  management commitment 225
  pollution prevention 224
  product control 224–5
  security control 224
loss of earnings claims 230–1
loss prevention 221
low-velocity displacement ventilation 207
lung cancer 66, 72, 227
  asbestos exposure-related

fibre type influences 423
risk assessment 422–3
lung fibrosis 308
health surveillance programmes 297–8
lung function tests 293–5, *294*, *295*
asbestos case study 426
isocyanates exposure case study 374, 375, 377

machinery hazards 92
UK legislation 460
major industrial hazard 101
FN curves 9
societal risk assessment 8–9
MAK Commission 125
Malaysia
asbestos industry case study *see* asbestos
legislation 5
malignant melanoma 66
Management of Health and Safety at Work Regulations (MHSWR) (1992) 5, 346, 348, 355, 392, 447
management systems assessment 317, 318, 334–41, *337*, *338*
criteria for managing compliance 339, *340*
ISO 14001 *335*, 336
occupational health programmes *337*
reports/recommendations 335, 339–41, *341*
manual handling 120
back injury risk 390
capability under standardized conditions 393
drum filling methods 199, *200*
ergonomic rating scales 393
exposure risk 197, 393
legislative requirements 392
risk assessment 392–5, *394*
risk management case study *see* back pain
Manual Handling Operations Regulations (MHOR) 392
materials safety data sheets (MSDS) 284
pesticides 364
relative evaporation rates 166
vapour pressure information 165
maximum exposure limits (MELs) 124, 126
isocyanates 372
mechanical hazards 92
consequence analysis 182
media
response in emergencies 262–4
risk communication 282
violent incidents reporting 448
median effective dose (ED_{50}) 42, *42*
median lethal dose (LD_{50}) 42
medical examination 288, 307
health surveillance procedures 293
mercury 44, 45, 308
health surveillance procedures 293
mesothelioma 227
fibre type influences 423
risk assessment 422–4
meta analysis 68, 70
metabolism toxicokinetics 43–4
methane diisocyanate (MDI) 369
microorganisms, hazard group classification **94**
microwave radiation (MW) 86, 87, 120
health surveillance procedures 292–3
mists 81
Mond Index 102, 103
monitoring exposure *see* atmospheric exposure monitoring; biological monitoring
Monte Carlo simulations 173, *173*
motor vehicle assembly
back pain risk management case study 390, 395–404
isocyanates exposure case study 369, 373–6
musculoskeletal problems 238, 390
display screen equipment hazards 405, 406–7
workstation design 406–7
mutagens 48
assessment tests 49, 51
exposure levels 12, 43
risk perception 270, 271

nested case control studies 67–8, *69*
nickel compounds 75
chest X-ray surveillance 297
NIOSH exposure monitoring sampling strategy 152
NOAEL (no observable adverse effect level) 11, 12, 42, 122, 128
noise 87, 120, 238
continuous exposure 87
direct reading instruments 116
exposure modelling 161–2, 163, 170, 172
impact and intermittent noise 87
noise action levels 185
Noise at Work Regulations (1989) 5, 219
noise-induced hearing loss 87–8, 226, 227, 296
non-ionizing radiation 86
exposure modelling 162, 163
Notification of New Substances (NONS) Regulations (1993) 49
Nuclear Electric 347

observational studies 63
occupational asthma *see* asthma
occupational exposure limits (OELs) 42–3, 54, 79, 119, 185
acute/chronic exposure 47
application 126–8

chemical mixtures 127, 133
epidemiological studies 57
indicative criteria 125–6
international developments 120
sample size selection for exposure monitoring 150, **150**
sampling frequency selection 151
standard setting process 122
types 119
UK definition 124–5
occupational hygiene instrumentation 115–16
Occupiers' Liability Acts (1957; 1984) 347, 353
odour thresholds 84, **85**
odour warning properties 84
Offshore Installations (Prevention of Fire and Explosion, and Emergency Response) Regulations (1995) 247
Oil Industry International Exploration and Production Forum guidelines 248–9
operational audits 317
orf 94
organization for occupational health management 22–6, *23*, 28, 30–1
audit 31
business quality management aspects 23–4
coordination 28, 30
documentation 27–8, *29*
employee competence 30–1
Health Management Systems 24
health programme elements 25–6, **26**
health risk assessment activities 30, 31–5
line management responsibility 22–3
purposes **26**, 28, 35, 36
structure 24–5, *25*
targeting resources 35–6
organizational health policy 26–7
organizing health risk assessment activities 30, 31–5
assessment procedure 33–4
benefits to organization 31–2
definition of purposes 31
exposure control improvement 35
implementation 34
resources 32
specialist support 33
training 34
organophosphate pesticides 362–4
biological/biological effect monitoring 364–5, *366*
exposure assessment and management 364–5, *366*
mode of action 362–3, *362*, *363*
slow release formulations 363
ozone 82, 164

paraquat 361
particle size 80–1
passive sampling techniques 132
path of emission modelling 162, 167–70
box models 168–9, *168*
diffusion models 169–70
peak expiratory flow rates 295, *295*
permissible exposure limits (PELs) 5
personal exposure monitoring 121, 131, 132, 144
ionizing radiation case studies 435
isocyanates exposure case study 374, 375–6
location of sampling devices 144, *145*
personal health assessment (PHA) 444
personal liability 315
personal protective clothing/equipment 172
asbestos case study 425
isocyanates exposure case study 376–7
Q fever case study 418
receiver exposure modelling 172
personal radiation dosimeters 435
pesticides 268, 361–8
biological effect monitoring 302
exposure assessment and management 364–5, *366*
toxicity 361–4
physical hazards 84–90
UK legislation 459
workplace inspections 112
Piper Alpha 4, 228, 232, 247, 252, 256
pneumoconiosis 227
pollutant flow visualization 115
polynuclear aromatic hydrocarbons 81
polyurethane formation 369, *370*
powdered raw materials 199
bulk bag delivery methods 199–200, *201*
precision casting process case study *see* hand-transmitted vibration
prevalence rate 59
prevention of exposure 197–217
probability plots 153–4, *154*, **155**
procedures documentation 27–8
product control 224–5
product labelling 284
Prohibition Notice breaches 348
prospective employee medical screening 391
psychosocial hazards 92–3, **93**
risk assessment 353, 354
public liability insurance 221, 231–2
pulmonary carcinogens, health surveillance 296–7, 304

Q fever 94
case study 417–19
quality assurance (QA), atmospheric monitoring 139, 141–2
Quality Management System 24
BS 8800 24

HSG (65) 24
ISO 9001 24
ISO 14001 335, 336
quantitative risk assessment (QRA)
asbestos exposure 423–4
lung cancer 423
mesothelioma 423–4
definition 12
violence at work 452–3

radiation protection 187
Radioactive Substances Act (1993) 430
radiofrequency radiation (RF) 86
random error 70, 138
receiver exposure modelling 162, 170–2
dermal exposure 171–2
protective clothing/equipment effects 172
recommended limits (RLs) 124
records 27–8, *29*
atmospheric monitoring 156, *157*, 158
back pain risk assessment study 404
compliance auditing 332–3
confidentiality 311
health risk assessment activities 34
health surveillance 310–12
management systems assessment reports 339–41, *341*
risk communication programmes 285
storage 312
ventilation system performance 214–17, *215*, *216*
relative humidity 89
relative risk 61–2
renal toxicity 45
repeated-dose toxicity tests 51
Reporting of Injuries, Diseases and Dangerous Occurrences Regulations (RIDDOR) 106–7, 347
Schedule 3 461–70
reports 28
reproductive risk
assessment tests 49, 52
risk perception 270, 271
respiratory disorders 94, 96
respiratory sensitizers 48, 238, **291**
exposure levels 43
health surveillance 304
retrospective employee grouping 143–4
risk
acceptable vs. unacceptable 9–11, **11**, 269–72
analysis 178
definition 7
extent 7
individual vs. societal 8–9, 272–3
tolerability 9–11
uncertainty of estimates 12
voluntary vs. involuntary 9, 268–9
risk acceptibility 9–11, **11**
communication of risk 279
perception of risk 269–72
risk assessment 3–20, 178–87, 237
aims 3–4, 13, 179
asbestos case study 421–7
audit *see* audit
consequence analysis 181–2
definition 7, 177
display screen equipment 405–12
emergencies 246–7, 249, 252
exposure monitoring 134
hand-transmitted vibration case study 383–4, **384**
hazard identification 179, 181
checklist *180–1*
ionizing radiation case study 428–37
isocyanates exposure case study 372–3, 375–6
legislative developments 4–6
manual handling case study 392–5, *394*, 397–402
models 17–20, *19*
occupational health programme 30, 31–5
pesticides case study 361–7
procedure 178, *178*
psychological hazards 353, 354
Q fever case study 418
quantitative *see* quantitative risk assessment (QRA)
risk calculator application 189–92, *191*, 192
statutory requirements 345–6, 348, 349, 354–5
stress 438–9
tuberculosis case study 415
vibration case study 379–89
violence at work 452–3
risk calculator 187–92, *188*
risk assessment example 189–92, *191*
risk characterization 17, 177–92
definition 177
pesticides 365
risk communication 15–16, 20, 266, 275–6, 278–86
barriers 285–6
case studies 361–456
communicators 282
crisis communication 280
definition 279
emergency response teams 254
legal requirements 283–4
perception of risk 275–6
process 278–80
professionals' credibility 280
programme development 280–3
communication methods 282
goal setting 280–1
information disclosure 283
role of media 282
target audience assessment 281
programme implementation and

evaluation 284–5
records 285
risk perception 278, 285, 286
target audience 285–6
terminology 280
toxicity information 54–5
risk control strategies 17, 33, 35, 220
risk avoidance 3, 220
risk reduction (loss control) 221
risk retention 220
risk transfer 220–1
risk criteria 15
risk evaluation 178, 185–7
risk management 225
aims 4
audit *see* audit
case studies 361–456
cost benefit analysis 240–2
definition 13–14, 219, 221
economic aspects 16–17
employer's needs 242–3
health surveillance 289
models 17–20, *18*, *19*
principles 219–21
strategies 14
stress 438–9
risk matrix 185, *185*, 187
risk measurement 184–5
risk perception 266–76
age differences 273
communication of risk 275–6
determinant factors 268–74
attribution of responsibility 269
hazard familiarity 269–70
hazard information 269
immediate vs. delayed consequences 270–1
major catastrophic incidents 271–2
personality factors 271
risk benefit balance 272
voluntary vs. involuntary exposure 268–9
expressed preference studies 267
gender differences 273
individual vs. societal 272–3
perceived trustworthiness of assessors 272
risk communication 278, 285, 286
social amplification 274–5
social group differences 273–4
study approaches 267
risk rating 7–8
risk reduction *see* loss control
risk retention 220
risk transfer 220–1
Russian standard setting 122–3, **123**

safety case reports 5
safety data sheets 54, 55
safety factors 11–12, 54, 128, 169
safety policies 346
sample size selection
epidemiological studies 150–1
occupational exposure levels (OELs) comparisons 150, **150**
statistical methods 148–50
estimated mean and standard deviation 149–50
NIOSH method 148–9, **148**
sampling strategies 142–51
duration of sampling 146–7
location of sampling devices 144–5
number of samples 147–51
epidemiological studies 150–1
occupational exposure levels (OELs) comparisons 150, **150**
statistical methods 148–50
population selection 142–3
sampling frequency 151
sampling variation 70
security control 224
selection bias 71
self-employed contractors 350
severity of harm evaluation 7
severity rates 60
Severn Water 349
Seveso 247
Seveso Directive 101, 284
SFAIRP (so far as is reasonably practicable) 187
short-term exposure limits (STEL) 121, 124
exposure sampling duration 146
shot blasting enclosures 204
sickness absence 60
statistics screening for workplace inspections 113
stress-related illness 442
silica 75, 308
chest X-ray surveillance 297, 298
'six-pack' of regulations 5, 346, 347
skin irritation test 50
skin lesions, self-examination 292
skin sensitization 48
assessment tests 49, 51
smoke tube 115
smoke 81
smoking policy 346
social amplification 274–5
social group differences in risk perception 273–4
societal risk 8–9, 272–3
software packages 473–7
solvents
acute/chronic toxicity 270
drum filling methods 199, *200*
elimination from surface coatings 198
evaporation suppression 201–2
exposure modelling 164, 173, *173*
box models 168
evaporation models 165–7
substitution by less toxic substances 198, 199, 220
soots 75

specialist audits 317
spirometry 293–4, *294*
spray booths 204
standard setting 118–28
  acute/chronic toxic effects 121, **121**
  European Union (EU) 123–6
  UK 123–6
  USA vs. Russian comparison 122–3, **123**
standardized mortality ratio 62, 63
standards 119–20, 185
  application 126–8
  evaluation 120–1
  exposure monitoring data comparisons 154, 156
static exposure monitoring 131, 144, 145
stress 438–47
  causes **443**
  coping skills training 442
  determinant factors 445–6, **446**
  display screen equipment hazards 405, 407
  employee assistance programme (EAP) 441
  epidemiological studies 441–2
  management policy 447
  personal health assessment (PHA) programme 444
  preventive measures 439–47, **439**
  risk assessment/management 438–9
stress management skills 440
stress questionnaire 444–5, **444**
stress-related disorders 353–4
  damages awards 231
structure–activity relationships (SAR) 52
styrene 75, 298
subcontractors 350, 352
substance abuse 440
substitution by less toxic substances 198–9, 220
  isocyanates exposure case study 376
  organophosphate pesticides 366
  solvents 198, 199, 220
SUBTEC model 167
suppression methods 200–2
symptom review 290–2, 307, 308

target organs 45, **46**
task analysis 105, 181
  ergonomics 90
temperature extremes 88–90
threshold concept 120, 121
threshold dose 42
threshold limit values (TLVs) 120, 122, 300
time-weighted averages (TWAs) 120, 121, 124
  calculation 131
  exposure sampling duration 146
  integrated monitoring 130–1
tobacco smoking 72, 75, 122
  asbestos synergism 298, 422
  smoking policy 346
tolerability of risk 15, 186–7, *186*, 187, 267
  definition 9–11
toluene 47, 75
  dilution ventilation 206–7
  risk assessment using risk calculator 189–92, *191*
toluene diisocyanate (TDI) 369, *370*
  automotive industry case study 371–2
  respiratory sensitization 371
  see also isocyanates
toxicity assessment 56–7
  evaluation of toxicity data 52–4
  existing substances 48, 52
  extrapolation from animal experiments 53–4, 122
  new substances 48, 49–52
  repeated-dose toxicity tests 51
  substances classification/labelling 50
  tests 49–50
toxicokinetics 43–5
toxicology 41–55
  complex mixtures 127
  dose–response relationship 42–3
  exposure patterns 46–7
  hazard identification 41, 48–54
    existing substances 48, 52
    new substances 48, 49–52
    structure–activity relationships (SAR) 52
  pesticides *see* pesticides
  target organs 45, **46**
  toxic effects 45
    acute/chronic exposure 46–7
    immediate/delayed 47
    local/systemic 47
    reversible/irreversible 47–8
transport of materials
  associated hazards 197
  product labelling 284
tuberculosis 290, 291, 299
  in AIDS patients 414
  antituberculous drug resistance 414
  case study 413–17
Tyndall beam dust lamp 115

UK
  legislation 344–5, 459–60
  standard setting 123–6
  tolerability criteria 186, *186*
ultrasound 88
ultraviolet radiation (UV) 86–7
unacceptable risk 9–11, **11**
unsafe acts 99, *100*
unsafe conditions 99, *100*
urine sample monitoring 300
USA
  communication of risk (OSHA Hazard Communication Standard) 16
  legislation 5, 344

health surveillance requirements 304
safety factors 11
standard setting 122–3, **123**

vapour density 83
vapour hazard ratio (VHR) 83
vapour pressure (VP) 82, 83
solvent substitution 199
theoretical prediction of emission rates 165–6
vapours 82–4
atmospheric monitoring 132
direct reading instruments 116
exposure modelling
instantaneous monitoring instruments 130
odour 84
variability of exposure 139, *140*
ventilation systems 208
box models 169
checking performance 213–14
records 214–17, *215*, *216*
control of exposure 202–3
canopies/hoods 204–5
dilution/general ventilation 205–7
displacement ventilation 207
partial enclosure with extract ventilation 204
total enclosure under negative pressure 203–4
costs 209
make-up air 207, 211
multibranched systems 211
reasons for faulty performance 210–13
workplace inspections 115
vibration 88
direct reading instruments 116
exposure modelling 163
tools associated with injuries **89**
see also hand-transmitted vibration
vibration white finger 63, 64–5, 227, 379, 380
vinyl chloride monomer 75, 133, 144
statutory medical surveillance 306
violence at work 448–55
audit 454–5
definitions 449, 450, 454
exposure assessment/modelling 450–2
hazard control/prevention 451–2, 453–4
hazard identification 449–50
health and safety policy 454
high-risk situation evaluation 450–1, 452
procedure following incidents 455
quantitative risk assessment 452–3
reporting of incidents 448–9, 450, 451
self-defence training 453
viruses 94
visual display unit (VDU) working *see* display screen equipment operators
visual problems 405, 407
volatile organic compounds (VOCs) 130
voluntary risk 9, 268–9

water as dust suppressant 200–1
whole body vibration 88
work-related upper limb disorders (WRULDs) 406
work station design 406–7
Working Group on the Assessment of Toxic Chemicals (WATCH) 124
working hours
standards setting 120, 121
workplace inspections 108–17, *110*
accident/sickness absence data screening 113
actions implementation 116–17
inspection procedure 113–15
materials inventory 111–12
occupational health services 113
occupational hygiene instrumentation 115–16
personnel 112–13
preparation 111
process inventory 112
records 116
site plan 111

zoning method 152–3
zoonoses 94
case study 417–19